W0253823

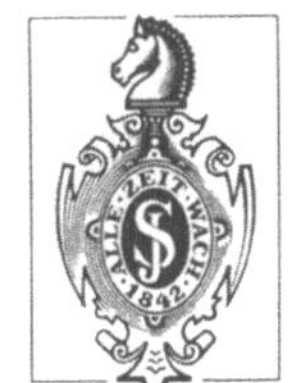
ALLE ZEIT WACH
1842

Michael M. Kochen (Hrsg./Ed.)

Rationale Pharmakotherapie in der Allgemeinpraxis

Möglichkeiten und Grenzen

Rational Pharmacotherapy in General Practice

Opportunities and Limitations

Springer-Verlag
Berlin Heidelberg New York
London Paris Tokyo
Hong Kong Barcelona
Budapest

Prof. Dr. med. MICHAEL M. KOCHEN, MPH
Leiter der Abteilung Allgemeinmedizin
der Georg-August-Universität Göttingen
Robert-Koch-Straße 40, W-3400 Göttingen,
Bundesrepublik Deutschland

Mit 46 Abbildungen und 55 Tabellen

ISBN-13: 978-3-540-54213-1 e-ISBN-13: 978-3-642-76731-9
DOI: 10.1007/978-3-642-76731-9

Die Deutsche Bibliothek – CIP-Einheitsaufnahme.
Rationale Pharmakotherapie in der Allgemeinpraxis:
Möglichkeiten und Grenzen; [mit 55 Tabellen]
= Rational pharmacotherapy in general practice / Michael M. Kochen (Hrsg.).
– Berlin ; Heidelberg ; New York ; London ; Paris ; Tokyo ;
Hong Kong ; Barcelona ; Budapest : Springer, 1991
ISBN-13: 978-3-540-54213-1
NE: Kochen, Michael M. [Hrsg.]; PT

Satz: Springer-TEX-Haussystem
19/3130-543210 – Gedruckt auf säurefreiem Papier

Vorwort

Das Verordnungsverhalten niedergelassener Allgemeinärzte (die über die Hälfte aller ambulant verordneten Medikamente verschreiben) wurde in den letzten Jahren zunehmender Kritik ausgesetzt: Die Kollegen und Kolleginnen hätten zu viele, zu teure und z. T. auch Arzneimittel mit ungesicherter Wirksamkeit in ihrer Feder.

Nur selten wird bei dieser Kritik berücksichtigt, daß die vielfältigen Einflüsse auf die Arzneimittelverschreibung von Primärärzten nicht immer etwas mit Pharmakologie, gelegentlich nicht einmal etwas mit Medizin zu tun haben.

Einen erneuten Beweis für diese These lieferte erst kürzlich eine Studie, die 1989 im renommierten *New England Journal of Medicine* publiziert wurde.[1] Darin ging es um einen Vergleich der unerwünschten Wirkungen von Captopril und Hydrochlorothiazid auf den Zucker- und Fettstoffwechsel bei Patienten mit Hypertonie. Bemerkenswert an dieser Untersuchung sind weder die offensichtlichen methodischen Mängel noch die wenig aufregenden Ergebnisse. Auch daß die Resultate keine Aussage über das koronare Risiko der so behandelten Patienten zulassen, soll nur am Rande bemerkt werden.

Entscheidend sind allein die Konsequenzen der Studie: Unmittelbar nach Publikation erschien eine Titelstory in der New York Times, gefolgt von weiteren Berichten in 200 US-amerikanischen Zeitungen und Zeitschriften. Mehrere größere Fernsehanstalten brachten sensationell aufgemachte Berichte in den Hauptsendezeiten. Vom Tag der Publikation im September 1989 bis zum Januar 1990, also in 4 Monaten, fiel die Anzahl von Diuretikaverordnungen um 13 %, was im wesentlichen auf den Wunsch besorgter Patienten zurückzuführen war.

Dieses Beispiel, das noch durch viele andere ergänzt werden könnte, zeigt exemplarisch, welchen Einflüssen z. B. von seiten der Medien oder von Patienten die Arzneimittelverordnung von Primärärzten unterliegen kann.

Damit wären aber die Besonderheiten der Pharmakotherapie in der Allgemeinpraxis noch keineswegs erschöpfend behandelt. Obwohl der Allgemeinarzt theoretisch dieselben Medikamente wie der Krankenhausarzt verschreiben könnte, sind die für Arzneimittelverordnungen maßgebenden „Umgebungsbedingungen" in der Allgemeinpraxis doch recht unterschiedlich. Das betrifft insbesondere

[1] Pollare T, Lithell H, Berne C (1989) A comparison of the effects of hydrochlorothiazide and captopril on glucose and lipid metabolism in patients with hypertension. N Engl J Med 321 : 868–873.

- das unterschiedliche Spektrum an Erkrankungen und Befindlichkeitsstörungen;
- die unterschiedliche Weiterbildung des Allgemeinarztes;
- die relative Isolation vieler Allgemeinärzte von Zentren der Forschung und Lehre;
- die in der Allgemeinpraxis häufig verspürte Notwendigkeit, geringfügige Befindlichkeitsstörungen symptomatisch zu behandeln;
- das Engagement des Allgemeinarztes bei der Dauertherapie chronischer Erkrankungen;
- die fehlende Möglichkeit, Patienten wie im Krankenhaus kontinuierlich zu überwachen und – wie schon erwähnt –
- die potentiellen Pressionen, denen jeder niedergelassene Arzt von Seiten des Patienten oder der Medien ausgesetzt sein kann.

Erwähnt werden muß auch, daß viele in der Allgemeinpraxis verordneten Arzneimittel an Patienten in Krankenhäusern – oft sogar in Universitätskliniken – getestet wurden. Und dies trotz der Tatsache, daß nur 0,3 % der Arzt-Patienten-Kontakte in einem gegebenen Jahr zu einem stationären Aufenthalt in der Universitätsklinik (und weitere 2,7 % in einem anderen Krankenhaus) führen.

Hinzu kommt, daß Arzneimittel für viele therapeutischen Probleme in der Allgemeinpraxis noch nie untersucht worden sind. Die Gründe liegen auf der Hand: entweder werden diese Probleme (meist von Klinikern!) als zu banal eingeschätzt, oder es mangelt an Geld bzw. interessierten Pharmafirmen.

Schließlich werden Primärärzte häufig mit Krankenhausverordnungen konfrontiert, die in keiner Weise die Situation der Allgemeinpraxis – z. B. in bezug auf die Festbetragsregelung oder das kassenärztliche Wirtschaftlichkeitsgebot – berücksichtigen.

Die gewählten Beispiele zeigen, daß Standards der klinischen Pharmakologie, die im wesentlichen für das Krankenhaus entwickelt wurden, nicht einfach der Allgemeinpraxis übergestülpt werden können. Für die primärärztliche Praxis werden neue Standards benötigt, die bislang noch nicht existieren, jedoch seit einigen Jahren auf europäischer Ebene erarbeitet werden. Daß vorwiegend Allgemeinärzte – und nicht etwas Kliniker – bei dieser Arbeit tätig werden müssen, wird klar, wenn man bedenkt, daß alle Allgemeinärzte einige Jahre in einem Krankenhaus verbracht haben, viele Krankenhausärzte jedoch noch nie in ihrem Leben einen Fuß über die Schwelle einer Praxis gesetzt haben.

Ich bin der Überzeugung, daß Allgemeinärzte für eine fruchtbare Zusammenarbeit mit klinischen Pharmakologen einiges anzubieten haben. Von seiten der klinischen Pharmakologie, die ihre wissenschaftlichen Bemühungen bislang kaum auf die Allgemeinpraxis gerichtet hat, könnte z. B. ein Angebot kommen, eine bestimmte Anzahl von Primärärzten in klinischer Pharmakologie weiterzubilden oder auf universitärer Ebene gemeinsame Lehrveranstaltungen mit der Allgemeinmedizin abzuhalten. Primärärzte könnten dann als „Botschafter" dienen, um die Ergebnisse der klinischen Pharmakologie in der Praxis umzusetzen.

Diesen notwendigen und konstruktiven Dialog zwischen Allgemeinmedizin und klinischer Pharmakologie auf den Weg zu bringen, ist eine wichtige Aufgabe des vorliegenden Buches, das die wesentlichen Vorträge des Kongresses „Rationale Pharmakotherapie in der Allgemeinpraxis"[2] enthält.

Mein Dank gebührt allen, die den Kongreß und die Herausgabe dieses Bandes ermöglichten: Den in- und ausländischen Referenten und Vorsitzenden, den Mitveranstaltern (European Formulary Group, WHO, Förderkreis Rationale Arzneimitteltherapie, Deutsche Gesellschaft für Allgemeinmedizin – DEGAM, Gesellschaft für Allgemeinmedizin – GAM und niedersächsische Akademie für ärztliche Fortbildung), den unterstützenden Firmen und Institutionen und nicht zuletzt den Mitarbeitern der Abteilung Allgemeinmedizin der Georg-August-Universität Göttingen.

Göttingen, im Sommer 1991 M.M. Kochen

[2] Dieser Kongreß fand am 15. und 16.03.1991 in Göttingen statt.

Preface

The prescribing behavior of general practitioners (who are, in the western part of Germany, responsible for over half of all ambulatory drug prescriptions) has been increasingly criticized in recent years. The critics say that general practitioners prescribe too many, too expensive drugs, and sometimes also medicines with undocumented efficacy. Only rarely, however, do the critics take into account that sometimes the factors influencing the prescribing habits of doctors in primary health care have nothing to do with pharmacology or even with medicine.

Renewed evidence for this thesis is provided by a study published in 1989 in the prestigious *New England Journal of Medicine* (Pollare T, Lithell H, Berne C, A comparison of the effects of hydrochlorothiazide and captopril on glucose and lipid metabolism in patients with hypertension. N Engl J Med 321 : 868–873). This investigation was remarkable neither for its obvious methodological shortcomings nor for its not very exciting results. Furthermore, it did not allow conclusions to be drawn about the coronary risks of the treated patients.

Despite all this, the consequences of the paper were wide-reaching: immediately after publication, the *New York Times* carried a front page story based on the paper, and this was followed by further reports in 200 US newspapers and journals. Several major television companies broadcast sensational news items at peak viewing times. In the four months from the date of the original publication in September 1989 to January 1990, the number of prescriptions for diuretics went down by 13 %, mainly at the request of concerned patients.

This example, which is by no means unique, shows how prescribing habits of primary care doctors can potentially be influenced by the media or by patients themselves.

However, this is by no means a complete picture of the peculiarities of pharmacotherapy in general practice. More generally important differences compared to drug treatment in hospitals are as follows:

1. Because of the different spectrum of diseases and conditions they encounter, and because of the frequently felt necessity to provide immediate help, general practitioners prescribe a broader repertoire of drugs.
2. Many drugs which are prescribed in general practice have only been tested in hospitals or even in university institutions. The strong selection of patients that occurs is shown by the fact that only 0.3 % of all doctor-patient contacts result in admission to a university institution (and another 2.7 % to other hospitals).

3. There are no drugs for many therapeutic problems in general practice. The reasons are clear: Either the problem is judged (mostly by hospital consultants!) as trivial, or there is no money, or no drug company is interested in it.
4. General practitioners are frequently confronted with prescriptions from hospitals that do not take into account the circumstances of general practices, e. g., with regard to drug costs.
5. As has been demonstrated by the example mentioned above, general practitioners are much more exposed to the economically very effective influence of patients and/or the media than their hospital colleagues.

This incomplete list indicates that the standards of clinical pharmacology which have been developed mainly for hospitals cannot simply be transferred to general practice. Practitioners need new and suitable standards for drug therapy, and these are currently being developed at a European level. When one considers that most general practitioners have spent some years in a hospital, but many hospital doctors have never set foot in a general practice, it seems clear that this work must be done mainly by general practitioners and not by hospital doctors.

I am thus convinced that general practitioners have much to offer in a constructive collaboration with clinical pharmacologists. Clinical pharmacology, which has seldom oriented its scientific endeavors to general practice, could contribute to this collaboration by training primary health care doctors in clinical pharmacology or by organizing joint teaching programs with departments of general practice. General practitioners who have been trained in this way could then be sent as "ambassadors" to their colleagues to help the results obtained by clinical pharmacology be put into practice.

To promote this necessary and constructive dialogue between general practice and clinical pharmacology is one of the important aims of this book, which contains most of the lectures and workshops from the congress on "Rational Pharmacotherapy in General Practice," held in Göttingen, March 15–16, 1991.

I am indebted to all those who made the congress and the publication of this book possible: The speakers and chairpersons from many European countries, the coorganizers (European Formulary Group, World Health Organization, Society for Promoting Rational Pharmacotherapy, German Society for General Practice, and Academy for Continuing Medical Education of Lower Saxony), the sponsoring companies and institutions, and, last but not least, my colleagues and collaborators from the Department of General Practice at Göttingen University Medical School.

Göttingen, Summer 1991 M.M. Kochen

Inhaltsverzeichnis

Plenum 1/Plenary Session 1

Strategies for Improving Drug Safety in Europe:
Can General Practitioners Contribute?
Andrew Herxheimer ... 3

Influence on Physicians' Prescribing Habits
by Drug Licensing Authorities: Norway as an Example
Gaut Gadeholt ... 7

Rational Pharmacotherapy in General Practice:
Education by Postgraduate Training
Theo P.G.M. de Vries ... 16

Plenum 2/Plenary Session 2

Erkenntnisse der klinischen Pharmakologie –
Erfordernisse der Praxis: Läßt sich beides verbinden?
Etzel Gysling ... 27

Arzneimittelmarkt (BR) Deutschland – eine kritische Bewertung
Gerd Glaeske ... 31

Probleme des Konsums und der Verfügbarkeit von Arzneimitteln
in Thüringen
Annemarie Hoffmann, Ina Blumöhr und Mechthild Knüpfer ... 49

Problemorientierte Workshops/Problem-Oriented Workshops
Hypercholesterinämie: Wen screenen, wen behandeln?
Hypercholesterolemia: Whom to Screen, Whom to Treat?

Cholesterinscreening: Die Irrationalität von Grenzwerten
und die Berücksichtigung des Gesamtrisikos für eine rationale Therapie
Johannes G. Schmidt ... 67

Hypercholesterinämie und kardiovaskuläre Risikofaktoren
Thomas Eisenhauer ... 82

Hypercholesterinämie und Myokardinfarktrisiko:
Ergebnisse der GRIPS-Studie
Rainer Muche, Olaf Gefeller, Dorothea Nagel und Peter Cremer ... 87

Cholesterinscreening: Vergleich verschiedener Strategien anhand der Daten der GRIPS-Studie
Olaf Gefeller, Rainer Muche, Dorothea Nagel und Peter Cremer 95

Schmerztherapie bei unheilbar Kranken
Analgesia in Terminal Care

Tumorschmerztherapie
Gerd-Gunnar Hanekop, Dirk-Bodo Eggebrecht, Ingrid Gutberlet und Jan Hildebrandt 107

Psychosoziale Probleme bei fortgeschrittenen Tumorerkrankungen aus der Sicht von Patienten, Angehörigen und Therapeuten
Dirk-Bodo Eggebrecht, Ingrid Gutberlet, Gerd-Gunnar Hanekop und Jan Hildebrandt 122

Respiratorische/grippale Infekte: Verschreiben oder nur beraten?
Upper Respiratory Infections: Prescription or Just Adivse?

Therapie bei „banalen" Erkrankungen
Adalbert Keseberg 129

Die Behandlung chronisch-obstruktiver Lungenerkrankungen in der Allgemeinpraxis
Chris van Weel, Constant van Schayck, Edward Dompeling, Hans Folgering, Cees van Herwaarden und Pierre van Grunsven 134

Arzneimittel mit zweifelhafter Wirkung:
Venentherapeutika, Lebermittel, Geriatrika
Therapeutics of Doubtful Efficacy:
Drugs for Varicose Veins, Liver Disease, "Old Age"

Daten zur Verordnungshäufigkeit von Lebermitteln, Venenmitteln und Nootropika
Gerd Glaeske 145

Der therapeutische Nutzen von Lebertherapeutika, Venenmitteln und Mitteln zur Behandlung von Hirnfunktionsstörungen aus der Sicht einer Allgemeinärztin
Christa A. Ossmann 150

Pharmakotherapieunterricht für Medizinstudenten – Neue Konzepte
Teaching Pharmacotherapy to Students – New Concepts

Teaching Pharmacotherapeutics: Experiences in Ghent
Luc Blondeel 163

Eigenverantwortliche Qualitätsprüfung ärztlichen Verordnungsverhaltens: Wann und wie?
Medical Audit of Prescribing: When and How?

Rational Prescribing: An Exemplar of Auditing Prescribing in Updating a General Practice Formulary
David A. Gregory ... 169

Medical Audit of Prescribing in General Practice
Philip M. Reilly ... 174

Plenum 3 / Plenary Session 3

A European Formulary for General Practice: State of the Art and Future Developments
George B. Grant ... 181

Rational Discussion as a Guide to More Cost-Effective and Scientific Prescribing in General Practice: 15 Years of Experience in Northern Ireland
Hugh McGavock ... 186

Möglichkeiten und Grenzen des Wirksamkeitsnachweises beim niedergelassenen Allgemeinarzt aus der Sicht der medizinischen Biometrie
Joerg Hasford ... 201

Plenum 4 / Plenary Session 4

Lebensalter, Geschlecht und Psychopharmaka
Ursula Sehrt ... 209

Allgemeinärztliche Therapiefreiheit – ein Mythos?
Ivan Nemitz ... 221

Drugs and Placebos in General Practice: The View of a Sceptic
James S. McCormick ... 227

Problemorientierte Workshops / Problem-Oriented-Workshops
Arzneimittelverordnung in Europa – Traditionen
Drug Prescribing in Europe: Can Traditions Be Overcome?

Drug Prescribing – Can Traditions Be Overcome?
Daniele Coën ... 235

Nootropika und „durchblutungsfördernde“ Pharmaka: Eine Pille für alle Alten?
Nootropics and Drugs “for Better Circulation”: A Pill for All Aged?

Hausärztliche Verordnungsweise von Nootropika und durchblutungsfördernden Pharmaka
Ulrich Rendenbach ... 243

Schlaflosigkeit – Benzodiazepine – Abhängigkeit
Sleeplessness – Benzodiazepines – Addiction

Über den Umgang mit Benzodiazepinen in der Allgemeinpraxis
Ursula Sehrt 251

Muskel- und Gelenkbeschwerden in der Allgemeinpraxis: Therapiemöglichkeiten
Muscle Pain and Arthropathies in General Practice: Which Treatments are Possible?

Pharmakologische Gesichtspunkte
Gerhard Schmidt 263

Moderne Phytotherapie
Medicinal Plants

Möglichkeiten und Grenzen einer modernen Phytotherapie
Volker Fintelmann und Claus-Peter Siegers 275

Diabetes mellitus: Therapiestandard in der Allgemeinpraxis
Diabetes mellitus: Treatment Standard in General Practice

Die Versorgung von Typ-II-Diabetikern in Hausarztpraxen
Joachim A. Szecsenyi und Michael M. Kochen 279

Therapiestandards aus der Sicht eines Klinikers
Eberhard G. Siegel 291

Arzneimittelberatung durch Ärzte
Drug Counseling by Doctors

Peer Review Groups Concerned with the Quality Assessment of Pharmacotherapy in Primary Health Care: An Instrument for Educational Advancement and Quality Improvement
Liselotte von Ferber, Luciano Alberti and Jutta Krappweis 303

Factors Influencing GP Prescribing Habits
Henk G. A. Mokkink, Jan de Maeseneer, and Richard Grol 312

Sachverzeichnis / Subject Index 321

Verzeichnis der erstgenannten Autoren sowie der Plenums- und Workshopvorsitzenden

Blondeel, Luc, Dr. med., Arzt für Allgemeinmedizin, Wiss. Mitarbeiter, Abt. Allgemeinmedizin, Universität Ghent, Mitglied der belgischen Arzneimittel-Zulassungsbehörde, Projekt Farmaka, J. Vervaenestr. 14, 9218 Gent, Belgien

Cöen, Daniele, Dr. med., Editor „Ricerca & Pratica", Istituto di Ricerche Farmacologiche Mario Negri, Via Eritrea 62, 20157 Milano, Italy

Eggebrecht, Dietmar, Dipl.-Psych., Abt. Anästhesiologie, Georg-August-Universität, Robert-Koch-Str. 40 W-3400 Göttingen, Bundesrepublik Deutschland

Eisenhauer, Thomas, Priv.-Doz. Dr. med., Oberarzt, Abt. Nephrologie und Rheumatologie, Georg-August-Universität, Robert-Koch-Str. 40, W-3400 Göttingen, Bundesrepublik Deutschland

Ernst, Andrea, Mag. phil., Soziologin und Publizistin, Ostenstr. 53, W-4000 Düsseldorf, Bundesrepublik Deutschland

Ferber, Liselotte von, Priv.-Doz. Dr. med., Forschungsgruppe Primärärztliche Versorgung, Zentrum für Medizinische Soziologie, Psychologie und Statistik, Universität Düsseldorf, Moorenstraße 5, W-4000 Düsseldorf, Bundesrepublik Deutschland

Fintelmann, Volker, Dr. med., Leitender Arzt, Medizinische Abteilung B, Deutsches Rotes Kreuz- und Freimaurer-Krankenhaus, Suurheid 20, W-2000 Hamburg 56, Bundesrepublik Deutschland

Gadeholt, Gaut, Prof. Dr. med, Department of Pharmacotherapeutics, University of Oslo, POB 1065, 0316 Oslo, Norwegen

Gefeller, Olaf, Dr. rer. nat., Abt. Medizinische Statistik, Georg-August-Universität, Humboldtallee 38, W-3400 Göttingen, Bundesrepublik Deutschland

Glaeske, Gerd, Dr. rer. nat., Leiter des Pharmakologischen Beratungsdienstes der AOK Mettmann, Dürerstr. 29, W-5620 Velbert 1, Bundesrepublik Deutschland

Grant, George, MB, BS, FRCGP, General practitioner, Senior Honorary Lecturer, Department of Primary Health Care, University of Newcastle/Tyne, Framlington Place, Newcastle NE20 9AH, Großbritannien

Gregory, David, MB, BS, FRCGP, Senior Lecturer,
Department of Primary Health Care, University of Newcastle/Tyne,
Framlington Place, Newcastle NE20 9AH, Großbritannien

Gundert-Remy, Ursula, Prof. Dr. med.,
Leiterin der Abt. Klinische Pharmakologie,
Institut für Arzneimittel des Bundesgesundheitsamtes, Seestr. 10,
W-1000 Berlin 65, Bundesrepublik Deutschland

Gutberlet, Ingrid, MR Dr. med., Ärztin für Allgemeinmedizin,
Leiterin der Abt. Allgemeinmedizin, Poliklinik Erfurt-Süd,
Uhlandstr. 10, O-5082 Erfurt, Bundesrepublik Deutschland

Gysling, Etzel, Dr. med., Internist FMH,
Herausgeber der „pharma-kritik", Bergliweg 17, 9500 Wil, Schweiz

Hanekop, Gerd-Gunnar, Dr. med., Oberarzt,
Abt. Anästhesiologie, Georg-August-Universität, Robert-Koch-Str. 40,
W-3400 Göttingen, Bundesrepublik Deutschland

Hasford, Jörg, Priv.-Doz. Dr. med., Wiss. Leiter,
Biometrisches Zentrum für Therapiestudien, Pettenkoferstr. 35,
W-8000 München 2, Bundesrepublik Deutschland

Herxheimer, Andrew, MB, FRCP, Senior Lecturer, Department of
Clinical Pharmacology, Charing Cross and Westminster Medical
School, Editor „drug and therapeutics bulletin",
77 Carthew Road, London W6 OD4, Großbritannien

Hildebrandt, Jan, Prof. Dr. med., Leiter der Schmerzambulanz,
Abt. Anästhesiologie, Georg-August-Universität,
Robert-Koch-Str. 40, W-3400 Göttingen, Bundesrepublik Deutschland

Hoffmann, Annemarie, Prof. Dr. sc. med.,
Direktorin des Instituts für Klinische Pharmakologie,
Friedrich-Schiller-Universität, Bachstr. 18, O-6900 Jena,
Bundesrepublik Deutschland

Holzer, Benedikt, Dr. med., DTMH, Arzt für Allgemeinmedizin/
Tropenmedizin, Mittlere Straße 3, 3600 Thun, Schweiz

Kahl, Regine, Prof. Dr. med., Abt. Pharmakologie II,
Georg-August-Universität, Robert-Koch-Str. 40,
W-3400 Göttingen, Bundesrepublik Deutschland

Keseberg, Adalbert, Prof. Dr. med., Arzt für Allgemeinmedizin,
Lehrbeauftragter an der Universität Bonn, Am Hohnacker 36,
W-5042 Erfstadt-Liblar, Bundesrepublik Deutschland

Kochen, Michael M., Prof. Dr. med., Arzt für Allgemeinmedizin,
Leiter der Abt. Allgemeinmedizin, Georg-August-Universität,
Robert-Koch-Str. 40, W-3400 Göttingen, Bundesrepublik Deutschland

König, Benno, Prof. Dr. med., Arzt für Allgemeinmedizin,
Lehrbeauftagter an der Universität Mainz, Prunkgasse 9,
W-6550 Mainz-Finthen 21, Bundesrepublik Deutschland

McCormick, James S., MD, FRCGP, Prof. and head,
Department of Community Health, Trinity College Medical School,
University of Dublin, 199 Pearse St., Dublin 2, Republic of Ireland
McGavock, Hugh, BSC, MD, Director, Prescribing Information Unit,
Department of Therapeutics and Pharmacology, Queens University,
Whitla Medical Bldg., Belfast BT9 7BL, Northern Ireland
Mokkink, Henk, PhD, Research Fellow, Department of General Practice,
University of Nijmegen, POB 9101, 6500 HB Nijmegen, Niederlande
Muche, Rainer, Dipl.-Stat., Abt. Medizinische Statistik,
Georg-August-Universität, Humboldtallee 38,
W-3400 Göttingen, Bundesrepublik Deutschland
Nemitz, Ivan, Dr. med., Arzt für Allgemeinmedizin FMH,
3 Chemin du Critet, 1470 Estavayer le Lac, Schweiz
Ossmann, Christa, Dr. med., Ärztin für Allgemeinmedizin,
Leitende Redakteurin „Arzneiverordnung in der Praxis",
Mitglied der Arzneimittelkommission der Deutschen Ärzteschaft
Rohrackerstr. 70, W-7000 Stuttgart, Bundesrepublik Deutschland
Reilly, Philipp, MD, FRCGP, Prof. and head, Department of General Practice,
Queens University, Dunluce Health Center, Belfast B57 7HR,
Northern Ireland
Rendenbach, Ulrich, Dr. med., Arzt für Allgemeinmedizin,
Lehrbeauftragter an der Georg-August-Universität Göttingen,
Marktstr. 23–25, W-3408 Duderstadt, Bundesrepublik Deutschland
Schmidt, Gerhard, Prof. Dr. med., Leiter der Abt. Neuropharmakologie,
Georg-August-Universität, Robert-Koch-Str. 40, W-3400 Göttingen,
Bundesrepublik Deutschland
Schmidt, Johannes, Dr. med., Praktischer Arzt, cand. MMSc.
(clinical epidemiology), Tödistr. 34, 8810 Horgen, Schweiz
Sehrt, Ursula, Prof. Dr. med., Ärztin für Allgemeinmedizin,
Lehrbeauftragte an der Ruhr-Universität Bochum,
Mitglied der Arzneimittelkommission der Deutschen Ärzteschaft,
Gneisenaustr. 37, W-4330 Mühlheim, Bundesrepublik Deutschland
Siegel, Eberhard, Priv.-Doz. Dr. med., Oberarzt,
Gastroenterologie und Endokrinologie,
Georg-August-Universität, Robert-Koch-Str. 40,
W-3400 Göttingen, Bundesrepublik Deutschland
Siegers, Claus-Peter, Prof. Dr. med.,
Institut für Toxikologie der Medizinischen Universität,
Ratzeburger Allee, W-2400 Lübeck, Bundesrepublik Deutschland
Szecsenyi, Joachim, Dr. med., Dipl.-Soz., Abt. Allgemeinmedizin,
Georg-August-Universität, Robert-Koch-Str. 40,
W-3400 Göttingen, Bundesrepublik Deutschland

Vries, Theo PGM de, Dr. med., Arzt für Allgemeinmedizin,
Senior lecturer, Division of Clinical Pharmacology,
Department of Pharmacology, WHO Collaborating Center for
Pharmacology and Drug Policy, University of Groningen,
Bloemsingel 1, 9713 Groningen, Niederlande
Weel, Chris van, Prof. Dr. med., Arzt für Allgemeinmedizin,
Head of the Department of General Practice, University of Nijmegen,
POB 9101, 6500 HB Nijmegen, Niederlande

Plenum 1 / Plenary Session 1

Strategies for Improving Drug Safety in Europe: Can General Practitioners Contribute?

Andrew Herxheimer

Of course the answer is yes: general practitioners (GPs) can contribute more to drug safety than any other group of doctors. Over 80% of all medicines prescribed are prescribed by GPs, and GPs have by far the most important educational role in relation to medicine-taking behaviour. They can contribute in a number of interrelated ways, which have to do with the quality of prescribing, the education of patients and the information they are given the monitoring of drug treatment, and clinical research.

Improving the Quality of Prescribing

Good prescribing requires organisation and systematic thought, but need not take extra time. Most doctors now in practice were not taught the elements of rational prescribing as students, and have not had adequate opportunities to learn them since. Every prescribing decision is or should be made up of series of decisions which are commonly not explicit and are not considered separately – both because time in the consultation is short and because they are not in doctors' minds. These components of the prescribing decision can be expressed as questions:

1. Does the patient's problem require drug treatment? It may require some other treatment, or only advice.
2. If yes, what drug effect is required?
3. What type of drug can best provide the required effect?
4. Which particular drug (i.e. active substance) of that type ist the most suitable? Here it is necessary to think about efficacy, safety, convenience and cost.
5. What route of administration, what preparation, what dose and frequency are best?
6. For how long should this treatment be continued?
7. How should the desired effects and any unwanted effects be monitored, when, and by whom?
8. What will be done if the effect is insufficient, or if unwanted effects occur?
9. What does the patient need to know about the treatment?
   What does he want to know? What can he understand about it?

It is clearly impossible to consider each of these questions in detail during a consultation, but that is not necessary. Nearly all of them can and should be answered beforehand: the answers should be part of a well thought out therapeutic

Rationale Pharmakotherapie in der Allgemeinpraxis
Rational Pharmacotherapy in General Practice
M. M. Kochen (Hrsg.)

policy. Only parts of question 5 above, namely the type of preparation and the dosage, need brief consideration in the consultation. Treatment policies are needed for all common medical problems met in practice, and all doctors evolve them – but often they evolve by accretion of undigested experiences and ill-defined ideas. The key point in developing conscious policies is to concentrate on the essentials, and to base them on independent professional sources of information: well designed and reliably performed clinical trials; a relevant formulary produced by GPs, clinical pharmacologists and pharmacists; good-quality drug bulletins; and focused discussion with experienced and knowledgeable colleagues and experts. And all this has to be a continuous process, taking place throughout a doctor's professional life.

Information from pharmaceutical companies is much less useful because its primary aim is to increase the sales of particular products. It is best used only to answer specific questions that a doctor may have about individual products. Medical representatives, promotional meetings and pharmaceutical advertising are a waste of time. They are designed to flatter doctors and make them feel clever and up-to-date. Medical representatives are drilled to make doctors focus on what the company wants them to consider, but the doctor has the professional task of setting his or her own agenda. When a GP has a substantive question about a product, e. g. about efficacy in a particular setting or some aspect of safety, dosage, or mode of use, it is best to write to the medical director, and not to ask a representative. Most representatives do not know enough, and if they admit that, say they will ask the medical department to send the details. They may think they know when they do not, and quite innocently give a misleading answer. It is better to deal directly with the professional colleague in the company who has the responsibility for the product.

Educating Patients

The second way in which GPs can contribute to drug safety is by educating and informing their patients, and indeed the community in which they practise. As Michael Balint liked to point out, the word "doctor" means "teacher", and every consultation is an opportunity for learning and for teaching. Note that learning will occur even in the absence of any conscious attempt to teach: a patient prescribed an antibiotic for a cold "learns" that it is effective and appropriate treatment, and will come back for it next time he has a cold – or take some left-over antibiotic that he finds in the bathroom cupboard. The doctor who is sympathetic, but convincingly explains that a cold does not require an antibiotic, and explains how particular symptoms can be eased without the need to see a doctor, is educating the patient (and partly his family and friends), giving him knowledge and confidence to deal with the problem himself in the future. This simple example shows that we also need what we might call teaching policies about common health problems, and that these can make an important contribution to the safe use of medicines.

Systematic Monitoring of Drug Treatment

We can consider monitoring under three headings: (a) monitoring that the drug is adequately effective, (b) watching for unwanted effects that are known to affect a proportion of patients, and (c) remaining alert to the possibility of rare or still unknown adverse effects. Although the first two tasks are easier than the last, they are often not very well done either in general or in specialist practice. I suspect that there are two reasons for this. One may be that "new" consultations, with the need for assessment and diagnosis, and a treatment decision, are felt to be more interesting than "repeat" or follow-up encounters; the other, that to be successful they require explicit and coherent policies which in many practices do not exist. In some conditions that are treated jointly by GPs and specialists, e. g. diabetes, asthma, peptic ulcer disease, epilepsy, rheumatoid arthritis, an effective policy for shared care has to be worked out and agreed upon jointly. That is still rare, but as such policies are developed and put into practice we can expect treatment to become more effective and safer.

Alertness to rare and possibly unkown adverse effects of drugs requires doctors to ask themselves whenever they are presented with something unexpected, "Could this symptom/phenomenon/disease possibly be due to a drug that the patient has taken?" If the answer is yes, then the doctor should not only investigate and treat the problem as necessary, but should also report it in sufficient detail to the local or national adverse reaction monitoring centre – in Germany, for example, to the *Arzneimittelkommission der Deutschen Ärzteschaft*. This is necessary with all serious adverse events, but it is especially important for those that may be related to new drugs. Many uncommon reactions to a new drug are unknown when the drug is first marketed, and therefore both doctors and patients must think of the possibility that an unexpected event could be due to it. In Britain the Committee on Safety of Medicines annually issues a list of new drugs for which it asks doctors to report all suspected adverse effects, not only serious ones. These drugs are identified in the British National Formulary, the industry's prescribing guide, and in advertisements, by a black triangle printed next to the drug name. It is unfortunate that most patients do not know when they are taking a relatively new "black triangle" drug and when they are taking a well-established old one. In my opinion patients have the right to know this. When a new drug, i. e. one that has been marketed for less than say 3 years, is prescribed, it should be explained to the patient that it might affect some people in ways which are still unknown, and that he should therefore report any unexpected happening to the doctor so that its possible relationship to the drug can be assessed. Of course the pharmaceutical industry dislikes this idea, and doctors may fear that it would waste time in consultations. That may explain why it has not yet been adopted anywhere, though it has been advocated repeatedly since 1983 [1]. I am sure that when enough patients understand the point it will be adopted. Doctors should always be prepared to justify using a new drug in preference to an older one. If a patient is not convinced, he can be prescribed an older alternative.

Clinical Research

There will always be important unanswered questions about the efficacy, safety and best ways of using drugs in general practice. They need well designed studies by GPs to answer them. Those who regularly take part in such work, and their patients, are making a substantial contribution to drug safety. I believe that patients who enter a good clinical trial are usually better cared for than those who receive routine care – because those who do trials are working according to a well thought out protocol and are more meticulous in their attention to detail. Further, by taking part in good clinical research GPs not only improve their own practice, but also general practice as a whole.

Conclusion

I have described various ways in which GPs can and should contribute to greater drug safety, but I know that many colleagues will sigh and say that they are already extremely busy and have no time to do any of the things I have suggested. My reply to them is that to have time to think properly about the drugs they use, they must make better, more discriminating choices, use fewer drugs, and prescribe them less often. That will save them time. To end with one of my favourite proverbs: God helps those who know what they are doing.

Reference

1. Anon (1983) Reporting adverse reactions: the black triangle and the patient (editorial). Drug Therapeut Bull 21 : 93–94

Influence on Physicians' Prescribing Habits by Drug Licensing Authorities: Norway as an Example

Gaut Gadeholt

Monitoring of Prescription Practices

The most readily available information about prescription practices in Norway are provided by the sales data [1] from the Norwegian Medicinal Depot (NMD), which has had monopoly on the wholesale of drugs. This organization issues annual reports on drug sales, divided into therapeutic classes and substances, expressed in defined daily doses per 1000 inhabitants per day. More long-term overviews, for example 1974–1976 (the first issue), and 1984–1988 (the most recent one) are also given. For drugs of special interest, the sales figures are given for each of 19 counties. No information is given about specific products when a substance is sold under different brand names. We thus have difficulties in assessing the effect of opening generic competition on prescription practices.

Variability of Prescription Practices

Norway has a population of 4 million in a total area larger than Germany. Neither natural conditions nor drug prescription practices are homogeneous. Some of the

Table 1. Utilization of systemic antiasthmatics in two counties in Norway in defined daily doses per 1000 inhabitants per day (1989)

	β_2-Stimulators	Theophylline
Hedmark	3.4	11.7
Sør-Trøndelag	1.2	2.6
National average	3.3	8.2

Table 2. Utilization of antiasthmatics for inhalation in four counties in Norway (1989). Values are defined daily doses per 1000 inhabitants per day

	β_2-Stimulators	Corticosteroids
Hedmark	25.8	14.9
Sør-Trøndelag	20.4	18.1
Sogn og Fjordane	15.1	9.6
Buskerud	20.4	22.9
National average	20.9	15.5

Rationale Pharmakotherapie in der Allgemeinpraxis
Rational Pharmacotherapy in General Practice
M. M. Kochen (Hrsg.)

differences between the regions can be illustrated by the utilization of antiasthmatics (Tables 1, 2) [1].

Influences on Prescription Practices

Prescription practices are influenced by rules of medical ethics, professional attitudes toward drug selection, public attitudes toward drug use, medical needs and demands (morbidity, population characteristics), local drug committees, and the structure and organization of health services. The Norwegian drug licencing authority may influence prescription practices by regulating:

1. Drug availability (registration of drugs, refusal of registration, restrictions on prescribing)
2. Marketing of drugs
3. Drug prices
4. Information
5. Reimbursement schemes (indirectly).

Areas Controlled by the Licencing Authorities

Drug Availability

The drug control authority (*Statens legemiddelkontroll*, SLK) receives an application for the registration of a drug, studies the documentation, and gives advice to the specialty commission, which takes the formal decisions whether or not to licence the drug. In cases where the SLK has no specific expertise, external consultants are used. Usually, these will be high-ranking members of specialties with special interest in the drug. These consultants are very influential.

Following are some of the guidelines for drug approval (the legal foundation for this was laid in 1928; the famous need clause came in 1938):

- Efficacy and safety must be satisfactory. Scientific documentation of reasonable quality is mandatory.
- Medical need must exist. There is always a need for breakthrough drugs for any important disease. The next new drugs within a class (so-called me-too-drugs) are often registered to allow for some competition. Subsequently added drugs within the class must show some important difference or advantage compared to those already on the market. Otherwise, registration will be refused because present drugs will cover the need.
- New combination products must be rational.
- Every drug on the market is re-evaluated every 5 years. This means that drugs may be removed from the market if they no longer are considered medically justified, and regulatory action can be taken to change the composition of drugs, as illustrated by the best-selling combination analgesic, Paralgin forte. Other

combination analgesics were subject to similar changes. (Norwegian physicians now only have access to combination analgesics with two components; table 3.)
- The drug must be technically acceptable (most important for "synonyms", i.e., competing products of well-known drugs). Bioavailability must be similar to that of products already on the market.

Table 3. The varying composition of Paralgin forte. Values are in mg per tablet

	Registered 1964	Changed 1968	Changed 1976	Changed 1979
Codeine	15	15	20	30
Paracetamol	250	250	400	400
Salicylamide	200	200		
Caffeine	50	50		
Mebumal	20			
Promethazine		5	5	

Limitations on Prescribing

Restrictions on Prescribers. Some drugs are registered with the limitation that only hospitals or specified specialists may prescribe them. This applies for example to drugs with undesirable side-effects requiring special follow-up, such as levodopa, amphetamine, methylfenidate, aminoglycoside antibiotics, amiodarone, ketoconazole, and omeprazole. Others may be continued by general practicioners if specialists or hospitals have initiated them: auranofin, penicillamine, or H_2-blockers for long-term use. Expensive treatments of uncertain long-term value such as lovastatin are also subject to restrictions.

Restrictions on Drugs. Technical obstacles may influence prescription practice of potential drugs of abuse. Common prescription drugs are in group C, requiring name of patient and prescriber, and name of drug. Drugs like benzodiazepines and codeine are in group B. After December 1979 [1], it was required that prescriptions for these drugs must also contain address and date of birth of the patient. The prescriptions are retained for 1 year by the pharmacy. Ordinary prescription forms can be used. Figures 1 and 2 show the impact of this restriction on the sales of benzodiazepines, compared to other psychotropic drugs. It can be seen that there was an almost immediate response to the change in prescription rules. The increase after 1984 reflects the commercial success of triazolam (Fig. 1).

Group A drugs are narcotics, e.g., methadone and morphine. In addition to the requirements of group B, special, numbered, and prescriber-identified forms have to be used for a valid prescription. The prescriptions are retained for 3 years. Both for group A and group B, prescription statistics are used to monitor the prescription practices of physicians. Those who overprescribe these drugs, receive a warning

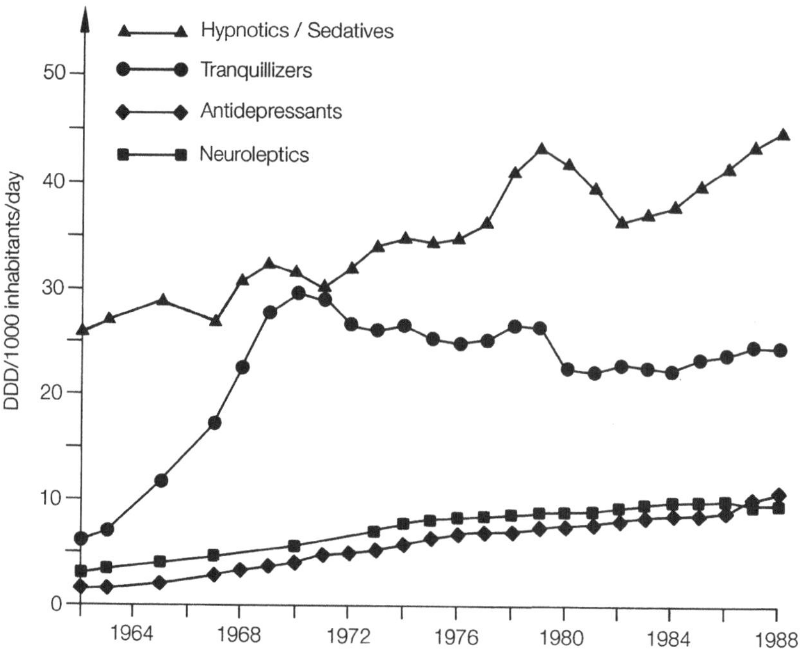

Fig. 1. Annual sales of psychotropic drugs in Norway. Source: NMD [1]

and may lose this right for a shorter or longer period. In 1981 dextropropoxyphene was moved from group B to group A. Immediately, there was a 50% decrease in the prescription of this drug. From 1983 to date the sales have been about one-third of the pre-1981 figures. Simultaneously, there was a considerable increase in the prescription of codeine-paracetamol combinations and pure paracetamol preparations (Fig. 2).

Nonregistered Drugs

Some useful drugs will not be registered, for medical, commercial or other reasons. If a doctor thinks a patient needs a nonregistered drug, the doctor may send an application for the patient to the drug control authority. Usually, these applications are granted quickly, and any drug available in the world may in principle be available to Norwegian patients. Applications are rejected for drugs that are routinely denied registration, for example, organ extracts and stimulants for slimming purposes (fenfluramine), and drugs that have been refused for registration when there are suitable alternatives already on the market, for example astemizole. Applications for drugs that have not been approved for safety reasons also run a risk of being rejected. The Norwegian Medicinal Depot has informed me that in 1989, 19 packs of lisinopril were sold (enalapril and captopril are registered), but 2500 packs of isotretinoin for acne were sold on prescription from dermatologists (no other retinoid for acne is available). Of standard drugs, the main volume of

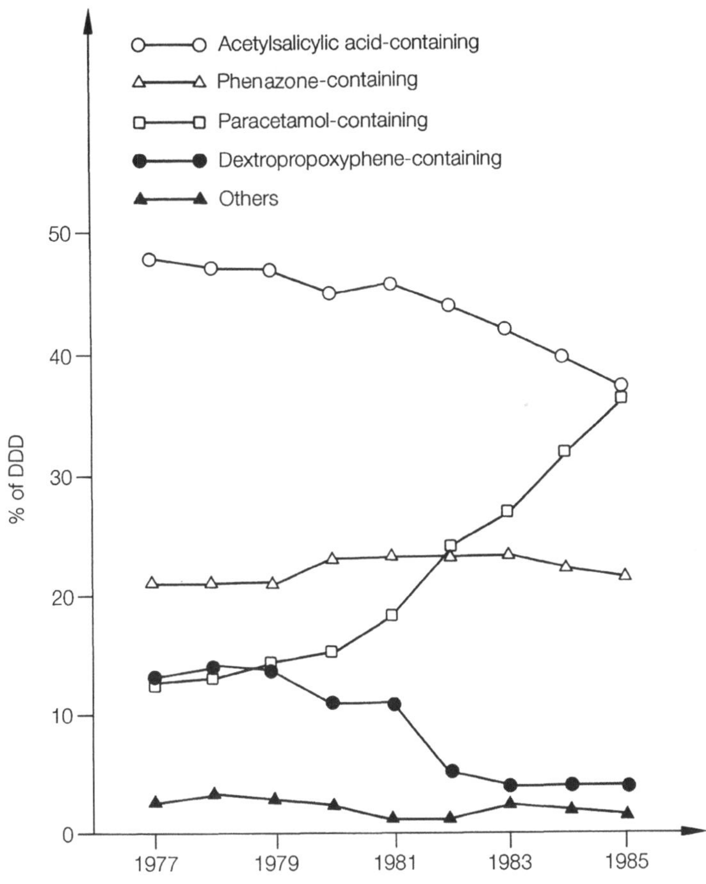

Fig. 2. Sales of analgesics in Norway. Source: NMD [1]

sales involves drugs that later become registered. The sales may thus to some degree reflect the marketing effects of preregistration clinical trials.

Marketing of Drugs

Only approved and registered drugs may be actively promoted by formal marketing such as advertising. Prescription drugs may not be advertised to the public, only to physicians. Some marketing to the public appears to take place through newspaper articles, even of unregistered drugs. When a new drug is approved, marketing to the target prescriber groups cannot start before the drug control authority and the supplier have agreed on a monograph for the *Common Drug Catalogue* (Felleskatalogen). All marketing information is required to comply with the monograph. Only the approved indications are permitted to be promoted. This is a limitation on the suppliers, not on the physicians. There is full freedom to prescribe a drug for a nonapproved indication if he or she thinks this drug could be useful. The prescriber, of course, still has to comply with the normal ethical rules concerning rational therapy.

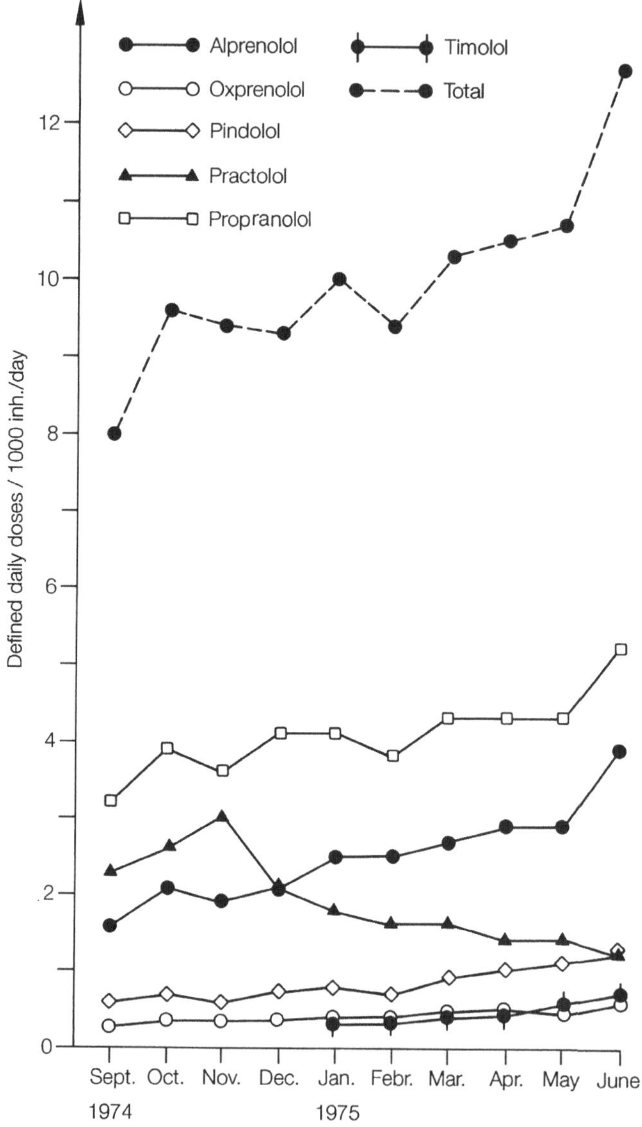

Fig. 3. Monthly sales of beta blockers in Norway September 1974 to June 1975. Source: NMD; taken from [2]

Drug Prices

Prices are negotiated by the drug control authority upon registration and then annually. Price appears to have little impact on prescription practices for reimbursed drugs; more so far drugs that are paid for by the patient for nonchronic conditions or nonapproved indications. Reimbursement is generally granted for all licensed drugs that are approved for reimbursable conditions, mainly chronic disesas. This is only indirectly influenced by the drug licencing authority.

Information

The drug licencing authorities may take action if new information appears on the safety of drugs. Figure 2 shows β-blocker sales in 1974 and 1975, the period when the oculocutaneous side effects of practolol were discovered. Warning against the side effects was issued 9 months prior to withdrawal. As can be seen from the graph (Fig. 3), the information caused a profound and selective drop in the prescription of practolol, in a period when the prescription of the other β-blockers was rising. When the drug was finally withdrawn, prescription ceased altogether.

Some of the effects of information can also be seen for dextropropoxyphene before 1981 and acetylsalicylic acid (Fig. 2).

Other Examples from some Therapeutic Classes

Cytotoxic Drugs

Lymphomas and leukemias are only treated in special centers. The drug licensing authority has had little influence on prescribing because of the investigational nature of these treatments. Until a few years ago, many of the most important drugs in the treatment programs of malignant diseases were not licensed or registered, but were still used according to medical need.

Hyperlipidemia

Dietary treatment is recommended, and drug treatment only if diet is unsuccessful. No drug treatment is recommended at cholesterol levels below 8–9 mmoles/liter. The contribution to a restrictive policy by the control authorities is to register only lovastatin among the statins, and confining the right of prescribing lovastatin to special and small groups of prescribers. For the drug treatment of hyperlipidemia, one can expect the strictness of the licensing authorities to limit prescription. The resins, cholestyramine, and colestipol, do not have such restrictions. Nevertheless, in 1989, lovastatin had half of the anticholesterol market, in terms of defined daily doses.

Hypertension

The effect of the previous generations of primary antihypertensives (mainly diuretics and beta blockers) on mortality has been disappointing. This has led to a rapid change towards angiotensin converting enzyme (ACE) inhibitors, α-blockers and calcium channel blockers for hypertension in the hope that they will improve the results of the treatment, even though there is no proof that these treatment principles constitute an improvement. Because all these drug principles are available to general practitioners, the effect of drug licensing is small. We now have six calcium blockers on the market: verapamil, nifedipine, nimodipine, diltiazem, amlodipine, felodipine. Some of them are marketed with profiles slightly different from the others. There is a risk that the liberal licensing of similar drugs will cause confusion in prescription practices.

Peptic Ulcer

Cimetidine, ranitidine and famotidine, and omeprazole, are registered. Omeprazole may only be prescribed by hospitals. This limits the availability of this very effective and very expensive drug, and in 1989 (it was registered in January of that year) it had only 5 % of the market, in terms of defined daily doses. When cimetidine was introduced, it was released only for hospitals. Later, specialists were permitted to prescribe it. Now cimetidine and the other H_2-blockers can be prescribed by general practitioners. Long-term treatment (with reimbursement) with H_2-blockers may still only be initiated by specialists. This ensures that the patients are adequately investigated prior to long-term therapy. There has been fear that treatable gastric cancers would remain undiagnosed if prescription rules for these drugs became too liberal.

Antipsychotic Therapy

There are 18 neuroleptic agents registered. The three agents perphenazine, haloperidol and zuclopentixol make up about 40 % of the sales, expressed in defined daily doses. The remainder is distributed quite evenly among the others. In this area, the licensing authority appears to have had little influence on prescription practices.

Conclusions

The Norwegian system of drug licensing has resulted in Norway having fewer drugs on the market than all other industrialized countries, except Iceland. The licensing system gives us rational drugs, and a possibility of weeding out irrational or dangerous ones. Laws and regulations are potentially effective means for decreasing the prescription of drugs and counteracting advertising and other marketing efforts by the industry. The strict rules for drug licensing are under pressure, and some relaxation seems inevitable as part of the adaptation to the internal market of Europe.

Acknowledgement. The author wishes to thank Professor P. K. M. Lunde for generously giving advice, suggestions and access to his material.

References

1. Legemiddelforbruket i Norge 1974–76; 1975–77; 1975–79; 1977–81; 1979–83; 1981–85; 1985–88; 1989. Øydvin K. (ed) Oslo: Norsk Medisinaldepot.
2. Lunde PKM. Differences in national drug-prescribing patterns. In: Clinical pharmacological evaluation in drug control. Copenhagen: World Health Organization, Regional office for Europe, 1976

Rational Pharmacotherapy in General Practice: Education by Postgraduate Training

Theo P.G.M. de Vries

Introduction

A recent article in the *European Journal of Clinical Pharmacology* had the following title: Clinical pharmacology and primary health care in Europe – a gap to bridge [1]. In this article, a group of senior European clinical pharmacologists state that clinical pharmacology has been developed in academic or other major hospitals, while 80% of all drugs are prescribed in primary health care (PHC). They state that this development is the major cause for this gap. In their opinion there might also be a relation between this gap and the major drug problems regarding the efficacy and safety of drug prescribing encountered in general practice.

The authors recommend at least two ways for bridging this gap: (a) an increasing volume of drug research and clinical trials should be carried out within PHC, and (b) general practitioners (GPs) should be informed about the results of this research through postgraduate training, in this way increasing their knowledge about drugs, and thus the rationality of prescribing.

These recommendations seem to emphasize knowledge about drugs. But should the aim of postgraduate training be more knowledge about drugs, and should there be more clinical pharmacology research in PHC to provide more knowledge?

Drug Knowledge

It is well known that in undergraduate training of doctors the emphasis is already on drug knowledge. In the first few years students have to learn many facts about drugs. In the last years of medical training, during their clerkships and internships, they are expected to learn how to use that knowledge in medical practice, e.g. in treating patients. After graduation and specialization, practising doctors keep their knowledge up to date by attending postgraduate training courses, reading journals, having contacts with colleagues, seeing pharmaceutical representatives, looking at advertisements, and so on. Most of this postgraduate training is, also, focused on obtaining (more) knowledge about drugs.

The results of the scarce studies on the drug knowledge of students and doctors affirm this view. The results of several multiple-choice examinations throughout the medical programme of two Dutch universities showed that the level of drug knowledge rises steadily during the first years of undergraduate medical training

Rationale Pharmakotherapie in der Allgemeinpraxis
Rational Pharmacotherapy in General Practice
M. M. Kochen (Hrsg.)

[2]. In the final years of undergraduate training the level of drug knowledge stabilises at approximately 60 % of the maximum possible score. After graduation this level seems to remain at the same level, if we may generalize the results of the only study that could be found in the Netherlands about drug knowledge of practising doctors [3]. Though it was not shown by the two studies, a few peaks in knowledge about drugs may be expected, the first two of these indicate regular exam periods in pharmacology. Each peak is usually followed by a rather huge dip in the level of knowledge, just after the exam period. Besides that, some small and short peaks may be expected after a postgraduate training course or the visit of a pharmaceutical representative.

In general, a 60 % level of knowledge is judged to be acceptable, though not ideal. But what is acceptable? It is not only the level that counts. Also, the content of knowledge is important; e.g. what kind of knowledge do students and doctors have. On the basis of the content of the questions it should be concluded that it is knowledge about generics, working mechanisms, pharmacokinetics, effects, side effects, indications, contraindications, and interactions. Laporte and Orme called this type of knowledge drug-oriented [4]. It is knowledge that is structured pharmacologically: from drug to indication, from drug to side effects, from drug to contraindications, and so on. So besides the level of knowledge about drugs, also the content seems to be acceptable, that is, from the pharmacological point of view.

However, having sufficient knowledge is no guarantee that doctors will use this knowledge rationally when prescribing drugs to patients. For that, practising students and doctors will also need the skills to use this knowledge rationally.

Prescribing Skills

In general, practising doctors need the skills to solve a patient's problem. What skills do they need for treating patients rationally with drugs?

When treating a patient in daily practice they will need enough skills (a) to make a rational drug choice (that is to choose a generic, a dosage form, a dosage schedule, and the duration which are expected to be effective, safe, and convenient to the patient, at the lowest possible cost), (b) to write a prescription accurately, (c) to give the necessary information and instructions accurately, that is in a way the patient can understand, and, some time later, (d) to correctly monitor the effectiveness, safety and convenience of the drug treatment.

It has already been shown that the level and content of drug knowledge of students and doctors seem to be reasonable. But do they have sufficient skills to use this knowledge accurately in solving patient problems with drugs? The results of the few studies on this subject can be summarized as follows. A study at the Medical Faculty in Groningen, the Netherlands, revealed that, without any systematic training in therapeutics, graduates make a rational drug choice in approximately 50 % of the patients problems they have to solve [5, 6]. The same goes for the choice of the dosage schedule. In 70 % of the cases they write a prescription accurately, and in approximately 30 % of the cases they give information and instructions to the patient correctly.

If the results of several studies on prescribing rationality of practising doctors in the last two decades are averaged, the scores are more or less the same as those of the graduates just mentioned before [7–20]. This holds except for those about 'information and instructions to patients'. This score is about 75 %. However, in 40 % of the cases the drug choice of practising doctors has been judged not to be acceptable. The same goes for the choice of the dosage schedule. And in 20 % of the cases the prescription lacks important information.

On the basis of the results of these studies it can be concluded that the level of these skills is not acceptable. So the lack of drug-prescribing skills – rather than a lack of knowledge – is probably the cause of irrational prescribing. But before searching for ways to improve these skills, it should be known why these drug prescribing skills are that poor.

Causes

Three important causes can be found for less optimal prescribing skills:

1. The knowledge that is taught does not meet practical use.
2. Students and doctors are not sufficiently trained in prescribing skills.
3. Non-teaching factors may negatively influence rational prescribing.

For all three of these causes enough proof can be found, or at least strong indications.

1. Concerning the first cause, it has already been mentioned that the teaching of pharmacology and clinical pharmacology is too drug-centred, from drug to indication. For practical use, this teaching should be more problem or indication centred: from patient problems to drugs. Or to put it differently: students and doctors should not only be told this drug can be used for this or that disorder because of these or other pharmacological properties. They also need to think the other way around – from indication to drugs. Or to put it differently again, for solving this problem these drugs are available, and, considering treating patients with one of them, you have to take its specific pharmacological properties into account.

2. A second cause is that students and doctors get too little practical training in prescribing skills. There is evidence that this training is very scarce. In 1987 a WHO working group sent an inquiry to the Deans of all 350 Medical Schools in WHO European Region to review pharmacology and therapeutic training [21]. The average number of total hours spent per year on basic pharmacology teaching was 96, on clinical pharmacology teaching, 28, and on therapeutics, only 18. These figures show that less time is spent on clinical pharmacology and therapeutics, if compared to pharmacology teaching. There is also a huge range in teaching hours; some medical schools do not have programmes on one or more of the teaching fields programs at all.

3. The third cause for poor prescribing skills is that non-teaching factors may influence rational prescribing negatively. Many studies have revealed that many factors may cause irrational prescribing [22–27]. For example: the pharmaceutical industry, its representatives and advertisements may influence rationality of prescribing negatively. Doctors who have large practices ususally prescribe drugs less rationally than their colleagues with smaller practices. Doctor and patient characteristics may also influence the rationality of prescribing. For example, if a doctor is very busy, or is annoyed for some reason, a drug may be prescribed to a patient that is not necessary at all, just as a sign to end the consultation.

Reaching this point it can be concluded that instead of transferring more knowledge to students and doctors, we had better see to it that (a) the knowledge we teach is practical, (b) students and doctors are trained in using this knowledge rationally when solving patients' problems, and finally (c) they are taught how to cope with factors that may negatively influence rational prescribing.

Recommendations

The Department of Pharmacology/Clinical Pharmacology of the University of Groningen has developed a problem-solving method for teaching students and doctors how to choose and prescribe drugs rationally. This method is based on the theories of diagnostic problem solving.

Part of this method will be described, namely, the way students and doctors can be taught how to make rational drug choices systematically. A rather simple example will be used to make the method more clear. It might be risky to give an example if it is meant to make something general clearer because people often react to the specific content of the example. So it is stressed that the 'game' and not the 'balls' are discussed here.

Problem-Solving Approach

Suppose we are thinking of treating a 36-year-old taxidriver for his cough. It is a dry and tickling cough that followed a cold. Besides this complaint he is perfectly healthy, does not smoke, and uses no drugs.

A drug treatment for this complaint can be found in two steps: (a) take your first-choice drug for the disorder or complaint (a first-choice drug is a drug that is generally most effective, safe, and cheap, for most patients); and (b) check if this first choice is suitable for this particular patient's problem. If no first-choice drug has been determined yet, this can be done in five steps:

1. Find out what is known about the *pathophysiology*, and/or define your *therapeutic objective.*
2. Make an *inventory* of possible groups of drugs that may influence pathophysiology the way you want, or that might help in reaching the therapeutic objective.
3. *Take* the *most effective group(s).*
4. *Compare drugs* on their efficacy, safety and cost.

5. *Choose* a (first-choice) *drug*.

1. The most likely cause for this kind of cough is that the mucous membrane of the bronchial tubes has been affected by the cold, and therefore is easily irritated. A slight irritation may cause a cough, that, in its turn, will affect the bronchus again. Hence the vicious circle is complete. There are various ways to break this vicious circle. The most important two are avoiding further irritation and suppressing the cough. For this last option drugs can be found.

2. There are three important groups of drugs for treating a cough: mucolytic agents, expectorants and suppressants.

Since we want to surpress a dry and tickling cough, the suppressants should be considered further.

3. In the group of suppressants, at least three drugs are important to consider: promethazine, codeine and noscapine. Next, information should be obtained according to three criteria: efficacy, safety and cost.

4. It is not fully known how these drugs exert their effect. Some studies have shown that patients prefer each of these drugs above placebo. But it has also been found that the frequency of the cough did not decrease when using the drug. So the conclusion might be that all three drugs are equally effective in suppressing the cough.

Concerning safety, the following is known: (a) promethazine, being an anticholinergic drug, is a strong sedating drug; (b) codeine might depress the respiratory centre and may cause little sedation; and (c) there are hardly any important side effects known about noscapine. Since the prices of these three drugs vary considerably from country to country, the differences in price found in the Netherlands are used.

5. On the basis of this information the three drugs can be compared, and the best one chosen. This drug will be the first-choice drug for treating a dry, tickling cough after a cold. It depends on the way the different information is valued what the first choice drug will be. For that reason different doctors may choose different drugs. But let us choose noscapine as the first-choice drug, and return to the patient.

The next thing to do is to check if this drug is suitable for this particular patient. This means that it has to be checked for contraindications, possible interactions, or possible inconveniences for this patient. For example, noscapine syrup should not be prescribed if the man is a diabetes patient, or a daily dosage of 4 × 1 suppository will not be a very convenient treatment for a cab driver. Noscapine can be prescribed to this patient if suitability has been checked thoroughly and if no reasons have been found for not prescribing it.

So, the first step is to find a first-choice drug for the disorder by making an inventory on the basis of pathophysiology, and to compare the drugs according to efficacy, safety and cost. For this comparison clinical pharmacology facts are of essential importance. The second step is to check if the first-choice treatment is suitable for the individual patient. So much for the example of choosing a drug systematically. However, drug-choice is only one part of the whole prescribing process. It is an important part, but only one part of the whole problem-solving process.

After having chosen a drug, this treatment has to be carried out, e. g. a prescription has to be written accurately, the patient has to be informed and instructed correctly, and the results have to be monitored. As has been shown before, these are the skills students and doctors have to learn concerning drug prescribing.

Teaching Materials

There are numerous books in which the necessary pharmacological facts about drugs can be found, but none about how these facts must be used when prescribing drugs. For that reason the department of clinical pharmacology in Groningen has developed teaching materials for therapeutic training. It consists of written and video material. *The Guide to Good Prescribing* describes all the steps of the problem solving process, with an emphasis on solving patients' problems with drugs. On request of the WHO in Geneva this book is being translated into English for medical students, and will be published this year. We also developed drug-choice schemes, in which the facts about drugs are ordered according to the four choice criteria: efficacy, safety, cost and suitability. This way students and doctors are trained to use pharmacology facts in a practical manner when defining their first-choice drugs. Besides, these schemes function as short references for facts which are forgotten. The third part of the teaching materials is an empty formular. Students have to fill this formulary with about 60 drugs they have chosen themselves. Filled with these so-called first-choice drugs it becomes their personal formulary. The students are expected to understand the properties of these drugs very well, and know when to prescribe them, know when not to prescribe them, be able to find alternatives, and be able to prescribe them accurately. Prescribing experience can be obtained by exercises, at first by solving written patient problems, later on by prescribing drugs to real patients, under supervision.

To illustrate some important aspects of drug prescribing a few videos have been produced. The first one, called 'Good thinking, Watson', shows how a rational drug choice can be made in a practice setting, that is, when treating a patient. This video has been subtitled in English and in Spanish.

Results

Up until now we only have the results of an undergraduate teaching course. Courses for general practitioners are being developed at the moment. Prescribing skills improve markedly for the patient problems that have been discussed with students during a training course in therapeutics. The only exception is the skill to give information and instructions to patients accurately; this level remains low. Further analysis revealed that either students did not know what to tell the patient, or did not know how to tell it accurately. Without training, students graduate with prescribing skills at a significantly lower level.

Conclusions

This presentation started with a question: Should students and doctors have more knowledge of drugs in order to bridge the gap between clinical pharmacology and PHC? If clinical pharmacology knowledge is distinguished from clinical pharmacology facts the answer is yes and no. Indeed, there should be more facts, more facts provided by clinical pharmacology research in PHC. Much is still unknown about the actual efficacy and safety of drug treatments in primary health care. But what is urgently needed is training in drug-prescribing skills, in using the known facts rationally. Only then might we reach a higher level of rational prescribing. Because what we really need is more rational prescribing!

References

1. Dukes MNG, Lunde PKM, Mclander A et al. (1990) Clinical pharmacology and primary health care in Europe – a gap to bridge. Eur J Clin Pharmacol 38 : 315–318
2. Cohen-Schotanus J (1983) Voortgangstoets in Groningen, Maastricht en Leiden, Rijks Universiteit Groningen
3. Bender W (1980) Opnemen en onthouden. Rijks Universiteit Groningen
4. Laporte JR, Orme M (1991) Drug utilization and teaching rational drug use. (in press)
5. Vries de, TPGM (1982) Pilot study; internal publication. Dept of Pharmacology/Clinical Pharmacology, University of Groningen
6. Vries de, TPGM (1989) Longitudinal assessment of prescribing drugs. Report Workshop Basic teaching in drugs and therapeutics (WHOPPER). University of Groningen
7. Achong MR, Hauser BA, Krusky JL (1977) Rational and irrational use of antibiotics in a Canadian teaching hospital. Can Med J 116 : 256–259
8. Ray WA, Federspiel CF, Schaffner W (1977) Prescribing of tetracycline to children less than 8 years old: a two-year epidemiological study among ambulatory Tennessee medicaid recipients. JAMA 237 : 2069–2074
9. Victoria CG, Facchini LA, Filho MG (1982) Drug usage in Southern Brazilian hospitals. Tropical Doctor 12 : 231–235
10. Walker G (1987) Introducing concepts of essential drugs/limited lists of drugs. Publication Role of Uni; E 19/370/2, Action Program of Essential Drugs, WHO, Geneva
11. Hasday JD, Karch FE (1981) Benzodiazepine prescribing in a family medicine center. JAMA 246 : 1323–1325
12. Ray WA et al. (1986) Reducing long-term diazepam prescribing in office practice. JAMA 256 : 2536–2539
13. Makela M (1989) Effect of latex agglutination test on prescribing for group A streptococcal throat disease in primary care. Scand J Infect Dis 21 : 161–167
14. Haayer-Ruskamp FM (1984) Het voorschrijfgedrag van de huisarts. Rijks Universiteit Groningen
15. Hohmann AA (1989) Gender bias in psychotropic drug prescribing in primary care. Med Care 27 : 478–490
16. Lawson DH, Jick H (1976) Drug prescribing in hospitals. An international comparison. Am J Public Health 66 : 644–648
17. Hasday JD, Karch FE (1981) Benzodiazepine prescribing in a family medicine center. JAMA 246 : 1323–1325
18. Monson RA, Bond CA (1978) The accuracy of the medical record as an index of out-patient drug therapy. JAMA 240 : 2182

19. Barnett GO, Winickoff RN, Morgan MM, Zielstorff RD (1983) A computer-based monitoring system for follow up of elevated blood pressure. Medical Care 21: 400–409
20. Bryan CK (1976) Patient information vs patient education. Drug Intell Clin Pharm 10: 314–318
21. Orme M, Sjoqvist F, Bircher J et al. (1990) The teaching and organisation of clinical pharmacology in European medical schools. Eur J Clin Pharm 38: 101–105
22. Haayer-Ruskamp FM, Hemminki E (1991) The social aspects of druguse. (in press)
23. Dukes MNG, Haayer-Ruskamp FM (1984) Drugs and money, a preliminary survey and research proposal. WHO regional office for Europe, Copenhagen
24. Barnett A, Creese AL, Ayivor ECK (1980) The economics of pharmaceutical policies in Ghana. Int J Health Serv 10: 479-499
25. Avorn J, Chen M, Hartley R (1982) Scientific versus commercial sources in influence on prescribing behavior of physicians. Am J Med 73: 4–8
26. Stolley PD (1972) The relationship between physician characteristics and prescribing appropriateness. Med Care 10: 17
27. Haayer-Ruskamp FM (1982) Rational prescribing and sources of information. Soc Sci Med 16: 2017–2023

Plenum 2 / Plenary Session 2

Erkenntnisse der klinischen Pharmakologie – Erfordernisse der Praxis: Läßt sich beides verbinden?

Etzel Gysling

Die klinische Pharmakologie ist eine Dienerin der praktischen Medizin. Wenn sich die Erkenntnisse der Wissenschaft *nicht* mit den Erfordernissen der Praxis verbinden ließen, so wären wohl einige Zweifel an dieser Wissenschaft anzubringen.

Nutzen der klinischen Pharmakologie für die tägliche Praxis

Die Anwendung klinisch-pharmakologischer Erkenntnisse hat eine Vielfalt von günstigen Auswirkungen auf die Praxis. Die wichtigsten Punkte lassen sich folgendermaßen zusammenfassen:

Wirkungsvergleich: Angelpunkt bei der Auswahl alter und neuer Arzneimittel

Die klinische Pharmakologie fordert einen Wirkungsnachweis für unsere medikamentösen Therapien. Wichtiger noch: sie bemüht sich um den Vergleich erwünschter und unerwünschter Wirkungen von Therapien, die bei den gleichen Symptomen oder Krankheiten angewandt werden. Wir sind heute mit einer Flut von ähnlichen Wirkstoffen konfrontiert. Der Wirkungsvergleich ermöglicht es, die Spreu vom Weizen zu trennen und für unsere Patienten die jeweils beste Therapie zu finden. Eine Verschreibungspraxis, die sich auf Autoritätsglauben und Gewohnheiten stützt, wird allmählich durch eine überlegte, optimierte Pharmakotherapie abgelöst. Auch bei der Frage nach den Vorteilen eines *neuen* Medikamentes ist der Wirkungsvergleich der Schlüssel zur besten Therapie.

Pharmakokinetik: Kein Stiefkind mehr

Je mehr wir über das Schicksal von Arzneimitteln im Körper und über Aufnahme und Ausscheidung pharmakologisch aktiver Stoffe wissen, desto besser setzen wir die Arzneimittel ein. Die Berücksichtigung der Kinetik stellt einen großen Fortschritt dar. So hätten sich z.B. viele Nebenwirkungen, die in der Vergangenheit auftraten, bei besseren kinetischen Kenntnissen vermeiden lassen. Die größte Aufmerksamkeit gilt heute der Wirkungskinetik, die nicht notwendigerweise mit der Plasmakinetik identisch sein muß.

Rationale Pharmakotherapie in der Allgemeinpraxis
Rational Pharmacotherapy in General Practice
M. M. Kochen (Hrsg.)

Unerwünschte Wirkungen: Auf dem Weg zu einer offenen Informationspolitik

Die klinische Pharmakologie hat uns Auge und Ohr für medikamentös bedingte Probleme geöffnet. Kranke, die sich über „ungewöhnliche“ Symptome beklagen, werden nicht mehr als Simulanten behandelt. Unsere Bereitschaft, auf arzneimittelinduzierte Probleme einzugehen, findet ihre Ergänzung in einer offeneren Informationspolitik der Industrie. Klinisch-pharmakologische Überlegungen sind insbesondere auch zum Verständnis der Interaktionen von großem Nutzen.

Klinische Pharmakologie und Pathophysiologie: Unzertrennlich

Bei der Auswahl des „besten“ Medikamentes sind pathophysiologische Erwägungen von großer Bedeutung. Der Zustand einer oder eines Kranken und ihrer/seiner Organsysteme ist oft maßgebend für therapeutische Entscheidungen. Diese Zusammenhänge sind in der täglichen Praxis ebenso wichtig wie im Krankenhaus.

„Spezielle“ Patienten: Ein besonderes Anliegen der klinischen Pharmakologie

Die intensive Beschäftigung mit den Wirkungen von Arzneimitteln hat zu Erkenntnissen geführt, die für „spezielle“ Patienten besonders wichtig sind. Bei kleinen Kindern, schwangeren Frauen und alten Leuten sind Arzneimittel oft problematischer als bei der „Durchschnittsperson“. In der Praxis ist man häufig mit diesen Problemen konfrontiert.

Nutzen der Beschränkung: Weniger ist oft besser

Die klinische Pharmakologie hat uns gezeigt, wie wichtig die Beschränkung im Bereich der Pharmakotherapie ist. Das Prinzip, möglichst wenige (aber gut dokumentierte) Medikamente so zurückhaltend wie möglich einzusetzen, ergibt in der Praxis einen direkt faßbaren Nutzen. Dieser Nutzen äußert sich in zuverlässigeren Wirkungen, geringeren Nebenwirkungen und reduzierten Kosten.

Der Praktiker: Im Idealfall der beste Pharmaexperte

Gute, auf unabhängigen Quellen beruhende Arzneimittelkenntnisse und der ständige Kontakt mit den Kranken verschaffen dem Praktiker eine Sicherheit im Umgang mit Medikamenten, wie sie sonst niemand erreichen kann. Ein Praktiker, der sich die klinisch-pharmakologische Denkweise angeeignet hat, wird nicht mehr von der Pharma-Werbung manipuliert. Er ist auch gegen das oft praxisferne Besserwissen einzelner Hochschullehrer gefeit.

Die Praxis als Herausforderung für den klinischen Pharmakologen

Die Tätigkeit als Praktiker bringt dem klinischen Pharmakologen eine Reihe von Anregungen. Er wird hier mit der Realität der trivialen Probleme vertraut, aus der sich immer wieder neu auch wissenschaftliche Fragestellungen ergeben, von denen nachfolgend einige Beispiele genannt werden.

Eigenverantwortung der Kranken

Anders als im Krankenhaus kommt in der ambulanten Praxis der Eigenverantwortung der Kranken ein hoher Stellenwert zu. Es ist oft möglich und kann sehr nützlich sein, Patienten an therapeutischen Entscheidungen teilhaben zu lassen. Die Non-Compliance, ein alltägliches Phänomen, hat nicht nur negative Seiten.

Anekdoten und Zufälle

In der Praxis erlebt man auch die statistisch weniger wahrscheinlichen Ereignisse. So kann z.B. der Entzündungshemmer, den man im allgemeinen für den am besten verträglichen hält, in einem Fall eine Magenblutung verursachen. Die Praxis demonstriert auch tagtäglich den Nutzen von Placebos und Pseudoplacebos. Das Erleben von Anekdoten und Zufällen erlaubt dem klinischen Pharmakologen, seine primär theoretischen Überlegungen zu nuancieren.

Genuß- und Suchtmittel, frei erhältliche Arzneimittel

Alkohol und Tabak sowie die vielen rezeptfreien Mittel spielen in der ambulanten Praxis eine große, meist verkannte Rolle. Sie sind nicht nur als Krankheitsursache, sondern auch als Interaktionspartner von ärztlich verordneten Medikamenten von Bedeutung.

Praktische Probleme

Einzelheiten, die mit den Arzneimittelwirkstoffen kaum oder gar nichts zu tun haben, sind im Alltag oft Anlaß zu Schwierigkeiten. So ist es z.B. tatsächlich wichtig, daß ein Medikament nur einmal täglich genommen werden kann, daß eine Tablette nicht zu groß (oder gut teilbar) ist oder daß ein Sirup den Kindern auch schmeckt. Ich halte es für sehr wichtig, daß der Industrie in diesen praktischen Fragen viel „Feedback" aus der Praxis zukommt.

Sonderfälle

Es gibt Personen, die zu fast unkontrollierbarer Polymedikation neigen und die sich ihre Mittel nötigenfalls von verschiedenen Ärzten verschreiben lassen und/oder in verschiedenen Apotheken beschaffen. Andererseits gibt es Menschen, die auch mit wiederholter, eindringlicher Schilderung möglicher Folgen nicht von ihrer Non-Compliance abzubringen sind. Ich halte es für nützlich, daß auch klinische Pharmakologen diesen frustrierenden Phänomenen ausgesetzt sind.

Zusammenfassung

Ich wünschte, daß alle Praktiker „klinische Pharmakologen" wären. Erfahrungen aus Doppelblindstudien, die Beobachtung von Placebo- und Nocebo-Effekten, die Beschäftigung mit der Kinetik, mit unerwünschten Wirkungen und Interaktionen, dies alles kann uns helfen, unseren Patienten die *beste* Therapie zu vermitteln.

Arzneimittelmarkt (BR) Deutschland – eine kritische Bewertung

Gerd Glaeske

Der Arzneimittelmarkt in der Bundesrepublik Deutschland galt für die pharmazeutischen Hersteller lange Zeit als eines der letzten Paradiese: Er sei, so schrieb der englische Informationsdienst Scrip in einem Spezialreport 1983 [14], hinter den USA und Japan weltweit der drittgrößte Markt, die freie Marktwirtschaft werde mit einem Minimum behördlicher Interventionen erhalten, es existierten keine staatlichen Preiskontrollen und kaum Einschränkungen bei der Erstattungsfähigkeit von Arzneimitteln. Außerdem bestehe relative Freiheit im Bereich des Marketing für Arzneimittel.

Diese hier beschriebenen paradiesischen Zustände decken in schöner Offenheit Defizite eines Arzneimittelmarktes auf, dessen Intransparenz, Qualitätsmängel und Kosten zu ausreichend Kritik Anlaß bieten. Diese Kritik soll nachfolgend anhand dreier Thesen zusammengefaßt werden.

These 1: Der Arzneimittelmarkt in der Bundesrepublik wurde einmal als „Apotheke der Welt" bezeichnet; er ist zu einem unaufgeräumten Kramladen verkommen!

Bereits die Zahlen sprechen für sich: Eine Aufstellung der verfügbaren Arzneimittel auf dem Arzneimittelmarkt der Bundesrepublik Deutschland zeigt im Vergleich zu anderen europäischen Ländern deutliche Unterschiede (s. auch Abb. 1):[1]

In der Bundesrepublik werden rund 130 000 Arzneimittel gezählt, in Großbritannien 25 000, in Frankreich 8 000, in Irland 7 500, in den Niederlanden 4 000, in Dänemark 3 000 [14].

Wenn auch diese Zahlen wegen der international z. T. unterschiedlichen Arzneimittelbegriffe nicht unbedingt einen verläßlichen Vergleich zulassen, so läßt sich doch für die Bundesrepublik Deutschland das Problem eines offensichtlich überladenen und damit intransparenten Marktes ableiten. Als 1978 ein neues Arzneimittelgesetz in Kraft trat, das zum ersten Mal für die Zulassung den Nachweis der Wirksamkeit („efficacy"), Unbedenklichkeit („safety") und Qualität verlangte, hatten viele gehofft, daß die damals bereits auf dem Markt befindlichen 140 000 Arzneimittel im Rahmen einer 12jährigen Übergangsbetimmung deutlich vermindert würden. Die Hoffnungen sind wahrscheinlich trügerisch, wir werden weiterhin

[1] Weiteres Datenmaterial zum europäischen Vergleich und zum Arzneimittelverbrauch in der Bundesrepublik Deutschland findet sich im Anhang.

Rationale Pharmakotherapie in der Allgemeinpraxis
Rational Pharmacotherapy in General Practice
M. M. Kochen (Hrsg.)

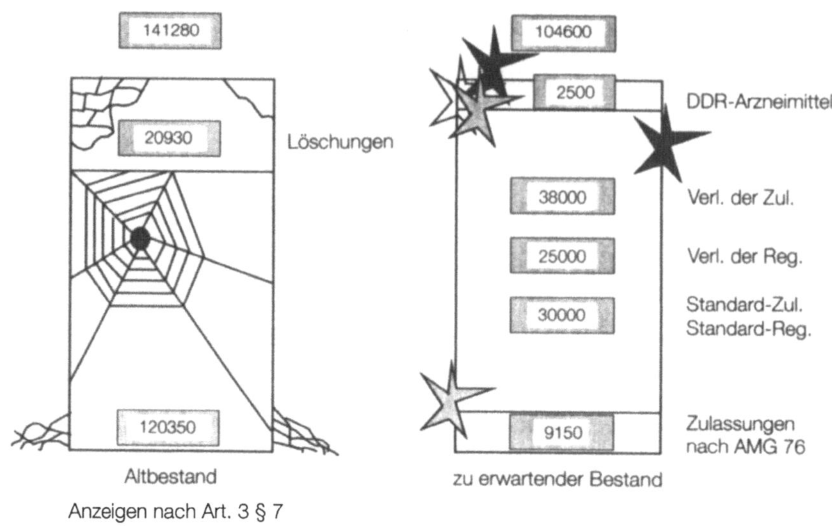

Abb. 1. Der Arzneimittelmarkt der BRD. (Aus Hagemann 1991, persönliche Mitteilung)

von ca. 100000 Arzneimitteln ausgehen müssen. Darunter sind dann allerdings bereits 9150 Arzneimittel, für die auf der Basis des neuen Arzneimittelgesetzes seit 1978 die Zulassung durch die zuständige Behörde, das Bundesgesundheitsamt (BGA), erteilt worden ist. Damit übertreffen die neu zugelassenen Präparate bereits die Zahl von Arzneimitteln, die auf anderen europäischen Märkten den Gesamtumfang des Sortiments darstellen.

Die hohen Zulassungszahlen werden die eher schlechte Tradition eines intransparenten Marktes perpetuieren. Allerdings kann ein Unterschied positiv vermerkt werden: Während sich der Altbestand in 19 % Monopräparate und 81 % Kombinationspräparate aufteilt, sind die Verhältnisse bei den neuzugelassenen Mitteln umgekehrt: 80 % der Zulassungen entfallen auf Monopräparate, nur noch 20 % auf Kombinationen (s. Abb. 2). Damit hat sich die Zulassungsbehörde die allgemeine Kritik an *Kombinationspräparaten* (ausgenommen einige Arzneimittelgruppen, z. B. Antihypertensiva oder Kontrazeptiva) zu eigen gemacht, die sich immer wieder gegen die bis dahin herrschende deutsche Liberalität gegenüber Kombinationsarzneimitteln gerichtet hatte. Seit 1986 ist die Zulassungsbehörde an einen Passus im Arzneimittelgesetz gebunden, der eine Begründung dafür erfordert, „daß jeder arzneilich wirksame Bestandteil einen Beitrag zur positiven Beurteilung des Arzneimittels leistet" (§22, 3 a) – eine Formulierung übrigens, die bereits 1983 vom Ministerrat der EG als Empfehlung ausgesprochen worden war [10]. Noch 1985, also schon in der Geltungszeit des neuen Arzneimittelgesetzes und 2 Jahre nach dieser EG-Empfehlung, wurde aber z. B. die *Schmerzmittelkombination Togal mit den Wirkstoffpartnern Acetylsalicylsäure, Lithiumcitrat und Chinindihydrochlorid* zugelassen, ein Arzneimittelfossil, das in dieser Zusammensetzung seit 1914 angeboten wird [5]. Auch Arzneimittelkombinationen zwei verschiedener Barbitursäu-

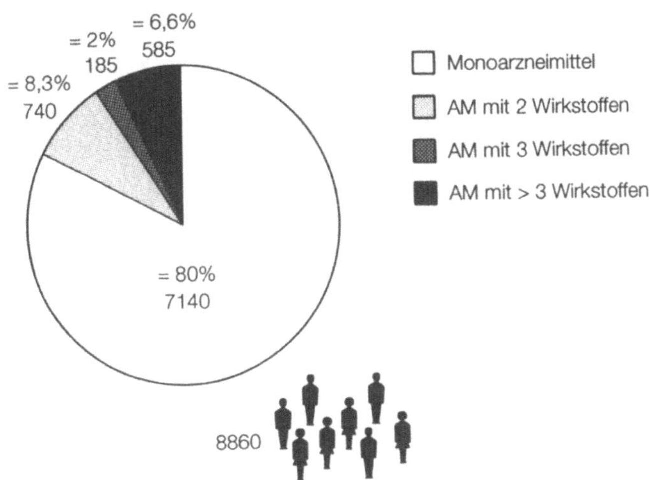

Abb. 2. Zugelassene Arzneimittel nach verschiedenen Aspekten. (Aus Hagemann 1991, persönliche Mitteilung)

rederivate mit einer anderen zentralnervös wirksamen Substanz, z. B. in *Vesparax mite (Secobarbital + Brallobarbital + Etodroxizin)* oder mit Benzodiazepinderivaten, z. B. in dem inzwischen wieder vom Markt genommenen *Psyton (Nomifensin + Clobazam)* fallen in diese Zeit. Dabei war z. B. seit 1980 die Empfehlung des britischen Committee on the Review of Medicines bekannt, Benzodiazepine nicht mit anderen Substanzen zu kombinieren. Standardlehrbücher wiesen bereits Mitte der 70er Jahre auf die unsinnige Kombination von Barbitursäurederivaten untereinander bzw. von Barbitursäurederivaten mit anderen zentralwirksamen Mitteln hin [9].

Aber auch im Bereich der Zulassung von Monopräparaten ist Kritik angebracht: Nur rund 15 % aller Zulassungen entfielen auf Arzneimittel mit neuen Wirkstoffen oder zumindest Strukturvariationen bekannter Substanzen; 1988 waren es 62 von 429 Humanarzneimitteln und 1989 148 von 1090 (Abb. 3). Von den 1988 zugelassenen „neuen" Arzneimitteln werden nach einem abgestuften Innovationsschema schließlich nur noch 4 Arzneistoffe als wirklich neuartige Wirkstoffe oder Wirkprinzipien bezeichnet, nämlich Taurolidin (Taurolin, ein lokales Chemotherapeutikum bei Knocheninfektionen), Gadopentetsäure (Magnevist, ein Kontrastmittel für die Kernspintomographie), kolloidales Bismutsubcitrat (Telen, Bismutsalz bei Gastritiden) und Propofol (Disoprivan, ein neuartiges Injektionsnarkotikum). 1989 bleiben nach dem gleichen Schema lediglich 8 Arzneistoffe übrig: Erythropoietin (Erypo, gentechnologisch hergestelltes Hormon zur Steuerung der Erythrozytenbildung), Flumazenil (Anexate, Benzodiazepinantagonist), Cicletanin (Justar, neuartiges Antihypertensivum), Corticoliberin (Corticobiss, für die endokrinologische Funktionsprüfung), Surfactant (Survanta, beim Atemnotsyndrom von Neugeborenen), γ-Interferon (Polyferon, bei chronischer Polyarthritis), Lovastatin (Me-

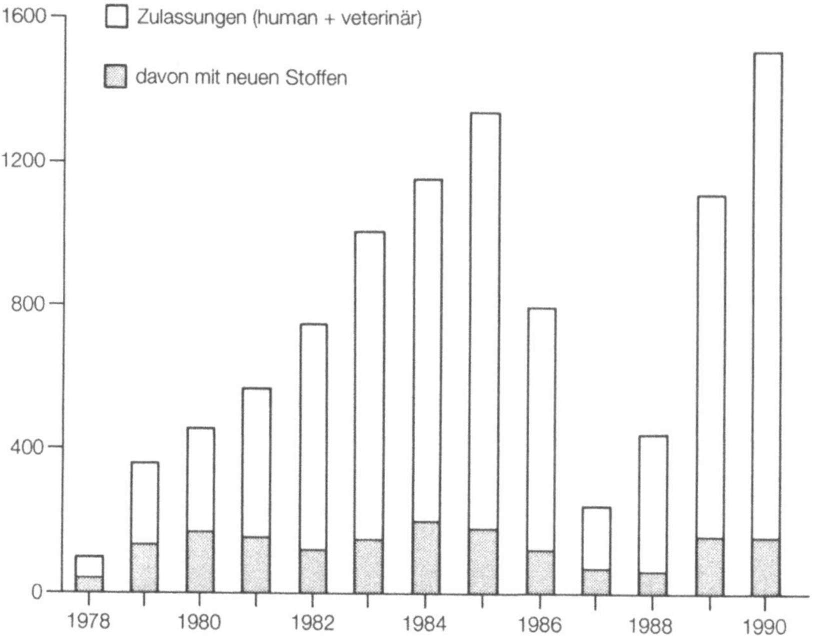

Abb. 3. Zulassung von Arzneimitteln. (Aus Hagemann 1991, persönliche Mitteilung)

vinacor, bei Hyperlipoproteinämie) und Omeprazol (Antra, bei Zollinger-Ellison-Syndrom sowie bei der Ulkustherapie) [3].

Eine andere Aufstellung kommt für die Zeit zwischen 1985 und 1989 zu dem Schluß, daß von den rund 3000 zugelassenen Humanarzneimitteln nur 112 wirklich neue Wirkstoffe enthielten. Die Autoren beurteilen lediglich 12 Wirkstoffe (= 11 % der Neuerungen bzw. 0,4 % der Zulassungen) als Innovation mit echten Vorteilen gegenüber bereits eingeführten Präparaten, 7 ohne Vorteil, während 32 zumindest pharmakokinetische oder pharmakodynamische Eigenschaften verbessern. Die größte Gruppe der Neueinführungen umfaßt 52 Analogpräparate, die keine oder nur marginale Unterschiede zu bereits eingeführten Präparaten besitzen. Vier Arzneimittel wurden als fragwürdiges Therapieprinzip bzw. als Mittel ohne erkennbaren therapeutischen Effekt eingestuft: das „Antirheumatikum" Ademetionin (Gumbaral); das „Kataraktmittel" Pirenoxin (Clarvisor), das „Antiphlogistikum" Serrapeptase (Aniflazym) und die als „Neuraltherapeutikum" angebotenen Ganglioside aus Rinderhirn (Cronassial), ein Präparat, das inzwischen wegen akuter Polyradikulitiden (im Sinne eines Guillain-Barré-Syndroms) vom Markt genommen werden mußte [1].

Insgesamt müßten also viele Arzneimittel bei einer Zulassungsprüfung, die ein medizinisches Bedürfnis als Kriterium hätte (z. B. die „need-clause" in Norwegen), vom Markt ferngehalten werden, weil sie weder einen therapeutischen Fortschritt

Tabelle 1. Indikationsbereiche der zugelassenen Arzneimittel 1989. (Aus bga-Tätigkeitsbericht)[a]

Herz- und Kreislaufmittel	191 (44)
Schmerz- und Rheumamittel	154 (36)
Chemotherapeutika	114 (2)
Dermatika	81 (4)
Bronchialmittel	84
Psychopharmaka	73 (6)
Antibiotika	54 (32)
Magen- und Darmmittel	42 (7)
Endokrinologische Präparate	36

[a] Es sind nicht alle 1090 Zulassungen des Jahres 1989 berücksichtigt.

gegenüber eingeführten Arzneimitteln noch eine Innovation im Sinne eines neuen Therapieprinzips darstellen.

Die Verteilung der Indikationsbereiche der zugelassenen Arzneimittel im Jahre 1989 gibt Tabelle 1 wieder.

Die Nennungen in Klammern beziehen sich auf Arzneimittel mit neuen Stoffen, alle anderen Mittel sind in gewisser Weise Nachahmerpräparate (sog. „Me-too-Präparate"), die in den meisten Fällen das bereits vorhandene Sortiment lediglich ausweiten, aber keinesfalls bereichern. Darunter sind vielfach auch Generikazulassungen, die zwar evtl. Kostenvorteile in der Verordnung mit sich bringen, letztlich aber eigene Probleme von Intransparenz schaffen: Vielfalt von Warenzeichennamen („branded generics") und Unsicherheiten hinsichtlich Bioäquivalenz und Bioverfügbarkeit [8].

Wem nutzen letztlich 269 zugelassene Zubereitungen und Stärken mit Diclofenac oder 243 mit Ibuprofen, 192 mit Nifedipin oder 181 mit Ambroxol, 93 mit Vitamin E und 86 mit Verapamil, 83 mit Propranolol und 44 mit Diazepam (Stand 10/90)?

Der Arzneimittelmarkt wird auch durch solche Zulassungen ständig erweitert; die Marktrücknahmen halten sich dagegen in Grenzen – zwischen 1978 und 1988 wurde eine Rücknahme durch das BGA lediglich für 1014 Arzneimittel angeordnet.

Die therapeutische Qualität des Angebots geht dabei augenscheinlich im Arzneimitteldschungel verloren:

So zeigen Studien zur vergleichenden pharmakologischen Bewertung der angebotenen Arzneimittel erschreckende Ergebnisse.

Die Übersicht in Tabelle 2 zeigt, daß ca. 50 % aller angebotenen Arzneimittel nach pharmakologischen Kriterien, die auf einer Risiko-Nutzen-Abschätzung basieren, nicht für die therapeutische Anwendung empfohlen werden können. Die immer wieder euphemistisch als Vielfalt angesprochene Intransparenz unseres Arzneimittelmarktes ist eher ein Sammelsurium von Altlasten, bestenfalls zweifelhaft wirksam, schlechtestenfalls auch noch gefährlichen Irrationalitäten neben einem großen Anteil unnötiger Diversifikationen und einem kleinen Anteil nützlicher

Tabelle 2. Vergleichende pharmakologische Bewertung einiger angebotener Arzneimittelgruppen

Indikationsgebiet	Wirksamkeit und/oder Sinn der Kombination erwiesen	umstritten
Angina pectoris	177	222[a]
Arterielle Hypertonie	502	156[a]
Arterielle periphere Durchblutungsstörungen	103	181[a]
Diabetes mellitus	190	87[a]
Fettstoffwechselstörungen	83	32[a]
Gicht	163	41[a]
Herzmuskelinsuffizienz	163	220[a]
Herzrhythmusstörungen	238	57[a]
Kreislaufinsuffizienz	243	159[a]
Periphere venöse Durchblutungsstörungen	209	647[a]
Antibiotika/Chemotherapeutika	346	108[b]
Hypnotika/Sedativa	76	261[b]
Psychopharmaka	172	126[b]
Analgetika/Migränemittel/ Antirheumatika (systemisch)	250	311[b]
Gesamt	2752 (51,3 %)	2608 (48,7 %)

[a] Aus: Dölle, Schwabe (1986) Internist 27 : 21–31.
[b] Aus: Greiser (1983) (Hrsg) Bewertender Arzneimittelindex, 1983, 1985 bzw. unveröffentlicht.

und wirksamer Arzneimittel. Diese herauszufinden, wird daher für jeden Arzt, der sich um eine rationale, d. h. indikationsbezogene, begründbare Pharmakotherapie bemüht, zur täglichen Herausforderung.

These 2: Die Arzneimittelversorgung kann qualitativ nicht besser sein als der Arzneimittelmarkt!

Hans Friebel, pharmakologischer Berter in einem Projekt zur Analyse von Verordnungsdaten in Dortmund („Dortmunder Arzneimittel-Transparenz-Modell“) drückt es zurückhaltend so aus:

> Der Angebotsvielfalt [des Marktes, d. V.] entspricht die Vielfalt ärztlicher Verordnungsprofile. [...] In Dortmund verordneten niedergelassene Internisten im Durchschnitt 767 Patienten im 1. Quartal 1985 585 verschiedene Fertigarzneimittel. Diese Daten induzierten die Frage, ob der zum Teil marktbedingte Umfang des ärztlichen Arzneimittelsortiments überhaupt theoretisch möglich erscheinen läßt, daß der Verordnende sich über die erwünschten und unerwünschten Wirkungen so zahlreicher Produkte ausreichend informieren kann. [...] am häufigsten verordneten Fertigarzneimittel wurden binnen Jahresfrist ausgewechselt, in der Regel ohne erkennbare Verbesserung der therapeutischen Qualität der Sortimente. Dieser rege Sortimentenwandel konnte demnach nur zu Verlusten an präparatbezogener therapeutischer Erfahrung führen. [...] Der Trend zur Ausweitung des Arzneimittelangebotes hält an – zum Wohle des Kranken [4]?

Wohl kaum! Diese neuen Analysen von ärztlichem Verordnungsverhalten mit Negativbewertung haben übrigens Tradition in der Bundesrepublik (s. Glaeske 1988 [8]).

Bereits 1977 kommt ein im Auftrag des Bundesverbandes der Ortskrankenkassen durchgeführtes Gutachten u. a. zu folgendem Ergebnis: „Arzneimittel, deren therapeutische Wirksamkeit im Sinne der vom Hersteller empfohlenen Indikation fraglich ist, stellen einen Kostenanteil von 16,2 v. H. an den Gesamtkosten dar. Arzneimittel, deren therapeutische Wirksamkeit nicht nur als fraglich, sondern als nicht erwiesen eingestuft wurden, machen 28,3 v. H. an den Gesamtkosten aus."

Eine Untersuchung in einer Allgemeinpraxis in Berlin kommt zu folgendem Ergebnis: „Die systematische Untersuchung ergab nach einer kritischen Bestandsaufnahme des „Arzneischatzes" eine reale Kostenersparnis von 22,1 v. H. Dabei zeigte sich, daß bei diplomatischer Umsetzung der Therapie so gut wie keine Schwierigkeiten bei den Patienten auftraten, nur 16 forderten, die ursprüngliche Therapie weiter verordnet zu bekommen."

In der richtungsweisenden Arbeit von E. Greiser und E. Westermann, die auf der Auswertung von Rezepten der RVO-Kassen (zu den Reichs-Versicherungs-Ordnungs-Kassen gehören z. B. AOK, IKK, BKK) aus Niedersachsen beruht, wird darauf hingewiesen, daß z. B. in der untersuchten Gruppe von Arzneimitteln zur Behandlung der Herzinsuffizienz 60,6 v. H. der Verordnungen im 1. Halbjahr 1974 bzw. 55,4 v. H. im Jahre 1976 den in der Arbeit aufgestellten Kriterien für eine rationale, pharmakologisch begründete Pharmakotherapie nicht entsprachen.

In einer weiteren Arbeit wird die Validität von Verschreibungen von Mitteln gegen hohen Blutdruck, gegen niedrigen Blutdruck und gegen Herzrhythmusstörungen untersucht. Als Ergebnis wird festgehalten, daß im Schnitt 50 % Kombinationspräparate verordnet wurden, ein Anteil, der als ungerechtfertigt hoch beurteilt wird. Weiter heißt es: „Die höchste Verordnungsfrequenz wiesen mit fast 40 v. H. die Kardiaka auf, gefolgt von zusammen 27,2 v. H. für durchblutungsfördernde Mittel einschließlich der Koronarmittel, die überwiegend Substanzen ohne gesicherten therapeutischen Nutzen für die angegebene Indikation enthalten."

Eine Untersuchung zur Validität der Verordnungen von herzwirksamen Medikamenten anhand eines auf pharmakologisch-wissenschaftlichen Kriterien beruhenden Bewertungsschlüssels kommt zu folgenden Ergebnissen: 60 v. H. der praktischen Ärzte und 54,7 v. H. der niedergelassenen Internisten verschrieben herzwirksame Arzneimittel, die nicht den pharmakologischen Kriterien einer adäquaten Pharmakotherapie genügten. In absoluten Zahlen: Bei den praktischen Ärzten und den Ärzten für Allgemeinmedizin entsprachen von 31 800 Verordnungen 19 000 nicht den vorgegebenen Kriterien hinreichender Validität. H. Herken hatte 1962 bereits ein ähnliches Ergebnis gefunden und vermutete seinerzeit, daß mehr als 60 v. H. der Verordnungen von „praktischen Ärzten" „nur im guten Glauben an eine Wirksamkeit verordnet" wurden.

In den ergänzenden Gutachten zur „Analyse zur Struktur und Entwicklung der Arzneimittelausgaben im Rahmen der Krankenversicherung der Rentner werden u. a. folgende Schlußfolgerungen gezogen:

a) Es ist dringend eine Verbesserung der Information der Ärzte über rationale und rationelle Verordnungsweisen erforderlich.
b) Ebenso dringlich ist die Herausnahme von Arzneimittel-Gruppen aus der Erstattungspflicht der gesetzlichen Krankenkassen, wenn der therapeutische Nutzen zweifelhaft ist.

Schließlich wird in der Einleitung des „Arzneiverordnungs-Report '90' [15], der einen Überblick über die Arzneimittelversorgung innerhalb der Gesetzlichen Krankenkassen (GKV) bietet, zusammenfassend gewertet:

Tabelle 3. Arzneimittelgruppen mit umstrittener Wirksamkeit. Verordnungen und Umsatz 1989. (Aus [15])

Arzneimittelgruppe	Verordnungen [Mio.]	Änderung zu 1988 [%]	Umsatz in [Mio. DM]	Änderung zu 1988 [%]
Antiallergika, topische	2,0	+12,2	19,8	+17,2
Antianämikakombinationen	2,1	+7,3	60,0	+13,7
Antiarrhythmikakombinationen	0,4	–4,8	35,9	–0,3
Antidiarroika (Sonstige)	2,9	+13,8	56,1	+18,9
Antiphlogistika (Sonstige)	4,1	–4,1	132,9	+3,7
Arterioskleroseminittel	0,2	–6,2	4,2	+0,6
Carminativa	2,9	+0,6	49,7	+7,4
Cholagoga	4,4	–9,9	141,2	–9,5
Chondroprotektiva	2,0	–3,8	78,5	–1,8
Dermatika (Varia)	0,8	–4,5	13,2	+3,6
Durchblutungsfördernde Mittel	19,2	–15,4	1195,3	–16,5
Expektoranzien	45,4	+5,6	713,7	+7,7
Glukokortikoidkombinationen	1,3	–15,0	19,7	–13,4
Grippemittel	4,2	–4,9	40,0	+0,4
Gynäkologika (Sonstige)	2,0	–7,8	44,0	–4,4
Hämorrhoidenmittel	4,9	–10,2	82,4	–6,0
Herzglykosidkombinationen	0,9	–20,5	27,9	–16,2
Pflanzliche Hypnotika und Kombinationen	4,4	–6,7	57,0	+3,0
Kardiaka (Pflanzenauszüge)	5,1	–5,2	96,4	1,3
Koronardilatatoren	1,7	–17,8	61,2	–10,5
Lebertherapeutika	2,6	–8,6	108,6	–11,5
Magnesiumpräparate	6,2	+0,5	122,9	+4,5
Migränemittel (Kombinationen)	4,6	+0,3	80,2	+11,7
Mund- und Rachentherapeutika	8,4	–8,7	79,7	–5,2
Muskelrelaxanzien (Kombinationen)	3,1	–7,1	97,0	–3,0
Nootropika	1,7	–6,9	103,6	–7,0
Ophthalmika (Sonstige)	4,4	–13,2	61,0	–12,3
Psychopharmaka (pflanzliche)	1,8	–8,3	42,9	–5,1
Rauwolfia-Extrakte	0,3	+47,8	7,0	+98,0
Rheumamittel (Externa)	24,4	–5,8	408,2	–5,2
Rhinologikakombinationen	4,5	–8,0	47,4	–5,5
Tetrazyklinkombinationen	0,4	–5,3	16,0	–5,4
Umstimmungsmittel	4,7	–5,4	88,7	+1,4
Urologika (Kombinationen und Sonstige)	10,8	–2,8	293,3	+0,7
Venenmittel	19,3	–8,8	578,2	–7,9
Verdauungsenzyme (Kombinationen)	3,0	–16,2	90,7	–11,9
Vitamin-B-Kombinationen	3,1	–0,3	70,6	–2,9
Xanthin-Kombinationen	1,0	–20,2	25,8	–13,5
Gesamt	215,0	–3,7	5250,9	–4,7

Einen relativ großen Anteil an den Arzneiverordnungen haben Arzneimittelgruppen, die auf bisher unsicheren oder umstrittenen therapeutischen Konzepten beruhen. Besonders häufig verordnete Gruppen sind die durchblutungsfördernden Mittel, Expektorantien, externe Rheumamittel und Venenmittel (s. Tabelle 3). In vielen Fällen sind tierexperimentell pharmakologische Wirkungen beschrieben. Ein klinisch relevanter therapeutischer Effekt ist jedoch häufig nicht überzeugend nachgewiesen worden. Da viele von diesen Arzneimittelgruppen in den USA, Großbritannien und den skandinavischen Ländern nicht erhältlich sind, wurde gefolgert, daß wir ohne Nachteil auf diese umstrittenen Arzneimittel verzichten können. Wenn dann noch unerwünschte Wirkungen hinzukommen, wie es kürzlich bei einigen durchblutungsfördernden Mitteln und Chondroprotektiva geschehen ist, wird ein vielleicht marginaler therapeutischer Nutzen sogar zum therapeutischen Risiko. Nutzlose Arzneimittel sind keine Placebos.

Zusammengenommen entfallen 1989 auf diese umstrittenen Arzneimittelgruppen 215,0 Mio. Verordnungen, was einem Anteil von 30,5 % am Verordnungsvolumen des gesamten Arzneimittelmarktes entspricht (703,8 Mio. Verordnungen 1989). Die Gesamtkosten für diese umstrittenen Arzneimittelgruppen betragen 5,3 Mrd. DM (von insgesamt 20,7 Mrd. DM (S. 10/11).

Diese Ausgaben sind aus pharmakologischer Sicht schwer verständlich. Es stellt sich bei den insgesamt weiter steigenden Kosten im Arzneimittelsektor daher durchaus die Frage, ob derartig hohe Summen nicht besser für wichtigere medizinische Aufgaben verwendet werden sollten als für die unspezifische und keineswegs immer risikolose Therapie mit Arzneimitteln, an deren Wirksamkeit und Nützlichkeit berechtigte Zweifel bestehen.

Neben dieser Auflistung von vielverordneten, aber nur zweifelhaft wirksamen Arzneimitteln können auch Angaben über die meistverkauften bzw. meistverord-

Tabelle 4. Arzneimittel mit den höchsten Umsatzwerten 1989

Rang	Präparat	Arzneistoff (INN)	Umsatz [Mio. DM]	Indikationsgebiet
1	Tebonin	Gingko-Extrakt	133	Durchblutungsstörungen
2	Sostril	Ranitidin	121	z. B. Ulzera
3	Zantic	Cimetidin	114	z. B. Ulzera
4	Cedur	Bezafibrat	107	Hyperlipidämie
5	Depot-H-Insulin	Schwein/Insulin	89	Diabetes
6	Adalat	Nifedipin	89	z. B. Bluthochdruck
7	Dusodril	Naftidrofuryl	88	Durchblutungsstörungen
8	Marvelon	Desogestrel/ Ethinylestradiol	79	Kontrazeptivum
9	Mevinacor	Lovastatin	72	Cholesterinsenker
10	Rytmonorm	Propafenon	72	Herzrhythmusstörungen
11	Beloc	Metoprolol	72	z. B. Bluthochdruck
12	Pepdul	Famotidin	70	z. B. Ulzera
13	Trental	Pentoxifyllin	67	Durchblutungsstörungen
14	Voltaren	Diclofenac	67	Rheuma
15	Capozide	Captopril/ Hydrochlorothiazid	65	z. B. Hochdruck
16	Isoket	Isosorbiddinitrat	63	Angina pectoris
17	Lopirin	Captopril	61	z. B. Hochdruck
18	Pulmicort	Budesonid	58	Asthma
19	Berodual	Ipatropium/Fenoterol	57	Asthma
20	Sandimmun	Ciclosporin	56	Immunsuppressivum

neten Arzneimittel einen Einblick in die Qualität der in der Bundesrepublik angewendeten Arzneimittel bieten.

In Tabelle 4 sind einzelne Arzneimittel aufgelistet, die 1989 die höchsten Umsatzwerte erzielt haben (Rangfolge nach Industrieumsatz, ohne Apothekenaufschläge).

Zu diesen umsatzstarken Arzneimitteln gehören v. a. Herzmittel, Mittel zur Behandlung von Durchblutungsstörungen oder zur Behandlung von Stoffwechselerkrankungen (zu hohe Blutfettspiegel, Diabetes mellitus u. ä.), Rheumamitel und Kalziumantagonisten sowie β-Rezeptorenblocker und ACE-Hemmer.

Tabelle 5 zeigt die innerhalb der gesetzlichen Krankenkassen im Jahre 1989 meistverordneten 20 Arzneimittel.

Eine Vergleichsstudie der Weltgesundheitsorganisation (WHO) hat die Auflistung der 50 meistverordneten Arzneimittel in unterschiedlichen Ländern analysiert und anhand pharmakologischer Kriterien qualifiziert [13]. Die im internationalen Vergleich hohen Verordnungsmengen von Mitteln gegen Durchblutungsstörungen (Tebonin, Dusodril), von Digitalisglykosid-haltigen Arzneimitteln (Lanitop, No-

Tabelle 5. 1989 am meisten verordnete Arzneimittel

Rang	Präparat	Arzneistoff (INN)	Verordnung [Mio.]	Kosten [Mio. DM]	Indikationsgebiet
1	Voltaren Gel	Diclofenac ext.	4,67	83,6	Rheuma
2	Novodigal	β-acetyldigoxin	4,40	59,9	Herzinsuffizienz
3	Olynth	Xylometazolin	4,14	22,0	Nasentropfen
4	ben-u-ron	Paracetamol	3,85	19,2	Schmerzen, Fieber
5	L-Thyroxin Henning		3,79	64,7	Schilddrüse
6	Lanitop	Metildigoxin	3,61	62,2	Herzinsuffizienz
7	Paracetamol-ratio		3,39	12,7	Schmerzen, Fieber
8	Tebonin	Gingko-Extrakt	3,34	218,9	Durchblutungsstörungen
9	Euglucon	Glibenclamid	3,04	102,5	Diabetes
10	Dusodril	Naftidrofuryl	2,93	148,4	Durchblutungsstörungen
11	Aspirin	ASS	2,92	15,7	z. B. Schmerzen
12	Imodium	Loperamid	2,89	51,4	z. B. Durchfall
13	Mucosolvan	Ambroxol	2,80	42,9	Husten
14	Isoket	Isosorbiddinitrat	2,78	124,3	Angina pectoris
15	Adalat	Nifedipin	2,72	195,3	z. B. Hochdruck
16	Diclophlogont	Diclofenac	2,66	33,6	Rheuma
17	Gastrosil	Metoclopramid	2,58	21,5	Magen-Darmmittel
18	Diclofenac-ratio		2,48	33,7	Rheuma
19	Maaloxan	Mg-/Al-Hydroxid	2,47	64,1	Magen/Antazidum
20	Sinupret	Phytotherapie	2,45	32,3	Erkältung

vodigal) oder externen Rheumamitteln (Voltaren Emulgel) bereits unter den 20 meistverordneten Arzneimitteln haben sicher dazu beigetragen, daß die „theoretische pharmakologische Validität" der in der Bundesrepublik am häufigsten angewendeten Arzneimittel zu der vergleichsweise schlechtesten gehörte: Während für Schweden (1,22), Großbritannien (1,29) und Norwegen (1,36) relativ gute „Zensuren" vergeben wurden, lag die Bundesrepublik (1,72) hinter Bulgarien (1,64) und Jugoslawien (1,66) und nur knapp vor Ungarn (1,89). Dies ist zumindest ein Hinweis für die Berechtigung der These 2, nach der die Qualität der Arzneimittelversorgung und die des Angebots nicht weit differieren.

Ein weiterer wichtiger Aspekt im Zusammenhang mit der Arzneimittelversorgungsqualität – die Verordnung von Arzneimitteln mit bekanntem Abhängigkeitspotential – soll hier aus Platzgründen nur erwähnt werden [6, 7].

Fazit dieses Abschnitts: Die Verordnungsrealität und -qualität wird durch die Qualität des Arzneimittelangebots beeinflußt. Die *Verfügbarkeit von Arzneimitteln* sowie die v.a. *arzneimittelherstellergebundenen Informationen sind wesentliche Determinanten für die Anwendung von Arzneimitteln.* Interventionen zur Verbesserung der Qualität in der Arzneimittelversorgung werden sich an dieser Analyse orientieren müssen.

These 3: Die Qualität der Arzneimittelversorgung in der Bundesrepublik läßt sich vor allem durch die Einschränkung der Verfügbarkeit bestimmter Arzneimittel und durch gezielte industrieunabhängige Informationsstrategien verbessern!

Der Hauptanteil aller Arzneimittel wird im Rahmen und zu Lasten der gesetzlichen Krankenkassen verordnet – was läge also näher, als hier nach Interventionsstrategien zu suchen, die das Regulierungsdefizit und den mangelnden Gestaltungswillen der Zulassungs- und Überwachungsbehörde Bundesgesundheitsamt auszugleichen versuchen. Die Bundesrepublik ist eines der wenigen übriggebliebenen europäischen Länder ohne umfangreiche, letztlich marktbeeinflussende Positiv- oder Negativlisten, mit denen den Ärzten pharmakologisch und medizinisch begründete Therapieempfehlungen zur Erleichterung ihrer Arzneimittelauswahl angeboten werden. Hier sei z. B. an die British National Formulary mit rund 2100 Einträgen erinnert. Solche Listen haben den Vorzug, daß sie aus einem bewertenden Vergleich heraus die Mittel der Wahl für bestimmte Indikationsbereiche bzw. die Mittel mit dem relativ günstigsten Risiko-Nutzen-Verhältnis zusammenstellen und dem verordnenden Arzt den *Überblick über therapeutisch gleichwertige Alternativen erleichtern.* Die Auswahl eines Arzneimittels aus therapeutisch gleichwertigen Arzneimitteln ist im übrigen Voraussetzung, um *Therapiefreiheit* reklamieren zu können. Alles andere wäre nur *Therapeutenfreiheit.*

In der Bundesrepublik wird mit dem 1. Juli 1991 zwar noch keine Positivliste in Kraft treten, eine Negativliste wird aber eine Reihe von Arzneimitteln aus der Leistungspflicht der gesetzlichen Krankenversicherung ausschließen. Die geplante

Negativliste umfaßt einerseits unsinnig kombinierte Arzneimittel, andererseits Arzneimittel mit zweifelhaft wirksamen Inhaltsstoffen.

Mit dieser Negativliste droht für viele Produkte die Ausgrenzung vom lukrativen Kassenmarkt, der doch einen bislang kalkulierbaren Gewinn sogar für solche Produkte versprach, die schon seit Jahren in pharmakologischen Standardbewertungen „negativ“ dargestellt werden. Ein 1,5-Mrd.-Segment ist z. Z. in Gefahr, durch die Negativliste ausgegliedert zu werden. Einige Beispiele:

- Antifibrillantien mit anderen Wirkstoffen (z. B. Cordichin: Chinidin + Verapamil);
- Benzodiazepine mit anderen Wirkstoffen (z. B. Persumbran: Oxazepam + Dipyridamol; Limbatril: Chlordiazepoxid + Amitriptylin);
- Chinin mit anderen Wirkstoffen (z. B. Togal: Chinin + Lithiumcarbonat + Acetylsalicylsäure);
- Herzglykoside mit anderen Wirkstoffen (z. B. Nitro-Novodigal: β-Acetyldigoxin + PETN).

In die Negativliste werden auch Wirkstoffe aufgenommen, für die von den zuständigen BGA-Kommissionen sog. Negativmonographien („therapeutischer Nutzen nicht erwiesen“) erstellt wurden. Hierunter fallen z. B. Wirkstoffe wie Bucetin, Cholin, Cinnarizin (bei Hirnleistungsstörungen im Alter), Clofezon, Crotamiton, Dantron u. a.

Der zuletzt vorgelegte Referentenentwurf für eine Negativliste der unwirtschaftlichen Arzneimittel betraf unter den 1000 meist verordneten Arzneimitteln 147 mit einem GKV-Kostenvolumen von 1,1 Mrd. DM [11]. Die Einsparungen betrügen rund 200 Mio. DM, wenn jede bisherige Verordnung weitergeführt und durch ein pharmakologisch sinnvolles Produkt ersetzt würde. Gewonnen wäre damit also weniger spektakulär im Kostenbereich als deutlich im Bereich der verordneten Mittel: Der gesicherte therapeutische Nutzen ist schließlich die erste Forderung für eine wirtschaftliche Arzneimittelversorgung.

Neben derartigen „Interventionen“ zur Sicherung der Versorgungsqualität kommt der Informationsvermittlung und deren Qualität größte Bedeutung zu: Ein Inhaltsstoff wird schließlich erst durch die indikationsbezogene Information zum Arzneimittel. Die Qualität der Arzneimittelinformation leidet in der Bundesrepublik wie in vielen anderen Ländern an der Industriegebundenheit und Marketingnähe. Die in einigen Krankenkassen und Kassenärztlichen Vereinigungen begonnenen pharmakotherapeutischen Beratungen sind dagegen ein möglicher und erfolgversprechender Weg, die *industrieunabhängige, individuell ausgerichtete Arzneimittelinformation* für die Verbesserung der Verordnungsqualität einzusetzen.

Ausblick

Die Ursachen mangelnder Qualität der Arzneimittelversorgung und damit verbunden auch mangelnder Arzneimittelsicherheit liegen zweifellos in der unüberschaubaren Vielzahl der auf dem Markt befindlichen Arzneispezialitäten, die – wie der

Berliner Pharmakologe Hans Herken schon 1972 auf der Jahrestagung der Deutschen Gesellschaft für Innere Medizin anmerkte – nur „von interessierter Seite als Arzneimittelschatz" bezeichnet würden. Schließlich finden sich bereits unter den 2000 am häufigsten verordneten Arzneimitteln innerhalb der gesetzlichen Krankenkassen, die 89,7 % aller Verordnungen und 90,1 % der Kosten ausmachen, rund 40 %, die nicht dem herrschenden medizinischen und pharmakologischen Kenntnisstand entsprechen. Offensichtlich ist dieser Zustand aber nicht auf eine Entwicklung der letzten Jahre zurückzuführen. Denn bereits vor einem halben Jahrhundert klagte Wolfgang Heubner, einer der Väter der Deutschen Pharmakologie, anläßlich seiner Antrittsvorlesung in Heidelberg:

> ... Übersicht und Erfahrung des Arztes zwecks richtiger Auswahl und Dosis eines Mittels im gegebenen Augenblick sind in vielen Fällen für die Wirkung bedeutsamer als die Möglichkeit, etwa unter 50 statt unter 5 verschiedenen Präparaten wählen zu können. Die Unübersichtlichkeit, die das Massenangebot notwendigerweise bedingt, verdirbt das Beste an jeder Arzneibehandlung. [...] Eine Überbewertung des Arzneimittels im ganzen Heilplan bedeutet eine Verminderung der Qualität ärztlicher Leistung. *[Daher]...ist es notwendig, viel von Pharmakologie zu verstehen, um wenig Arzneimittel zu brauchen* ([12]; Hervorhebung von mir).

Die Stärkung der pharmakotherapeutischen Kompetenz bei verordnenden Ärzten durch eine bessere pharmakologische und pharmakotherapeutische Ausbildung und individuelle Arzneimittelberatungen oder interventionistische Regulationen, z.B. mit Positiv- oder Negativlisten, erscheinen mir daher als Mittel der Wahl, den „Krankheitssymptomen" ansteckende Diversifikation, chronische Überladenheit und idiopathische Intransparenz des „Patienten" Arzneimittelmarkt in der Bundesrepublik begegnen zu können.

Literatur

1. Becker-Brüser W, Glaeske G, Heeke A, Schulz-Schalge T (1990) Die neuen Arzneimittel – Wirkungsweise und therapeutischer Stellenwert. Offizin 2 : 129–132
2. Dölle W, Schwabe U (1986) Ist Transparenz auf dem Arzneimittelmarkt möglich? Internist 27 : 21–31
3. Fricke U (1989, 1990) Arzneimittelmarkt 1988 bzw. 1989. Was war wirklich neu? Dtsch Apoth Ztg 129 : 881–892; 130 : 1107–1122
4. Friebel H, Rummel W (1991) Wandel in der Arzneiverordnung – Determinanten und Trends. Dtsch Ärztebl 88 : 19–22
5. Glaeske G (1986) Zulassung eines Arzneimittelfossils. Dtsch Apoth Ztg 126 : 541–542
6. Glaeske G (1988) Die Exposition der Bevölkerung mit suchtstoffhaltigen Arzneimitteln. In: Arnold W, Poser EW, Möller MR (Hrsg) Suchtkrankheiten. Springer, Berlin Heidelberg New York Tokyo, S 126–136
7. Glaeske G (1988) Medikamentstatistik 1988: Schätzungen zur Abhängigkeit von Arzneimitteln. In: DHS (Hrsg) Jahrbuch '90 zur Frage der Suchtgefahren. Neuland-Verlag, Hamburg, S 175
8. Glaeske G, Schefold D (Hrsg) (1988) Positivliste für Arzneimittel. Nomos, Baden-Baden
9. Greiser E (Hrsg) (1983) Arzneimittel-Index, Bd 2: Hypnotika, Sedativa, Psychopharmaka. Medpharm, Wiesbaden Stuttgart

10. Hart D, Reich N (1990) Integration und Recht des Arzneimittelmarktes in der EG. Nomos, Baden-Baden
11. Heeke A, Müller M (1989) Auswirkungen der Negativliste. Pharm Ztg 134:22–23
12. Heubner W (1931) Arznei als Wert (Text der Antrittsvorlesung vor der medizinischen Fakultät der Universität Heidelberg 1930). Springer, Berlin
13. Laporte JR (1988) Comparison of consumption patterns in the European region: A study of the most prescribed drugs in European countries. Report of the Meeting of the WHO Drug Utilization Research Group, Oslo 1987. WHO, Copenhagen (ICP/DSE 127, December)
14. NN (1983) The pharmaceutical market in West Germany. A scrip special report. PJB Publications, London
15. Schwabe U, Paffrath D (Hrsg) (1990) Arzneiverordnungs-Report '90. Fischer, Stuttgart New York

Anhang: Vergleich einiger Daten zum Arzneimittelmarkt

Der Umsatz auf dem Arzneimittelmarkt lag im Jahre 1989 bei ca. 15 Mrd. DM, gemessen am Apothekenumsatz bei 27,6 Mrd. DM und zuzüglich der hier üblichen 14 % MWSt. bei 31,5 Mrd. DM.

Der *weltweite ambulante Arzneimittelmarkt* hatte 1988 auf der Basis von Herstellerabgabepreisen einen Gesamtwert von 112 Mrd. $, die sich wie folgt aufteilten (ati, Berlin, persönliche Mitteilung):

EG: 32,4 Mrd. $ (= 29 %; in diesem Wert sind Dänemark und Luxemburg nicht enthalten, weil z.Zt. keine Daten vorliegen);
USA: 24,7 Mrd. $ (22 %);
Japan: 14,2 Mrd. $ (13 %).

Innerhalb der EG verteilte sich der *Umsatz* von 32,4 Mrd. $ folgendermaßen:

- Bundesrepublik Deutschland: 8,49 Mrd. $ (26,2 %),
- Frankreich:7,87 Mrd. $ (24,3 %),
- Italien: 6,87 Mrd. $ (21,2 %),
- Großbritannien: 3,66 Mrd. $ (11,3 %),
- Spanien: 2,49 Mrd. $ (7,7 %),
- Belgien: 0,97 Mrd. $ (3,0 %),
- Niederlande: 0,88 Mrd. $ (2,8 %),
- Portugal: 0,55 Mrd. $ (1,7 %),
- Griechenland: 0,45 Mrd. $ (1,4 %),
- Irland: 0,16 Mrd. $ (o,5 %).

Aus diesen Ergebnissen lassen sich die Pro-Kopf-Ausgaben für Pharmazeutische Produkte in den unterschiedlichen EG-Ländern im Jahre 1988 ableiten:

Bundesrepublik Deutschland:	173 $,
Frankreich:	137 $,
Italien:	123 $,
Belgien:	110 $,
Dänemark:	72 $,

Niederlande: 67 $,
Großbritannien: 66 $,
Spanien: 62 $,
Irland: 57 $,
Portugal: 54 $,
Griechenland: 39 $.

Arzneimittelverbrauch

Der Verbrauch an Arzneimitteln ist in Tabelle 6 als Summe aller verkauften Packungen bzw. – noch genauer – aus der Summe der einzelnen Dosierungseinheiten (Tabletten, Zäpfchen, Kapseln, Dragees, Tropfen- oder Safteinheiten, Salbendosierungseinheiten, Ampullen) errechnet worden.

Tabelle 6. Arzneimittelverbrauch in der Bundesrepublik Deutschland[a]

Jahr	Anzahl der Packungen [Mrd.]	Änderung [%]	Anzahl der Einzeldosen [Mrd.]	Änderung [%]
1982	1,219	–2,2	60,469	–0,8
1983	1,169	–4,1	58,614	–3,1
1984	1,168	±0	60,366	+2,9
1985	1,161	–0,6	60,777	+0,7
1986	1,198	+3,2	63,321	+4,2
1987	1,228	+2,5	65,992	+4,2
1988	1,288	+4,9	68,805	+4,3
1989	1,270	–1,4	67,600	–2,1

[a] Quelle: 1982–89 pharma daten 90 (herausgegeben vom Bundesverband der pharmazeutischen Industrie, BPI, Frankfurt am Main).

Danach entfielen 1989 auf jeden Bundesbürger, ob Kleinkind oder Greis, im Durchschnitt 21 Packungen Medikamente mit insgesamt ca. 1100 Arzneimitteldosierungen, also rund 3/Tag.

Die durchschnittliche Pro-Kopf-Menge liegt in benachbarten europäischen Ländern noch höher, 1989 z. B.

- in Belgien bei 1264 Dosierungen,
- in Italien bei 1598 Dosierungen,
- in Großbritannien bei 1767 Dosierungen,
- in Frankreich bei 1687 Dosierungen.

Lediglich für Österreich wird ein niedrigerer Wert angegeben: 1043 Dosierungen.

Fraglich ist allerdings, ob die Zahlenwerte wirklich vergleichbar sind, weil z. T. nicht vergleichbare Dosierungsmengen pro Zähleinheit verglichen werden.

Tabelle 7 listet aus dem Gesamtmarkt die umsatzstärksten Arzneimittelgruppen des Jahres 1989 auf.

Tabelle 7. Marktvolumen von 15 Arzneimittelgruppen im Vergleich

Basis	Umsatz in Mio. DM (exklusive MWSt.)	Marktanteil [%]
Gesamtmarkt		
– mit Apothekenaufschlägen	27 600	
– ohne Apothekenaufschläge (Herstellerabgabepreise)	14 980	100
Teilmarkt von 15 großen Arzneimittelgruppen	8 683	58,0
Herztherapeutika	882	5,9
Psychopharmaka (inklusive Hypnotika/Sedativa)	804	5,3
Vasodilatanzien	749	5,0
Antirheumatika (inklusive Rheumasalben)	720	4,8
Antiinfektiva	666	4,4
Hustentherapeutika (inklusive Erkältungsmittel)	586	3,9
Sexualhormone (inklusive Antikontrazeptiva)	562	3,7
Kalziumantagonisten	524	3,5
Antiasthmatika	520	3,5
Analgetika	504	3,4
Vitamine und Mineralien	473	3,1
β-Rezeptorenblocker	470	3,1
Ulkustherapeutika	454	3,0
Vasoprotektoren	411	2,7
Diuretika	358	2,4

Auf diese 15 aufgelisteten Arzneimittelgruppen entfielen rund 58 % des Industrieumsatzes. Sie geben damit zumindest Anhaltspunkte auf die in der Bundesrepublik meistbehandelten Erkrankungen bzw. Krankheitssymptome und Befindlichkeitsstörungen.

Die meistverkauften Arzneimittel

Die Top 20 der im Jahre 1989 am häufigsten verkauften Präparate sind in Tabelle 8 zusammengestellt (ati, Berlin, persönliche Mitteilung).

Die Schmerzmittel „beherrschen" diese Aufstellung der meistverkauften Arzneimittel; sie sind die „Renner" der Selbstmedikation. Auffällig ist dabei nach wie vor die führende Position von Schmerzmitteln mit einem Koffeinanteil, z. B. Thomapyrin und Spalt N, obwohl seit Jahren auf das mögliche Mißbrauchspotential solcher Schmerzmittel mit leicht anregenden Bestandteilen hingewiesen wird: Beide genannten Präparate haben auch von der Menge her ihre Position halten können. Daran hat auch eine gesetzliche Regelung vom 01. 07. 1989 nichts ändern können, die Rückgang der vieldiskutierten koffeinhaltigen Schmerzmittel bringen sollte: Diese Regelung besagt, daß jede Tablettenmenge eines koffeinhaltigen Schmerzmittels mit mehr als 10 g Schmerzwirkstoff(en) insgesaamt oder mehr als 0,5 g pro Einzeldosis nur noch auf Rezept verordnet werden darf. Aber selbst diese Verfügbarkeitsbeschränkung, die als Signal einer eingeschränkten Unbedenklichkeit gewertet werden darf, konnten Verbraucher, aber auch Fachleute wie Apotheker, nicht davon abhalten, weiterhin in hoher Menge solche Produkte zu kaufen bzw. zu verkaufen. Dieses Beispiel zeigt aber auch die Fragwürdigkeit einer halbherzigen Marktintervention: Potentiell bedenkliche, nicht rezeptpflichtige Arzneimittel sollten grundsätzlich von ihrer leichten Verfügbarkeit innerhalb der Selbstmedikation ausgeschlossen werden, Marktrücknahme oder Rezeptpflicht sind dabei die einzig wirksamen Regulatorien.

Tabelle 8. Die Top 20 bei den Arzneimitteln. *SM* nicht rezeptpflichtig, v. a. Selbstmedikation; *Rp* rezeptpflichtig

Rang	Präparat	Packungsmenge	Anwendungsbereich	
1	Thomapyrin	21,8 Mio.	SM	Schmerzen
2	Spalt N	12,8 Mio.	SM	Schmerzen
3	Aspirin	11,0 Mio.	SM	Schmerzen
4	Aspirin + C	8,6 Mio.	SM	Schmerzen
5	Benu-u-ron	6,8 Mio.	SM	Schmerzen, Fieber
6	Olynth	6,8 Mio.	SM	Nasentropfen
7	Bepanthen	6,7 Mio.	SM	z.B. Wundheilung
8	Voltaren	6,7	Rp	Rheuma
9	ph-5-Eucerin	5,9 Mio.	SM	Hautpflege
10	Paracetamol-ratio	5,5 Mio.	SM	Schmerzen, Fieber
11	Kwai	5,0 Mio.	SM	Knoblauch
12	Otriven	4,9 Mio.	SM	z.B. Nasentropfen
13	Novodigal	4,8 Mio.	Rp	Herzinsuffizienz
14	Marvelon	4,7 Mio.	Rp	„Antibaby-Pille“
15	Sinupret	4,7 Mio.	SM	z.B. Schnupfen
16	Vivimed	4,6 Mio.	SM	Schmerzen
17	Mucosolvan	4,4 Mio.	SM	Husten
18	Tebonin	4,1 Mio.	SM	Durchblutung
19	L-Thyroxin Henning	4,1 Mio.	Rp	Schilddrüsenmittel
20	ASS-ratio	4,0 Mio.	SM	Schmerzen

Verordnungsmengen

Weltweit wurden 1988 11,2 Mrd. Verordnungen registriert, davon 29 % (3,3 Mrd.) in der EG. Innerhalb der EG verteilen sich die Verordnungen (VO) nach den Angaben des Institutes für medizinische Statistik wie folgt:

- 766 Mio. (23,2 %) auf Italien (je Einwohner der 57,2 Mio.: 13,4 VO),
- 695 Mio. (21,0 %) auf die Bundesrepublik Deutschland (61: 11,4),
- 640 Mio. (19,4 %) auf Frankreich (55,3: 11,6),
- 518 Mio. (15,7 %) auf Spanien (38,7: 13,4),
- 413 Mio. (12,5 %) auf Großbritannien (56,7: 7,3),

- 122 Mio. (3,7 %) auf Belgien (9,9: 12,3),
- 66 Mio. (2,0 %) auf Portugal (10,3: 6,4),
- 53 Mio. (1,6 %) auf die Niederlande (14,6: 3,6).

Eines der auffälligsten Ergebnisse der Zusammenstellungen ist die hohe Verordnungsquote in Spanien (15,7 %) bei einem relativ geringen Kostenanteil (7,7 %) und der sehr niedrige Verordnungsanteil in Holland (1,6 %) bei einer relativ hohen Kostenstruktur (2,8 %).

Diese Zusammenhänge basieren auf der bislang bekannntesten Beobachtung beim Vergleich europäischer Länder:

Die *Arzneimittelpreise* in der EG weisen beträchtliche Unterschiede auf, beträchtlichere übrigens, als bei anderen Produkten, z. B. Autos, Haushaltsgeräten, Audio- und Videoausrüstungen, festgestellt wurden.

Die letztveröffentlichte Studie von BEUC aus dem Jahre 1989 bestätigte diese Unterschiede erneut:

Während die Einkäufe eines 125 Arzneimittel umfassenden Warenkorbes in Portugal den Index 100 ergab, in Frankreich 111, in Spanien 112 und in Griechenland 127, betrug der mit der gleichen Methodik zustandegekommene Index in den Niederlanden 214, in Dänemark 231 und in der Bundesrepublik den Spitzenwert von 239.

Übrigens endet jede dokumentierte Kontaktaufnahme mit einem niedergelassenen Arzt in der Bundesrepublik – zumindest im Durchschnitt – mit der Verordnung eines Arzneimittels. Dies ist in europäischen Nachbarstaaten und den USA anders; dort enden viele Konsultationen ohne die Verordnung eines Arzneimittels (die folgenden Prozentangaben beziehen sich auf Arztbesuche, die ohne die Verordnung eines Medikaments enden):

in Belgien	8 %,
in Italien	8 %,
in Spanien	16 %,
in Frankreich	22 %,
in Großbritannien	26 %,
in den USA	37 %,
in den Niederlanden	44 %.

Probleme des Konsums und der Verfügbarkeit von Arzneimitteln in Thüringen

Annemarie Hoffmann, Ina Blumöhr und Mechthild Knüpfer

Einleitung und Problemstellung

Arzneimittelverbrauchsanalysen sind unverzichtbar für Aussagen über Trendentwicklungen beim Verbrauch in verschiedenen Indikationsgruppen, der Aufdeckung von Möglichkeiten zur Einschränkung unzweckmäßiger Therapiegewohnheiten und der Analyse der Kostenentwicklungen [7]. Mit der DDD (definierte Tagesdosis, „defined daily dose") wurde eine für Gebrauchsanalysen geeignete und zweckmäßige Größe gefunden [4]. Sie gibt an die während eines Tages im Durchschnitt zu applizierende Menge eines Arzneimittels für die jeweilige Hauptindikation in Bezug auf einen Erwachsenen als Masse des Wirkstoffes oder bei Arzneimitteln mit mehreren Wirkstoffen als Anzahl der Einzeldosen. Wird der Verbrauch auf die Bevölkerung bezogen, nimmt die Aussagekraft der Verbrauchsanalysen zu. Es ist dann möglich, den durchschnittlichen Teil aus der Bevölkerung zu errechnen, der mit dem entsprechenden Arzneistoff behandelt wird [2].

Ziel der vorliegenden Studie war es, den Arzneimittelverbrauch ausgewählter Indikationsgruppen zweier thüringischer Kreise unter Nutzung der Vergleichseinheit DDD aus ärztlicher Sicht zu analysieren und Möglichkeiten der Einflußnahme auf die Durchsetzung einer wissenschaftlich begründeten Pharmakotherapie zu zeigen.

Material und Methode

Es wurden Arzneimittelverbrauchsanalysen zweier bezüglich Bevölkerungsstruktur und vorhandener Industrie relativ ähnlich strukturierter Territorien (Kreis Pößneck und Kreis Rudolstadt) über einen Zeitraum von 5 Jahren (1984–1988) durchgeführt. Die dazu notwendigen Verbrauchsangaben wurden aus den entsprechenden Inventurlisten der Kreisapotheken entnommen (Inventurlisten der Kreisapotheken Pößneck und Rudolstadt 1984–1988). Die Analyse des Arzneimittelverbrauchs erfolgte mittels Anwendung definierter Tagesdosen (DDD, „defined daily dose"), einer Vergleichseinheit, die durch die Drug Utilization Research Group (DURG) der WHO und den Nordic Council on Medicines kreiert wurde. Die für die Berechnungen notwendigen DDD entstammen dem Nordic Drug Index der Nordic Statistics on Medicine [5] und den Berechnungen des Institutes für Apothekenwesen der ehemaligen DDR in Leipzig.

Für den jeweiligen Kreis wurden mittels der Verbrauchszahlen und der DDD für 80 Arzneimittel aus 10 Indikationsgruppen – entsprechend der Inventurlisten

Rationale Pharmakotherapie in der Allgemeinpraxis
Rational Pharmacotherapy in General Practice
M. M. Kochen (Hrsg.)

der Kreisapotheken – die Kennziffer „Anzahl DDD pro 1000 Einwohner (EW) pro Tag" nach folgender Formel errechnet [6]:

$$\frac{\text{Anzahl DDD}}{\text{1000 EW} \cdot \text{Tag}} = \frac{\text{Anzahl Op} \cdot \text{Stück} \cdot \text{Stärke} \cdot 100}{\text{DDD} \cdot 365 \cdot \text{Einwohnerzahl}}$$

Für die Einwohnerzahl wurden die vom Amt für Statistik der jeweiligen Kreise überlassenen Zahlen von 53 605 Einwohnern im Kreis Pößneck und 69 242 Einwohnern im Kreis Rudolstadt im Jahr 1988 verwendet. Bei Arzneimitteln, die in verschiedenen Packungsgrößen und/oder unterschiedlichen Dosierungen pro Stück (z. B. Tabletten) vorhanden sind, erfolgt die Summierung der Kennziffer DDD/1000 EW/Tag.

Zur Bewertung der Ergebnisse wurden ausgewählte demographische Kennziffern aus den Kreisen (nach Angaben aus den jeweiligen Statistischen Jahrbüchern) herangezogen, die in den Tabellen 1–3 dargestellt sind.

Im Zeitraum von 1984 bis 1988 ist die Gesamtzahl der Ärzte im Kreis Pößneck annähernd gleich geblieben, im Kreis Rudolstadt von 97,9 auf 110,1 Voll-

Tabelle 1. Anteil der Bevölkerung im arbeitsfähigen und nichtarbeitsfähigen Alter an der Wohnbevölkerung (Statistischer Jahresbericht 1989)

	Von 100 der Wohnbevölkerung waren:		
Kreis (Stand 1988)	im arbeitsfähigen Alter	Rentner	Kinder
Pößneck	64,1	17,1	18,8
Rudoltstad	64,8	17,0	18,1

Tabelle 2. Ambulant tätige Ärzte (in Vollbeschäftigungseinheiten nach ausgewählten Fachabteilungen 1988. (Statistischer Jahresbericht 1989)

		Zahl der Ärzte					
Kreis	Zahl der Einwohner pro ambulant tätigen Arzt	Gesamt	Allgemeinmedizin	Innere Medizin	Chirurgie	Gynäkologie Geburtshilfe	Pädiatrie
Pößneck	1240,8	43,2	26,8	2,7	0,3	2,5	4,7
Rudolstadt	935,0	74,0	35,2	7,6	3,0	4,6	8,1

Tabelle 3. Stationär tätige Ärzte (in Vollbeschäftigteneinheiten nach ausgewählten Fachabteilungen 1988. (Statistischer Jahresbericht 1989)

		Zahl der Ärzte				
Kreis	Zahl der Einwohner pro stationär tätigen Arzt	Gesamt	Innere Abteilung	Chirurgische Abteilung	Abt. für Gynäkologie und Geburtshilfe	Pädiatrische Abteilung
Pößneck	2335,0	23,0	5,0	13,0	5,0	–
Rudolstadt	1915,0	36,1	13,8	9,0	5,0	4,0

beschäftigteneinheiten angestiegen. Vergleicht man die Anzahl der Krankenhausbetten im Jahr 1988, zeigt sich auch dabei ein Unterschied zwischen beiden Kreisen (Kreis Pößneck: 313 Krankenhausbetten, Kreis Rudolstadt: 435 Krankenhausbetten).

Die Anzahl der Arzneimittel, die in der DDR zur Verfügung gestanden haben, ist Tabelle 4 zu entnehmen.

Wegen der besseren Übersichtlichkeit der Ergebnisse erfolgte deren graphische Darstellung in Säulendiagrammen als Gegenüberstellung der errechneten Kennziffern ausgewählter Arzneimittel verschiedener Indikationsgruppen der 2 Kreise für das jeweilige Jahr. So wird der territoriale Vergleich zwischen den Kreisen Pößneck und Rudolstadt ermöglicht und eine zeitliche Analyse innerhalb eines Kreises im Zeitraum von 5 Jahren realisiert.

Tabelle 4. Arzneimittelzulassungen in der DDR vor dem Beitritt zur Bundesrepublik Deutschland (Stand 02. 10. 1990; *AM* Arzneimittel)

Herstellerland	Arzneifertigwaren	Standardrezepturen
DDR	1471 (65,1 %)	348
BRD	210 (9,3 %)	–
Andere EG-Staaten	27 (1,2 %)	–
RGW-Staaten	212 (9,4 %)	–
Andere Nicht-EG-Staaten	74 (3,3 %)	–
Gesamt (ohne homöopathische und radioaktive AM)	1994	
Homöopathische AM (DDR)	201 (8,9 %)	
Radioaktive AM (DDR)	45 (2,0 %)	
Radioaktive AM (Import)	18 (0,8 %)	
Gesamt	2258 (100,0 %)	
Registrierte Gesundheitspflegemittel: (ohne Körperpflegemittel)	318	

Ergebnisse und Diskussion

Indikationsgruppen

Aus den Inventurlisten der Apotheken der Kreise Pößneck und Rudolstadt wurden für die Jahre 1984–1988 die Indikationsgruppen Kardiaka, Vasodilatanzien, Antihypertensiva, Diuretika, Antitussiva und Sekretolytika, Antiasthmatika, Chemotherapeutika und Antibiotika sowie Antirheumatika analysiert. Es werden Teile der Analyse dargestellt.

Herzglykoside (Abb. 1)

In beiden Kreisen ist der Verbrauch an Herzglykosiden von 1984 bis 1988 kontinuierlich gesunken, bei Digoxin auf 44 (Pößneck) bzw. 38 % (Rudolstadt), bei

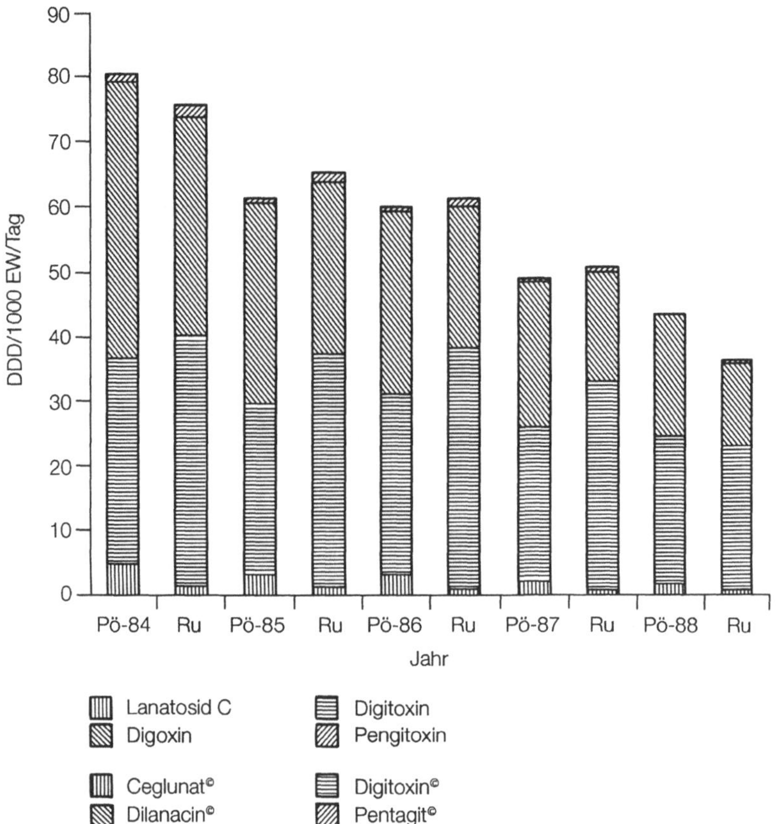

Abb. 1. Vergleich ausgewählter Arzneimittel der Indikationsgruppe *Herzglykoside* in den Kreisen Pößneck (*Pö*) und Rudolstadt (*Ru*) von 1984 (*84*) bis 1988 (*88*). Es werden jeweils die Arzneistoffe (*INN*) sowie die Präparatenamen der DDR genannt (durch ° nach dem Präparatenamen gekennzeichnet). Die Angaben erfolgen als definierte Tagesdosen pro 1000 Einwohner pro Tag (*DDD/1000 EW/Tag*)

Digitoxin auf 72 (Pößneck) bzw. 57 % (Rudolstadt). Der Rückgang an Glykosiden ist durch eine wissenschaftlich begründete Verordnungsweise erklärbar, zunehmend werden sie nur noch bei Herzinsuffizienz und Tachyarrhythmia absoluta (wobei auch hier der Antiarrhythmikaeinsatz zunimmt) angewendet.

Die deutliche Rückläufigkeit beim Digoxinverbrauch im Vergleich zu Digitoxin ist darauf zurückzuführen, daß bei älteren Patienten mit nicht exakt bestimmter Nierenfunktion wegen der Gefahr der Kumulation und des dadurch bedingten Auftretens von Nebenwirkungen in der ambulanten Praxis zunehmend Digitoxin bevorzugt wird [3, 8].

Beim Vergleich mit dem Glykosidverbrauch der Bundesrepublik 1988 [9] fällt auf, daß in Thüringen zu mehr als 50 % Digitoxin verordnet wird, während in den alten Bundesländern 1988 nur 13,9 % des Marktes durch Digitoxin abgedeckt wurden, 53,8 % durch Digoxin. Die Anzahl der DDD/1000 EW/Tag in den Kreisen Pößneck und Rudolstadt entsprechen denen der Bundesrepublik, wenn die Glykoside insgesamt betrachtet werden.

Diuretika (Abb. 2)

Die Triamteren-Hydrochlorothiazid-Kombination Triampur° ist vor Furosemid in beiden Kreisen führend.[1] Im Unterschied zur Bundesrepublik 1988 ist hier der Verbrauch an Thiaziden als Monopräparat sehr niedrig und nimmt weiter ab; es wird fast ausschließlich die Kombination mit dem kaliumsparenden Triamteren eingesetzt, wenn Thiazide verordnet werden.

Das Schleifendiuretikum Furosemid wurde 1988 in beiden thüringischen Kreisen etwa im gleichen Ausmaß wie in der Bundesrepublik verordnet.

Der Diuretikaverbrauch ist insgesamt steigend, Rudolstadt hat einen höheren Verbrauch pro 1000 EW als Pößneck.

Die steigende Tendenz im Diuretikaverbrauch ist auch in der Bundesrepublik zu verzeichnen, entspricht akzeptierten Therapieempfehlungen. Aldosteronantagonisten, von denen in der BRD 1988 64,4 Mio. DDD verordnet wurden [9], unterlagen im Untersuchungszeitraum in der DDR den Nomenklatur-C-Bestimmungen, durften also nur zur sehr hochspezialisierten Versorgung eingesetzt werden. Das erklärt die sehr niedrige Verordnungsrate.

β-Rezeptorenblocker (Abb. 3)

Im Kreis Rudolstadt wurden von 1984 bis 1988 bei leicht steigender Tendenz doppelt so viele β-Rezeptorenblocker verordnet wie im Kreis Pößneck. Hauptsächlich der β_1-selektive Blocker Talinolol steht hier in der Verordnungshäufigkeit mit 19,8 DDD/1000 EW/Tag gegenüber dem nichtselektiven Blocker Propranolol mit 13,3 DDD/1000 EW/Tag im Vordergrund und bedingt im wesentlichen den Mehrverbrauch im Vergleich zu Pößneck.

[1] ° = registrierte Arzneifertigware der DDR.

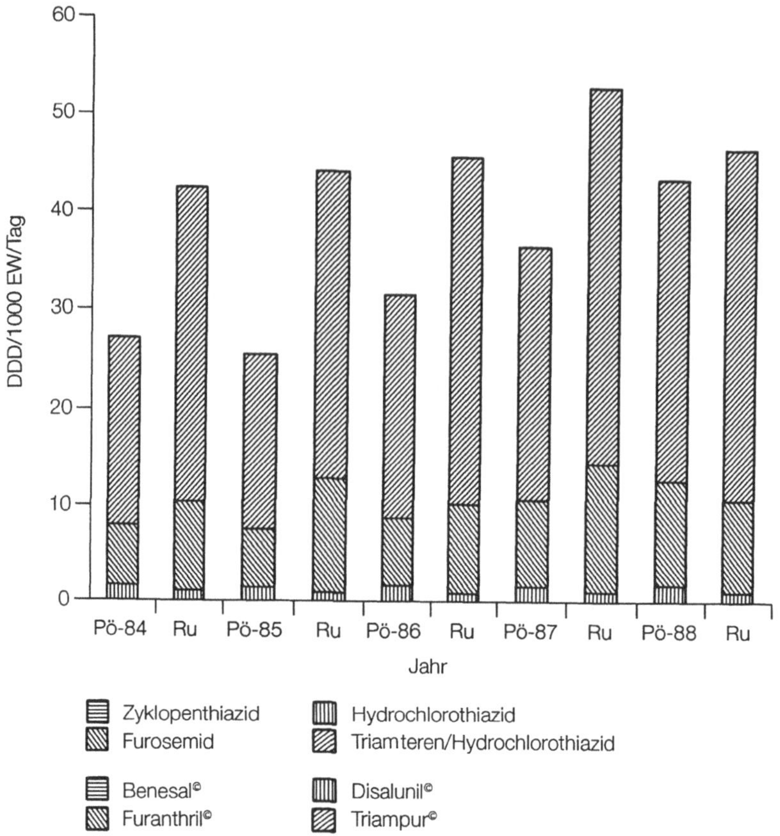

Abb. 2. Vergleich ausgewählter Arzneimittel der Indikationsgruppe *Diuretika* (Erläuterungen s. Abb. 1)

In der Bundesrepublik wurden 1988 398,6 Mio. DDD Monopräparate aus der Gruppe der β-Rezeptorenblocker verordnet, das liegt pro 1000 Einwohner zwischen dem sehr hohen Verbrauch in Rudolstadt und dem niedrigen Verbrauch in Pößneck. Schwabe u. Paffrath [9] erwähnen dabei den zunehmenden Trend zur Verordnung von β_1-selektiven Blockern, auf die im Jahre 1988 in der Bundesrepublik schon 70 % der verordneten Tagesdosen fielen.

Bei den β-Rezeptorenblockern muß der Unterschied zwischen BRD- und DDR-Markt erwähnt werden. In der Bundesrepublik waren unter den 2000 verordnungshäufigsten Arzneimitteln 22 β-Rezeptorenblocker, davon 9 β_1-selektive Präparate. Reduziert man diese Zahl auf die Wirkstoffe, sind das 9 nichtselektive und 6 β_1-selektive, denen in der DDR 1 nichtselektiver und ein β_1-selektiver β-Rezeptorenblocker gegenüberstanden. Daß eine reduzierte Palette nicht eine geringere Verordnungshäufigkeit bedingt, zeigt sowohl die Gesamtmenge der verordneten Monopräparate/1000 EW aus der Gruppe der β-Rezeptorenblocker in

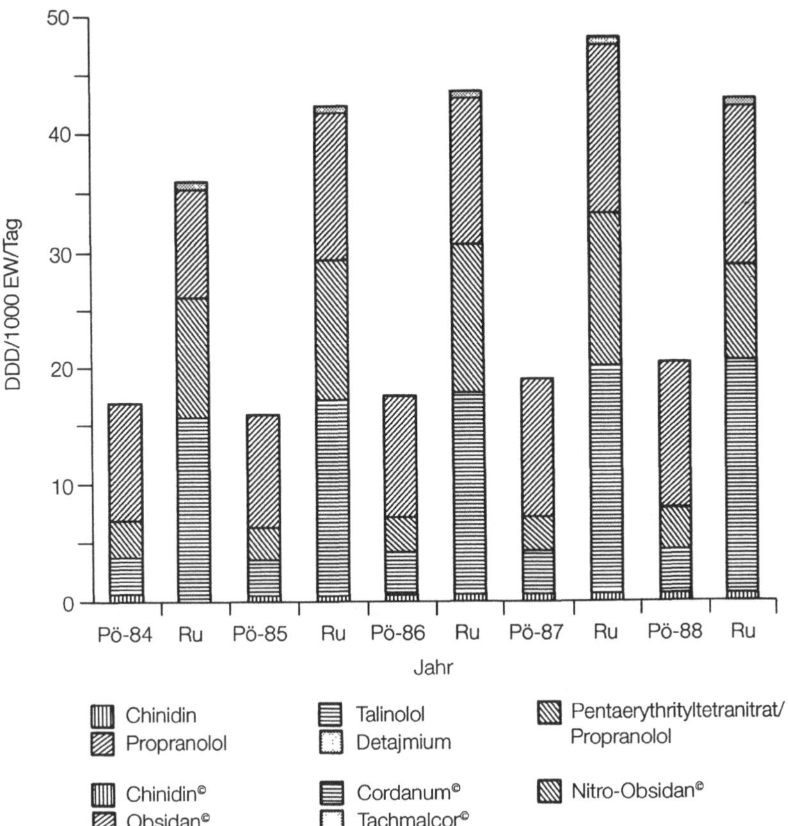

Abb. 3. Vergleich ausgewählter Arzneimittel der Indikationsgruppe *β-Rezeptorenblocker* (Erläuterungen s. Abb. 1)

Thüringen als auch die Trennung nach nichtselektiven und β_1-selektiven Blockern. Es unterstreicht die Aussage Lemmers (zit. nach [9]), daß grundsätzlich die verschiedenen therapeutischen Ziele mit allen β-Rezeptorenblockern erreicht werden können.

Kalziumantagonisten (Abb. 4)

In der DDR waren 3 Kalziumantagonisten auf dem Markt – in der Bundesrepublik befanden sich unter den 2000 verordnungshäufigsten Präparaten 1988 26 Kalziumantagonisten mit einer Verordnungshäufigkeit von 611,8 Mio. DDD, was gegenüber 1987 einer Zunahme von 17,8 % entspricht [9]. Diese über Jahre steigende Tendenz ist auch in den Kreisen Rudolstadt und Pößneck zu beobachten. Wie schon bei den β-Rezeptorenblockern, wird auch bei Kalziumantagonisten in Rudolstadt deutlich mehr pro 1000 EW verordnet als in Pößneck. Mit 2,2–5,1

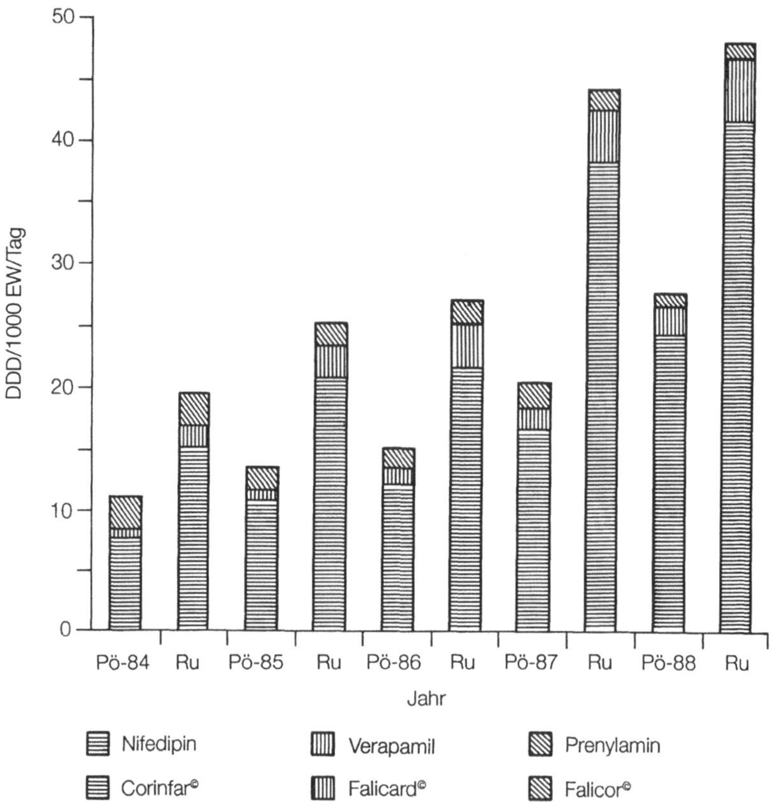

Abb. 4. Vergleich ausgewählter Arzneimittel der Indikationsgruppe *Kalziumantagonisten* (Erläuterungen s. Abb. 1)

DDD/1000 EW/Tag ist 1988 die Verordnung von Verapamil/1000 EW/Tag in den thüringischen Kreisen etwa gleich hoch wie in der BRD mit 113 Mio. DDD. Bei der Verordnung von Nifedipin überragt Rudolstadt bei Bezug auf DDD/1000 EW/Tag deutlich die Bundesrepublik (1988: 405 Mio. DDD) und den Kreis Pößneck. Gezieltere Analysen wären erforderlich, um die Ursache für die deutlich höhere Verordnungshäufigkeit für β-Blocker und Kalziumantagonisten im Kreis Rudolstadt herauszufinden. Da beide Arzneimittelgruppen unter verschiedenen Indikationen verordnet werden, sagt hier die Anzahl DDD/1000 EW/Tag nichts darüber aus, ob z. B. Hypertonie oder koronare Herzkrankheit häufiger mit den Arzneimittelgruppen behandelt werden.

Nichtsteroidale Antirheumatika, intern (Abb. 5a, b)

Nichtsteroidale Antirheumatika (Antiphlogistika) wurden mit 29,0 bzw. 38,8 DD/1000 EW/Tag in Pößneck und Rudolstadt häufiger verordnet als 1988 in der

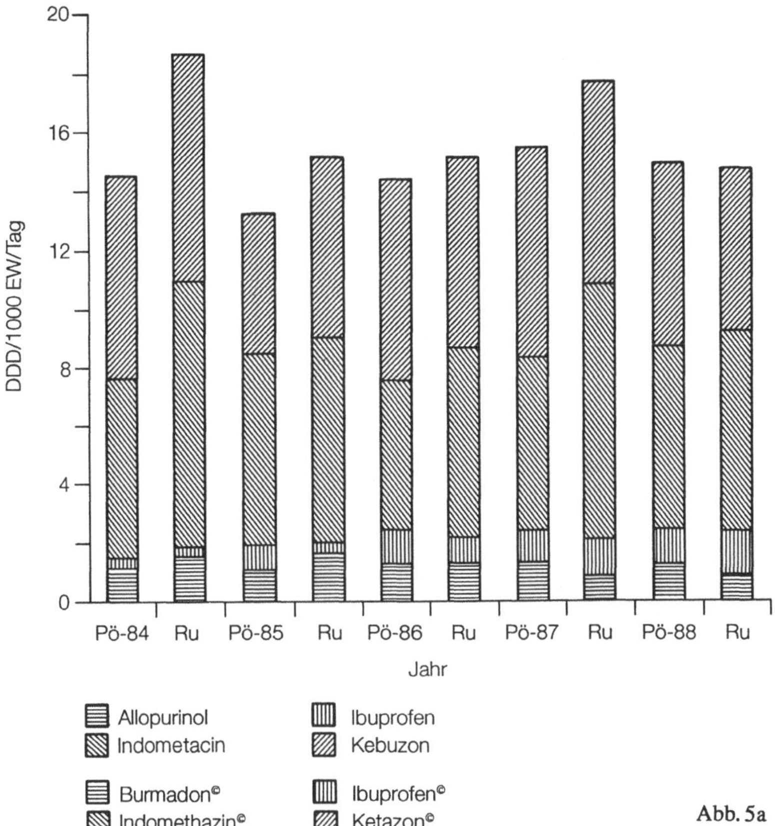

Abb. 5a, b. Vergleich ausgewählter Arzneimittel der Indikationssgruppe *Antirheumatika* (Erläuterungen s. Abb. 1)

Bundesrepublik mit 354 Mio. DDD [9]. Dabei führte 1988 Diclofenac in Thüringen ebenso wie in der BRD. Indometazin wurde in den beiden untersuchten Kreisen um das Mehrfache häufiger pro 1000 EW/Tag verordnet als in der Bundesrepublik, wo für 1988 31 Mio. DDD genannt werden. Ibuprofen und Piroxicam entsprechen sich in ihrer Verordnungshäufigkeit in Ost und West etwa. Im Fall der nichtsteroidalen Antirheumatika ist der im Kreis Rudolstadt deutliche Mehrverbrauch damit zu erklären, daß sich in Etzelbach (Kreis Rudolstadt) eine Spezialklinik zur Behandlung Rheumakranker befindet.

Während 1984 in beiden Kreisen noch Kebuzon und Indometacin die dominierenden Antirheumatika waren, verschiebt sich bis 1988 die Relation zugunsten von Diclofenac. Piroxicam ist erst seit 1986 verfügbar, seine Verordnungshäufigkeit steigt in Rudolstadt deutlich rascher als in Pößneck.

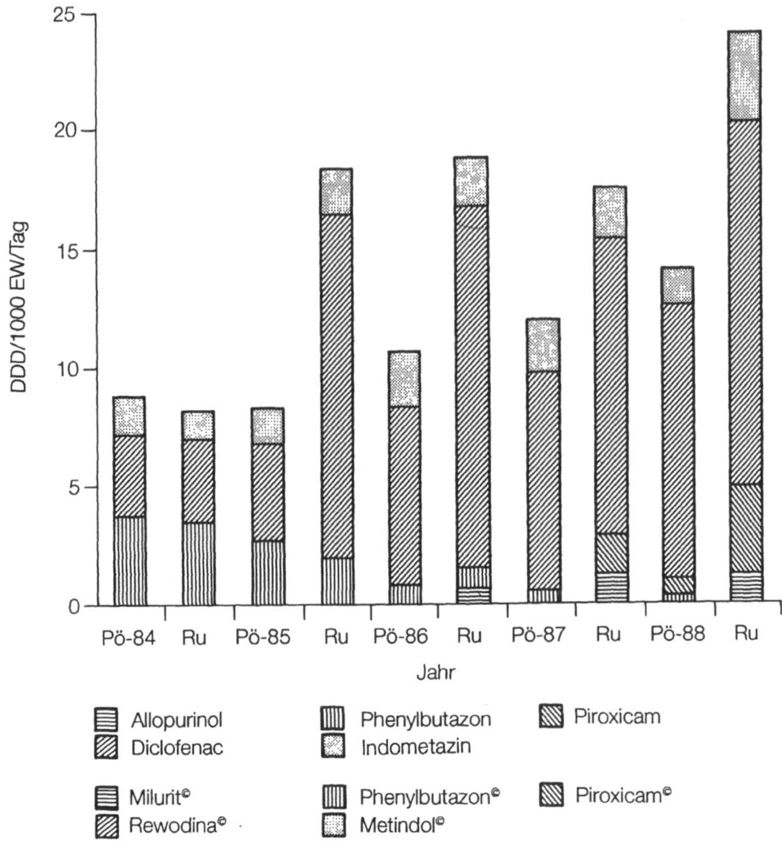

Abb. 5b

Chemotherapeutika (Abb. 6)

Hier gibt es bei gleichbleibender Tendenz keine Unterschiede zwischen den beiden untersuchten Kreisen. Die Sulfonamid-Trimethoprim-Kombination Berlocombin° dominiert. Mit 3,8 DDD/1000 EW/Tag wird diese Kombination mit breitem antibakteriellem Wirkungsspektrum in beiden untersuchten Kreisen mehr als doppelt so häufig verordnet wie in der BRD, wo für 1988 31,1 Mio. DDD angegeben sind [9].

Antibiotika (Abb. 7a, b)

Oralpenicilline werden bei gleichbleibender Tendenz in den Kreisen Pößneck und Rudolstadt etwa gleich häufig verordnet, etwa 2,2 DDD/1000 EW/Tag entsprechend der 1988 für die Bundesrepublik angegebenen Menge von 45,7 Mio. DDD.

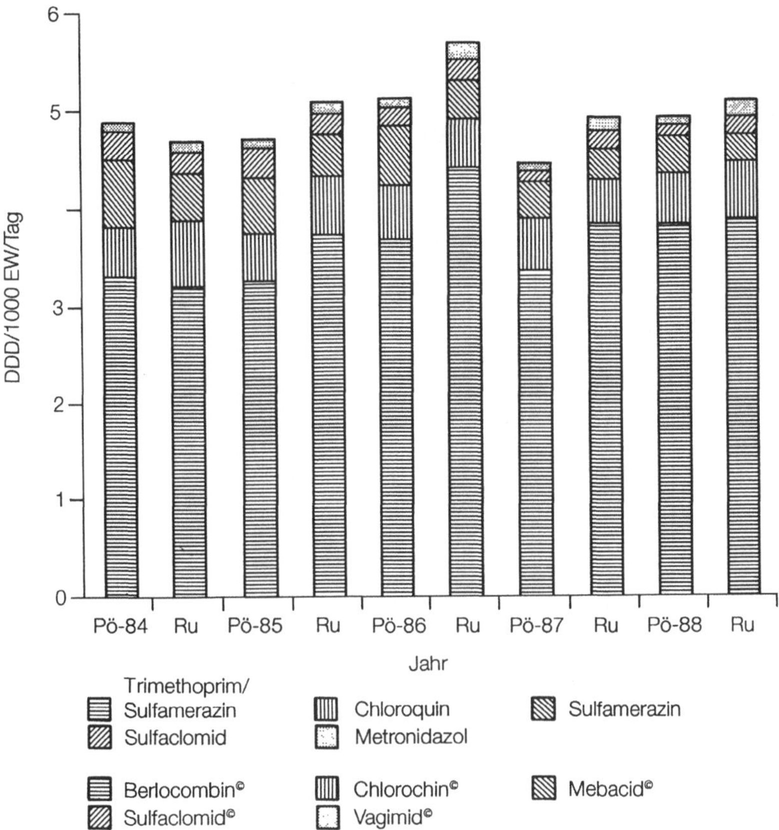

Abb. 6. Vergleich ausgewählter Arzneimittel der Indikationsgruppe *Chemotherapeutika* (Erläuterungen s. Abb. 1)

Ampicillin wird in Pößneck fast doppelt so häufig verordnet wie in Rudolstadt. Bei Ampicillin ist ein Vergleich mit dem Verbrauch in der Bundesrepublik nicht sinnvoll, wo in der Gruppe der Aminopenicilline 1988 Amoxicillin 10mal mehr als Ampicillin verordnet wurde, während in der DDR Amoxicillin nicht zur Verfügung stand.

Erythromycin ist in den untersuchten Kreisen etwa gleich und dabei deutlich geringer verordnet worden als in der BRD 1988 mit 11,4 Mio. DDD. Bei den Tetrazyklinen steht seit 1986 in der DDR auch Doxyzyklin zur Verfügung – zunächst über die Nomenklatur C noch begrenzt – hier steigt der Doxyzyklinverbrauch, während der OTC-Verbrauch zurückgeht. Dabei liegt auch 1988 in Thüringen der OTC-Verbrauch noch um das Mehrfache über dem des Doxyzyklins, während in der Bundesrepublik von 82,7 Mio. DDD 62,0 auf Doxyzyklin und nur noch 1,6 auf OTC entfallen [9]. Hier ist mit der Änderung des Sortiments für die untersuchten Kreise in Thüringen eine rasche Änderung zu erwarten.

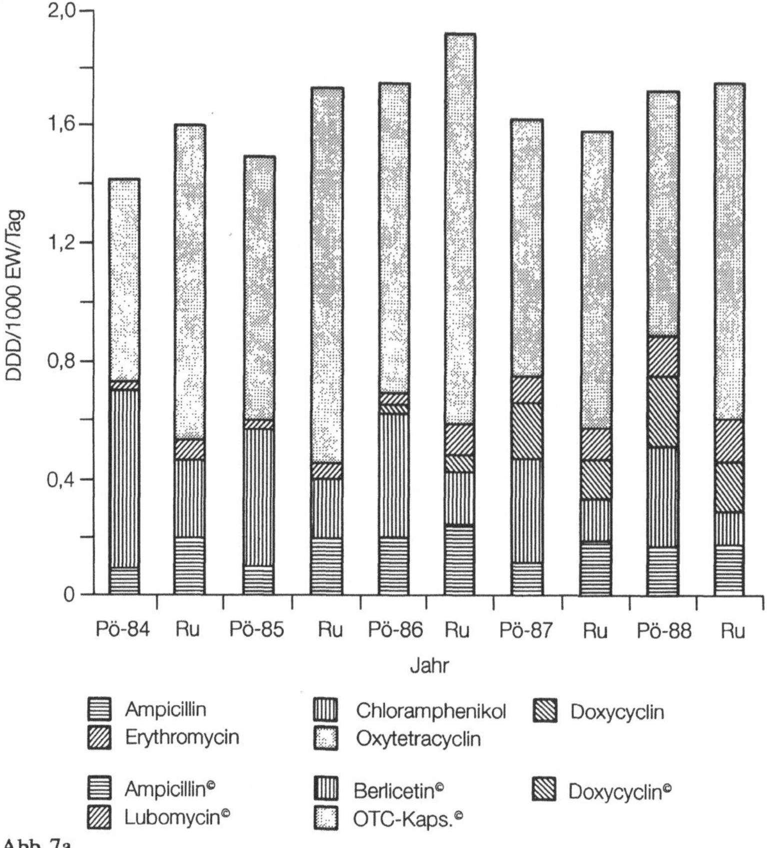

Abb. 7a

Abb. 7a, b. Vergleich ausgewählter Arzneimittel der Indikationsgruppe *Antibiotika* (Erläuterungen s. Abb. 1)

Darstellung der den Arzneimittelverbrauch beeinflussenden Faktoren

Eine ganze Anzahl von Vorgängen, Maßnahmen und Erscheinungen beeinflußt den Arzneimittelbedarf objektiv und subjektiv, gesetzmäßig und stochastisch, quantitativ und qualitativ, zeitlich und örtlich [1]. Als besonders wichtig erscheinen folgende Faktoren:

- Zahl der Ärzte und ihre Therapiegewohnheiten (fachärztlicher Versorgungsgrad, Facharztzugehörigkeit, Fluktuation von Ärzten im Untersuchungszeitraum);
- Struktur der medizinischen Versorgung (Spezialisierte Einrichtungen, Profil der Einrichtungen, Verhältnis ambulanter – stationärer Sektor);
- Bevölkerungsstruktur;
- Krankheitsgeschehen (Epidemie etc.);

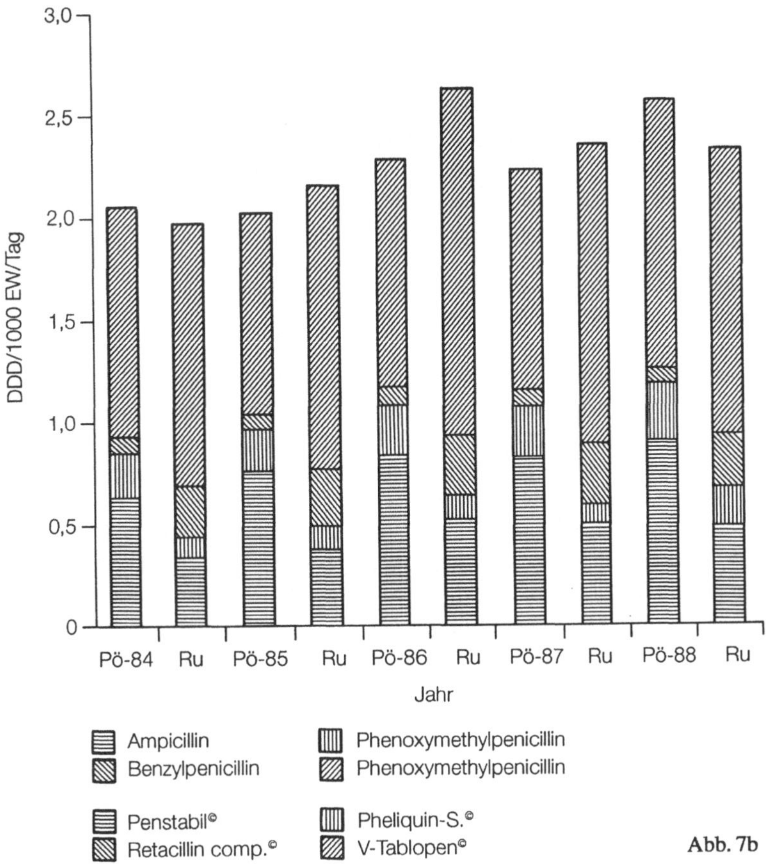

Abb. 7b

- Umweltbedingungen (Umweltbelastung durch Industrie, Berufskrankheiten, Witterungseinflüsse);
- Arzneimittelversorgung (Einflüsse neuer Arzneimittel, Veränderungen der Pakkungsgrößen, Arzneimittelinformationen, Therapierichtlinien, Veränderungen von Therapieauffassungen).

Die den Arzneimittelbedarf beeinflussenden Faktoren sind nur teilweise quantitativ erfaßbar, z. B. Bevölkerungsstruktur und Anzahl der Ärzte. Faktoren, die v. a. territorial den Arzneimittelverbrauch entscheidend beeinflussen können (Umweltbedingungen, Vorhandensein von Spezialeinrichtungen), werden im großen Maßstab unwesentlich, sind aber bei einer Betrachtung zweier kleiner Territorien wie der Kreise Rudolstadt und Pößneck unbedingt zu berücksichtigen (z. B. bei der Indikationsgruppe Antirheumatika das Vorhandensein der Rheumaklinik im Kreis Rudolstadt). Neu eingeführte Arzneimittel wirken als „Störfaktoren" bei Arzneimittelverbrauchsanalysen, dabei unterliegt jedes Präparat einer gewissen Eigengesetzlichkeit in der Phase seiner Einführung in die Therapie.

Bezüglich demographischer Faktoren konnte zwischen den betrachteten Kreisen Rudolstadt und Pößneck kein nennenswerter Unterschied festgestellt werden. Umweltbedingungen und Arzneimittelversorgung unterschieden sich ebenfalls nicht.

Die größere Arztdichte pro Einwohner in Rudolstadt und der größere Prozentsatz ambulant tätiger Internisten könnte eine Erklärung für den dort höheren Verordnungsgrad von β-Rezeptorenblockern und Kalziumantagonisten sein; zur Bestätigung wären gezielte Analysen erforderlich.

Mögliche Aussagebeschränkungen der vorliegenden Arzneimittelverbrauchsanalyse

Unsere Untersuchung läßt Rückschlüsse auf den Gesamtverbrauch von Arzneimitteln verschiedener Indikationsgruppen zu. Durch das Vorhandensein polyvalenter Arzneimittel wie β-Rezeptorenblocker und Kalziumantagonisten kann keine Aussage getroffen werden, welcher Anteil eines solchen Arzneimittels für welche Indikationsgruppe verordnet wurde.

Da die Apothekeninventurlisten die Berechnungsgrundlage für die DDD/1000 EW/Tag bildeten, können zwar Schlußfolgerungen über die Bevorzugung bestimmter Wirkstoffstärken und Packungsgrößen gezogen werden, jedoch sind keine Aussagen über konkrete Dosierungen möglich.

Das Verordnungsverhalten des einzelnen Arztes kann anhand unserer Analyse nicht beurteilt werden, ebenso ist keine Analyse über die den Verbrauch verursachenden Einrichtungen oder Fachrichtungen möglich.

Weiterhin ist zu beachten, daß im Untersuchungszeitraum durch länger anhaltende Versorungsdefekte Arzneimittel durch unbefriedigten Bedarf im Verbrauch scheinbar absinken, die dafür zur Substitution eingesetzten Arzneimittel überdurchschnittlich hoch verbraucht wurden. Als Beispiel sei der 1987/88 stark angestiegene Verbrauch an Indometacin-Suppositorien als Ersatz für die zu dieser Zeit nicht lieferbaren Indometacin-Kapseln zu nennen.

Bei Arzneimittelverbrauchsanalysen anhand von Inventurlisten, aber auch anhand von Rezepten, darf man nicht vergessen, daß aufgrund mangelnder Compliance des Patienten auch bei korrekter Verordnung durch den Arzt der wirkliche Verbrauch nur annähernd widergespiegelt wird.

Vorschläge zur Weiterführung der Untersuchungen

Nach der Wiedervereinigung Deutschlands eröffnet sich auch für Thüringen der Arzneimittelmarkt der alten Bundesländer. Außerdem wird es zu einer Umstrukturierung im Gesundheitswesen kommen. Von seiten der Krankenkassen als auch der Kassenärztlichen Vereinigungen werden ökonomische Aspekte in den Blickpunkt gerückt werden, z. B. wieviel Geld pro verordneter DDD aufgewendet werden muß und welche Fallkostendurchschnitte entstehen. Die Zusammenstellung der Indikationsgruppen, die in Ost und West z. T. Unterschiede aufwies, wird vereinheitlicht.

In Anbetracht dieser gegenwärtigen Umwälzungen sollten weiterführende Untersuchungen in den beiden Landkreisen Pößneck und Rudolstadt stattfinden, für die durch unsere Analyse Ausgangsdaten vorliegen. Sie sollten ergänzt werden durch Ranglisten der verordnungsstärksten Indikationsgruppen und der am häufigsten verordneten Arzneimittel dieser beiden Territorien, sollten preisliche Aspekte beinhalten. Rezeptanalysen ausgewählter niedergelassener Ärzte, ähnlich einem in Hessen schon existierenden Projekt, sollten angefügt werden, um durch das Aufzeigen individueller Verordnungsunterschiede die Ärzteschaft zur kritischen Selbsteinschätzung zu motivieren und gezielte Weiterbildungsmaßnahmen zu ermöglichen.

Literatur

1. Baumann D (1973) Untersuchungen zum Arzneimittel-Bedürfnis und zum Bedarf an Arzneimitteln unter besonderer Berücksichtigung der Bedarfsvorhersage mit Hilfe von Bestimmungsfaktoren – eine methodologische Studie zur Arzneimittel-Markt-Forschung. Dissertation, Universität Greifswald
2. Faerber L von (1988) Die ambulante ärztliche Versorgung im Spiegel der Verwaltungsdaten einer Ortskrankenkasse. Enke, Stuttgart, S 118–121
3. Görlt H, Lohmann D (1984) Wissenschaftlich begründeter effektiver Arzneimitteleinsatz in der medizinischen Betreuung auf der Grundlage von Analysen des Arzneimittelverbrauchs: – Ziel und Inhalt von Verbrauchsanalysen, – Nutzung der Analyseergebnisse in der Zusammenarbeit von Apothekenwesen und medizinischen Betreuungsbereichen. Z Ärztl Fortbild 73:661–666
4. Möller H, Hampich B (1988) Zur Arzneimittelverbrauchsanalyse unter Nutzung der defined daily dose – DDD. Medicamentum 29:146–147
5. Nordiska Läkemedelsnämnden (1988) Nordic Council on Medicines, Uppsala
6. Schaefer M (1989) Verbrauchsstatistiken für Arzneimittelschlüssel zu vergleichenden Untersuchungen. Pharmazie 44:390–393
7. Schaefer M, Audien H (1987) Vergleich zwischen verordneten und definierten Tagesdosen (DDD) ausgewählter Antihypertonika – Probleme und Schlufolgerungen. Pharmazie 42:850–853
8. Scholz H (1989) Kardiaka. In: Schwabe U, Paffrath D (Hrsg) Arzneiverordnungs-Report '89. Fischer, Stuttgart, New York, S 255–264
9. Schwabe U, Paffrath D (Hrsg) (1989) Arzneiverordnungs-Report '89. Fischer, Stuttgart New York

Problemorientierte Workshops
Problem-Oriented Workshops

Hypercholesterinämie: Wen screenen, wen behandeln?

Hypercholesterolemia: Whom to Screen, Whom to Treat?

Cholesterinscreening: Die Irrationalität von Grenzwerten und die Berücksichtigung des Gesamtrisikos für eine rationale Therapie

Johannes G. Schmidt

Einleitung

In Forschung und Praxis wird das Problem prophylaktischer Maßnahmen und Behandlungen meist ausschließlich auf die Frage reduziert: kann eine Früherkennung bzw. eine frühzeitige Risikofaktorbehandlung die Folgekrankheit kausal beeinflussen? Von einer praktischen Sichtweise wäre allerdings *die* Frage wichtig: Überwiegen die erwünschten Auswirkungen solcher prophylaktischen Maßnahmen die unerwünschten Auswirkungen, und durch welche Parameter sollen solche Wirkungen gemessen werden?

Obschon die zweite Fragestellung für die Nutzenbeurteilung einer Screeningmaßnahme leicht als die entscheidendere erkannt wird, werden Früherkennung und Screening heute mit wenigen Ausnahmen nach der ersten Fragestellung beurteilt.

Dies kommt daher, daß die Faszination der klinisch-akademischen Medizin einerseits sich vorrangig auf Wirkungsmechanismen innerhalb ihrer pathogenetischen Modelle ausrichtet mit der Folge, daß aus möglichen pathogenetischen Zusammenhängen – wie der sog. Lipidtheorie – schnell auch eine Behandlungs- und Screeningnotwendigkeit abgeleitet wird. Die *quantitative* Bedeutung solcher Interventionen bleibt dabei unberücksichtigt. Andererseits richtet sich die Faszination des praxisfern arbeitenden Epidemiologen und Präventivmediziners hauptsächlich auf Hochrechnungen der theoretischen volksgesundheitlichen Ausbeute, welche aus der Prävention einer häufigen Krankheit entstehen könnte. Bei dieser quantitativen Beurteilungsweise bleibt die *individuelle* Perspektive der gesundheitlichen Auswirkungen auf den potentiellen Patienten unberücksichtigt.

Beim Cholesterinscreening berufen sich die meisten Autoren und Kommissionen in ihren Empfehlungen auf die einfache Formel der Lipidtheorie, die popularisiert etwa lautet: „Eine 10 %ige Cholesterinreduktion führt zu einer Senkung der Infarktrate um 16 %". Daraus allein wird eine Screening- und Behandlungsnotwendigkeit der Hypercholesterinämie abgeleitet. Die Lipidtheorie ist zwar gut belegt und kann heute als erwiesen gelten, die Problematik liegt jedoch in der Frage, was diese Theorie *praktisch* bietet.

Die entscheidende Frage, ob bei Berücksichtigung aller für den Patienten relevanten oder in der Praxis sichtbaren erwünschten und unerwünschten Auswirkungen ein Cholesterinscreening und eine Hypercholesterinämiebehandlung einen „Nettonutzen" aufweisen, wird deshalb fast nie gestellt und beantwortet. Bei einer kritischen Analyse ist der Nutzen eines Massenscreenings denn auch eher fragwürdig, und ein Gesamtnutzen ist nicht belegt (vgl. [28]).

Rationale Pharmakotherapie in der Allgemeinpraxis
Rational Pharmacotherapy in General Practice
M. M. Kochen (Hrsg.)

Die Problematik und Aussagekraft von Cholesteringrenzwerten

Die geringe praktische Bedeutung von Cholesteringrenzwerten ergibt sich schon, wenn man sich wieder einmal daran erinnert, daß *die meisten Infarkte bei Menschen mit normalem Cholesterinspiegel* auftreten und daß ein unbehandelter hoher Cholesterinspiegel noch lange nicht zwingend zu einem Infarkt führen muß. Dieses praktische Dilemma wird in Abb. 1 verdeutlicht.

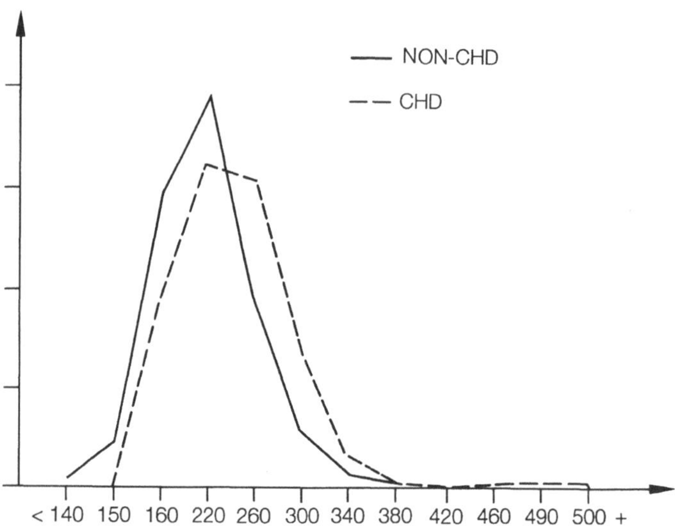

Abb. 1. Verteilung der Cholesterinwerte bei 30- bis 49jährigen Männern, die in den folgenden 16 Jahren infarktfrei (*Non-CHD*) blieben bzw. einen Infarkt (*CHD*) erlitten. (Framingham-Studie [15])

Was wir recht genau voraussagen können, sind *Gruppenrisiken*. So werden innerhalb von 6 Jahren von einer Gruppe von 100 nichtrauchenden, normotonen 50jährigen Männern mit einem Cholesterinwert von beispielsweise 7,3 mmol/l (285 mg/dl) *6* einen Infarkt erleiden, von 100 nichtrauchenden normotonen 50jährigen Männern mit einem Cholesterinwert von 5,4 mmol/l (210 mg/dl) werden *4* einen Infarkt erleiden (vgl. [1]). 94 der Männer mit hohem bzw. 96 der Männer mit normalem Cholesterinwert werden somit infarktfrei bleiben. Welche der Männer im *Individualfall* infarktgefährdet sind, läßt sich anhand des immerhin deutlich unterschiedlichen Cholesterinspiegels jedoch überhaupt nicht voraussagen. Wenn man also etwas einigermaßen Vernünftiges über den Gesundheitszustand ganzer Gruppen bzw. Bevölkerungen mit hohem oder tiefem Durchschnittscholesterinwert aussagen kann (in unserem Beispiel hätte die eine Gruppe eine 50% höhere Infarktinzidenz), so enthält diese Aussage im Individualfall fast nur Belangloses: Im Individualfall ist es doch praktisch ungefähr das gleiche, ob die Chance, infarktfrei zu bleiben, 96 oder 94% bzw. das Infarktrisiko 6 oder 4% beträgt.

Wie schwierig und willkürlich generelle Grenzwertfestlegungen bleiben, kann anhand der Aussagekraft solcher Grenzwerte dargelegt werden (Tabelle 1).

Tabelle 1. Cholesterin als Infarktprädiktor. (Pooling Project, 10 Jahre Follow-up [28])

Grenzwert [mmol/l]	[mg/dl]	Spezifität [%]	PPV [%]	Sensitivität [%]	NPV [%]
7,7	300	92,1	13,6	14,8	92,8
7,1	275	83,5	12,5	28,2	93,3
6,5	250	69,2	11,7	48,5	94,1
5,8	225	55,8	11,4	68,0	95,4
5,2	200	25,3	8,6	83,5	94,8
4,5	175	9,5	8,1	94,6	95,5

PPV „positive predictive value": Infarktrisiko der mit dem entsprechenden Grenzwert definierten Hypercholesterinämiker.
NPV „negative predictive value": Chance der Infarktfreiheit bei mit dem entsprechenden Grenzwert definierten Normocholesterinämikern.

Setzen wir als Grenzwert beispielsweise 6,5 mmol/l (250 mg/dl) fest, so erzielen wir eine *Spezifität* von rund 70 % in der Voraussage eines künftigen Infarktereignisses. Dies bedeutet, daß 70 % der Infarktfreien richtig als risikofrei klassifiziert worden sind, 30 % aller Infarktfreien werden zu „Risikopatienten". Würden wir den Grenzwert auf 5,2 mmol/l (200 mg/dl) festlegen, so betrüge die Spezifität 25 %, d. h. nur noch 25 % der Infarktfreien würden richtig als risikofrei klassifiziert, 75 % aller Infarktfreien würden zu „Risikopatienten". Je tiefer der Grenzwert, um so größer wird der Anteil der Bevölkerung, welcher fälschlich und unnötig zu Risikopatienten gemacht wird.

Entscheidend für das Individuum ist der *positive Vorhersagewert* („positive predictive value"): Mit einem Grenzwert von 6,5 mmol/l wird bei 12 % der so definierten Hypercholesterinämiker ein Infarkt in den nächsten 10 Jahren korrekt vorausgesagt, mit einem Grenzwert von 5,2 mmol/l ist dies nur noch bei 8 % der Fall. Bei einem Grenzwert von 6,5 mmol/l wird somit bei 88 % der gescreenten Hypercholesterinämiker fälschlich ein Infarktrisiko unterstellt, bei einem Grenzwert von 5,2 mmol/l werden 92 % der „Risikopatienten"*falsch-positiv* klassifiziert.

Bei diesen Daten handelt es sich um Untersuchungen an Männern. Frauen, v. a. in jüngerem Alter, haben bekanntlich bei gleicher Ausprägung der Risikofaktoren ein ca. 50 % geringeres Infarktrisiko als Männer (vgl. [1]). Dies bedeutet, daß bei Frauen der positive Vorhersagewert eines Cholesteringrenzwertes noch um die Hälfte reduziert ist. Hinzu kommt, daß eine identische Risikofaktorausprägung bei verschiedenen Völkern mit einem deutlich unterschiedlichen Infarktrisiko verbunden ist. So haben Europäer bei gleichen Cholesterinspiegeln, Blutdruckwerten und Nikotinkonsumgewohnheiten nur etwa ein halb so großes Infarktrisiko wie US-Amerikaner [16].

Der *negative Vorhersagewert* („negative predictive value") vermittelt die Wahrscheinlichkeit, bei einem entsprechend „normalen" Cholesterinwert keinen Infarkt zu erleiden. Wird der Grenzwert mit 6,5 mmol/l festgesetzt, so beträgt diese „Sicherheit" für einen Normocholesterinämiker 94,1 %, beim Grenzwert 5,2 mmol/l 94,8 %; praktisch besteht hier kein Unterschied.

Die *Sensitivität* bemißt den Anteil der Infarktgefährdeten, der durch einen bestimmten Grenzwert erfaßt wird. Bei einem Grenzwert von 6,5 mmol/l wären dies nicht ganz 5 % der Männer, die einen Infarkt erleiden werden; bei einem Grenzwert von 5,2 mmol/l 84 %. Je tiefer der Grenzwert ist, um so größer wird der Anteil aller prospektiven Infarktpatienten, die als Risikopatienten erfaßt werden.

Als praktische Folgerung läßt sich aus diesen Zahlen herauslesen, daß im Individualfall bei beliebiger Grenzwertfestlegung bis hinauf zu 7,7 mmol/l (300 mg/l) immer ein Risiko von 80–90 % besteht, Risikopatienten fälschlich zu klassifizieren und zu behandeln. Gleichzeitig hat ein als „normal" klassifiziertes Individuum ein Risiko von wenigstens 4 und höchstens 7 %, einen Infarkt zu erleiden, wie tief oder hoch der Grenzwert (zwischen 4,5 und 7,7 mmol/l) auch festgelegt wird.

Kann man da einen Patienten aufgrund eines – von wem und wie hoch auch immer – festgelegten Grenzwertes mitteilen, er sei infarktgefährdet und deshalb behandlungsbedürftig bzw. „es sei alles in Ordnung"?

Weiter gilt es, unvermeidliche Ungenauigkeiten in der alltäglichen Laborpraxis zu berücksichtigen. Ein Bericht über eine Quote von 10 % Fehlklassifikationen mit dem Reflotronsystem entspricht bereits einer ausgezeichneten und im Alltag kaum realisierbaren Laborgenauigkeit [3]. Eine *zuverlässige Cholesterinbestimmung* ist somit *in der Praxis nicht gegeben*, das Problem einer zuverlässigen Cholesterinbestimmung *nicht gelöst.*

Nicht genug damit: Der individuelle Cholesterinspiegel ist eine so schwankende Größe, daß auch unter konstanter Diät Standardabweichungen vom Mittelwert von 5–10 % die Regel sind [13]. In 95 % der Zeit schwankt der Cholesterinspiegel 10–20 % vom Mittelwert nach oben und unten, gelegentlich (in 5 % der Zeit) sogar noch weiter. Eine Studie fand bei Nachbestimmungen innerhalb der nächsten 5 Tage – trotz doppelter Bestimmung im Labor – beträchtliche Unterschiede von über 20 % bei der großen Mehrheit der Probanden; bei 40 % erfolgte eine falsche Risikogruppenzuteilung, bei 10 % ergaben sich gar intraindividuelle „Bewegungen" von einem Hochrisiko- zu einem Niedrigrisikostatus oder umgekehrt [23]. Dies bedeutet, daß die durch eine Therapie zu erzielenden Cholesterinunterschiede geringer sind als die natürlichen Schwankungen. Andere Autoren, die in einer großen Untersuchung mit nahezu 15 000 Probanden praktisch gleiche Ergebnisse fanden, kommen denn auch zu dem Schluß, daß eine Cholesterinspiegelbestimmung als Therapiekontrolle eine Illusion ist oder sogar irreführend sein kann [30]. Somit können Daten, die auf Bevölkerungsebene noch einigermaßen aussagekräftig und für die Beweisführung der Lipidtheorie geeignet sind, ihre individuelle Aussagekraft praktisch vollständig verlieren.

Risikokonstellationen mehrerer Risikofaktoren

Die individuelle Infarktgefährdung läßt sich schon etwas genauer vorausssagen, wenn weitere Risikofaktoren hinzukommen (s. Abb. 2).

So hat z. B. ein 35jähriger Mann mit einem sehr hohen Cholesterinwert (335 mg/dl) und einem gleichzeitig niedrigen Blutdruck das gleiche Infarktrisiko (rund 4 ‰ in 8 Jahren) wie ein Mann mit sehr niedrigem Cholesterinwert (185 mg/dl), der jedoch gleichzeitig hyperton ist und eine pathologische Glukosetoleranz aufweist. Hätte letzterer zusätzlich eine Linkshypertrophie im EKG und wäre er Raucher, dann wäre sein Infarktrisiko trotz niedrigem Cholesterinwert mehrfach höher als das des ersten mit der schweren Hypercholesterinämie. Während der absolute

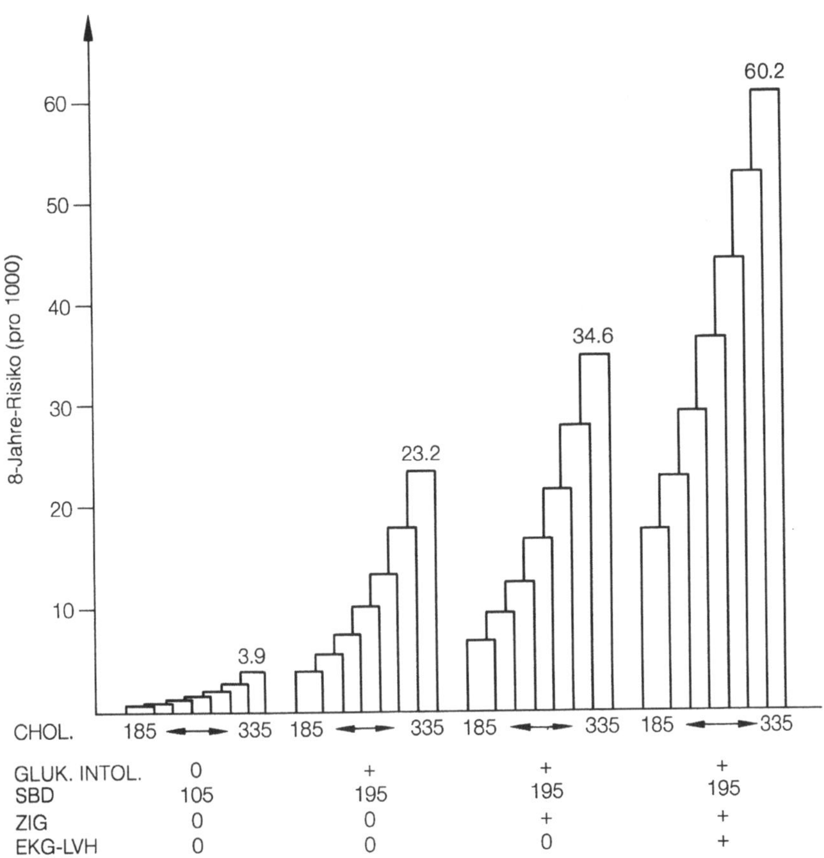

Abb. 2. Kardiovaskuläres Erkrankungsrisiko in 8 Jahren in Abhängigkeit vom Cholesterinspiegel und von verschiedenen weiteren Risikofaktoren bei 35jährigen Männern. *CHOL.* Cholesterinspiegel; *GLUK. INTOL.* Vorliegen einer pathologischen Glukosetoleranz (0 = nein; + = ja); *SBD* systolischer Blutdruck; *ZIG* Raucher (0 = nein; + = ja); *EKG-LVH* Vorliegen einer Linkshypertrophie im EKG (0 = nein; + = ja). (Framingham-Studie [14])

Risikounterschied zwischen 2 gesunden Männern mit oder ohne Hypercholesterinämie bescheiden ist (etwa 3 ‰) in 8 Jahren zwischen einem Mann mit einem Cholesterinwert von 335 mg/dl und einem mit 185 mg/dl), ist diese Differenz bei Vorliegen weiterer Risikofaktoren beträchtlich (über 40 ‰ in 8 Jahren, falls Linkshypertrophie, pathologische Glukosetoleranz und Nikotinkonsum vorliegen). Da nach der Lipidtheorie jeder Cholesterinanstieg unabhängig vom Ausgangswert ein Risikoanstieg bedeuten soll, ist ein allgemeingültiger Grenzwert somit gar nicht plausibel. Ein Hypercholesterinämiker ohne andere Risikofaktoren kann durch eine *Cholesterin*senkung sein individuelles Risiko weit weniger senken als ein Normocholesterinämiker, welcher gehäuft andere Risikofaktoren aufweist. Bei diesem *Normo*cholesterinämiker könnte eine Cholesterinsenkung deshalb weit mehr bringen als bei einem solchen *Hyper*cholesterinämiker. Das Nebenwirkungsrisiko einer lipidsenkenden Therapie dürfte hingegen bei beiden identisch sein. Somit wäre das Nutzen-Risiko-Verhältnis einer lipidsenkenden Therapie beim Normocholesterinämiker mit weiteren Risikofaktoren *günstiger* als beim Hypercholesterinämiker ohne weitere Risikofaktoren. Dies zeigt, daß ein genereller Cholesteringrenzwert als Indikation einer Therapiebedürftigkeit nicht rational ist.

Beurteilungsparameter in der Praxis oder was kann die Cholesterinsenkung leisten?

Autoren, die die Theorie der *klinischen Epidemiologie* mitbegründet haben [7], wiesen bereits seit 10 Jahren auf den wichtigen Unterschied zwischen *relativem* und *absolutem Risiko* hin. Dieser Unterschied wird anhand der Ergebnisse der Hyperlipidämie-Behandlung klar.

Heutige Screening- und Behandlungsempfehlungen stützen sich weitgehend auf die Studie der *Lipid Research Clinics* [19] und die *Helsinki Heart Study* [9]. In der ersten Studie erlitten nach 7 Behandlungsjahren von 1900 Probanden in der Placebogruppe 187 einen Herzinfarkt, verglichen mit 155 der 1906 mit Colestyramin Behandelten. Nach 5 Behandlungsjahren erlitten in der Helsinki-Studie 84 von 2030 Probanden in der Placebogruppe einen Herzinfarkt, verglichen mit 56 der 2051 mit Gemfibrozil Behandelten. Somit konnten 1,7 bzw. 1,4 % der behandelten Hypercholesterinämiker im Zeitraum von 7 bzw. 5 Jahren einen Behandlungsnutzen in Form eines verhüteten Infarkts erfahren. Die Chance, ohne Infarkt – sagen wir – die nächsten 5 Jahre zu überleben, erhöht sich also von 93,0 % ohne Behandlung auf 94,2 % (Colestyramin-Studie) bzw. von 95,9 % auf 97,3 % (Gemfibrozil-Studie). Diese Ergebnisse sind in Tabelle 2 zusammengefaßt.

Entscheidet man sich im Einzelfall für eine Behandlung (und damit indirekt auch für ein Screening), so sind die Studienergebnisse in dieser Form, d.h. in *absoluten Risiken*, am aussagekräftigsten. Die oben erwähnten Autoren [7] weisen denn auch darauf hin, daß die beiden unterschiedlichen Parameter *relatives* und *absolutes Risiko* (und gleichermaßen ein absoluter oder relativer Nutzen) grundsätzlich verschiedene Fragestellungen beantworten. Das relative Risiko ist ein Maß für die Strenge eines statistischen Zusammenhangs und damit ein Element für die Beur-

Tabelle 2. Infarktreduktion in den Langzeitstudien zur medikamentösen Cholesterinsenkung

				Infarkte (alle, inklusive nichttödliche)			
	Durchschnitts-alter (Jahre)	Durchschnittlicher Cholesterin-spiegel	Cholesterin-senkung	Inzidenz Kontroll-gruppe	Reduktion relativ	Reduktion absolut	Signifikanz
WHO-Studie (Clofibrat) (n = 10627)	46	6,5 mmol/l (250 mg/dl)	9 %	7,4 (pro 1000 jährlich)	20 %	1,5 (pro 1000 jährlich)	p = 0,03
Lipid Research Clinics (Colestyramin) (n = 3806)	48	7,5 mmol/l (290 mg/dl)	8,5 % (im Vergleich zu Placebo)	14,1 (pro 1000 jährlich)	17 %	2,4 (pro 1000 jährlich)	p = 0,07 (n.s.)
Helsinki-Studie (Gemfibrozil + Diät) (n = 4081)	47	7,4 mmol/l (289 mg/dl)	9 %	8,2 (pro 1000 jährlich)	34 %	2,8 (pro 1000 jährlich)	p = 0,01
Alle 3 kombiniert (n = 18514)	46,6	6,8 mmol/l (262 mg/dl)	9 %	8,8 (pro 1000 jährlich)	23 %	2,0 (pro 1000 jährlich)	$p < 0,01$

teilung der ätiologischen bzw. pathogenetischen Bedeutung eines Faktors. Je höher das relative Risiko ist, um so wichtigere ätiologische Bedeutung hat ein Faktor. Das relative Risiko eines Infarkts in bezug auf den Risikofaktor Cholesterin ist zweifellos statistisch signifikant über 1 (d.h. die Infarkthäufigkeit bei Hypercholesterinämikern ist satistisch signifikant größer als bei Normocholesterinämikern), was eine *kontributorische* Rolle des Cholesterins erkennen läßt. Andererseits ist dieses relative Risiko so gering, daß ein erhöhter Cholesterinspiegel weder notwendig noch hinreichend ist für die Entstehung eines Infarkts. Der Risikofaktor Cholesterin unterscheidet sich deshalb auch grundlegend von den *kausalen Faktoren* wie sie z.B. der Vitamin-C-Mangel für die Skorbut darstellen. Während diese Stoffwechselstörung notwendig und hinreichend für eine Skorbutentstehung ist und eine entsprechende einfache Intervention (ausreichend Vitamin C) diese Krankheit vollständig verhindert, trägt das Cholesterin nur geringfügig zur Infarktentstehung bei. Ein erhöhter Cholesterinspiegel erklärt denn bekanntermaßen auch nur etwa 20% der Infarkte. Der größte Teil der Infarkte entsteht immer noch aus unklarer Ursache. Als Maß für die praktische und therapeutische Bedeutung eines Risikofaktors muß deshalb das *absolute Risiko* gelten.

Wenn man sich die Resultate der Lipidsenkerstudien vergegenwärtigt, so stellt sich bei der Nutzenbeurteilung die Frage, ob 1 verhinderter Infarkt allfällige Nebenwirkungen bei 50 10 Jahre lang umsonst Behandelten mehr als aufwiegen kann.

Tatsächlich konnte bisher keine der Langzeituntersuchungen zur Cholesterinsenkung eine Senkung der *Gesamtmortalität* durch eine Hypercholesterinämiebehandlung aufzeigen. Im Gegenteil, eine frühere Langzeitstudie mit Verwendung von Clofibrat zeigte gar einen dramatischen *Anstieg der Gesamtmortalität um 44% unter der Behandlung* [27]. Die Zahl zusätzlicher Todesfälle in der Clofibrat-Gruppe war sogar größer als die Anzahl der verhinderten (meist nichttödlichen) Infarkte.

Auch ein Wirkungsnachweis einer *diätetischen* Cholesterinsenkung bei asymptomatischer Hypercholesterinämie auf die Infarktrate konnte bislang nicht erbracht werden [8,31]. Der Cholesteringehalt der Nahrung scheint ein Pseudogesundheitsparameter zu sein. So weiß man inzwischen, daß z.B. die cholesterinarme Margarine eine Lipidzusammensetzung aufweist, die nach heutigem Wissen ungünstiger als die von Butter sein dürfte [21]. Im Unterschied zur unsicheren Rolle des Nahrungscholesterins existieren epidemiologisch härtere Daten, die auf eine günstige Rolle einer faserreichen und fischreichen Diät hinweisen [10,17,18,24].

Die Wirkung einer Cholesterinsenkung auf die Infarktrate bei Frauen sowie bei den über 60jährigen ist ebensowenig belegt [6,31]. Mit zunehmendem Alter überleben diejenigen infarktfrei, bei denen ein hoher Cholesterinwert offenbar kein individuelles Risiko darstellt. Damit findet eine Selektion dieser sog. „Escaper" statt.

Eine Extrapolation der Ergebnisse von Studien an Männern mittleren Alters auf andere Gruppen scheint deshalb nicht zulässig.

Unerwünschte Auswirkungen des Cholesterinscreenings

Obwohl die Studienpopulation der 3 Langzeituntersuchungen insgesamt 18 500 Probanden ausmachte und 9300 davon „gegen zu hohes Cholesterin" behandelt wurden (in rund 52 000 Behandlungsjahren), ist eine statistisch signifikante Senkung der *Infarktsterblichkeit* (auch in einer gepoolten Analyse) ausgeblieben (Tabelle 3).

Tabelle 3. Kombinierte Analyse der Lipidstudien

	3 Studien gepoolt[a]		2 Studien gepoolt[b]	
	Veränderung	Signifikanz	Veränderung	Signifikanz
Infarktmortalität	16 % Senkung	$p = 0,24$	28 % Senkung	$p = 0,10$
Nichtinfarkt-mortalität	54 % Anstieg	$p < 0,01$	34 % Anstieg	$p = 0,12$
Gesamtmortalität	20 % Anstieg	$p = 0,06$	1 % Senkung	$p > 0,5$

[a] Alle 3 erwähnten Studien (s. Tabelle 2).
[b] Gemfibrozil-Studie + Cholestyramin-Studie.

Selbst ohne Einbezug der „ungünstigen" Clofibrat-Studie ist festzustellen, daß der Reduktion der Infarktmortalität um 28 % ein ebenso deutlicher Anstieg der übrigen Todesfälle um 34 % gegenübersteht. Beide Beobachtungen beruhen auf einem etwa identischen statistischen Vertrauen (p = 0,10 bzw. 0,12).

Eine detaillierte Analyse der Clofibrat-Studie zeigt bisher wenig beachtete Resultate: Während der aktiven Studiendauer war die Mortalität unter Clofibrat 44 % höher (5,7 zu 4,0 pro 1000 und Jahr), in der Nachbeobachtungsphase ohne Behandlung fand hingegen wieder ein Angleich an die Mortalität in der Kontrollgruppe statt (Tabelle 4).

Wenn in einem kontrollierten Experiment ein zugeführter Studienfaktor mit einer erhöhten Mortalität einhergeht, nach Wegnahme des Faktors die Mortalität sich der Kontrolle jedoch wieder angleicht, so ist mit großer Wahrscheinlichkeit eine kausale Rolle dieses Faktors gegeben. Praktisch alle klinisch-epidemiologischen Kausalitätskriterien sind erfüllt [26]. Zudem wurde eine erhöhte Mortalität unter Clofibrat auch in anderen Studien beobachtet [5, 22].

Die neuen Reduktasehemmer zeigen zwar stärker cholesterinsenkende Eigenschaften als die Fibrate und Ionenaustauschharze, die Wirkung auf Infarkt- und Gesamtmortalität in Langzeitstudien ist jedoch überhaupt nicht untersucht. Ob sich diese neuen Substanzen, die häufig zu Leberenzym-Anstiegen führen, günstiger als Clofibrat verhalten, läßt sich heute noch nicht voraussagen.

Hinzu kommen noch weitere mögliche Mortalitätseffekte einer Lipidtherapie: Aufgrund neuer, qualitativ guter Studien ist z. B. die Beziehung zwischen einem niedrigen Cholesterinwert und einer erhöhten Krebsrate noch immer ein seriöses Argument [14]. In einer kürzlich erschienen Metanalyse ist ebenfalls auf den

Tabelle 4. Mortalitätsentwicklung in der WHO-Clofibrat-Studie (jeweils altersstandardisiert, pro 1000 pro Jahr)

	Studienphase (5,3 Jahre)	Nachbeobachtungsphase 0–2 Jahre	2–4 Jahre	4–6 Jahrek	6–8 Jahre	8–11 Jahre	Gesamt	Gesamt (13,2 Jahre)
1. Gesamtmortalität								
Clofibrat	5,7	8,8	9,1	9,7	10,4	11,4	9,7	8,6
	1,13 – 1,81[a]	0,73–1,28	0,82–1,46	0,80–1,39	0,89–1,17	0,72–1,17	0,91–1,18	0,98–1,21
Placebo	4,0	9,2	8,3	9,2	8,9	12,5	9,4	7,9
2. Infarktmortalität								
Clofibrat	1,5	4,0	3,6	4,7	4,7	5,7	4,4	3,6
	0,61–1,41	0,71–1,08	0,76–1,95	0,73–1,61	0,73–1,61	0,61–1,20	0,87–1,31	0,86–1,22
Placebo	1,6	3,7	2,9	4,3	4,3	6,7	4,2	3,5
3. Mortalität ohne Infarkt								
Clofibrat	4,2	4,8	5,4	5,0	5,7	5,8	5,3	5,0
	1,31 – 2,37	0,60–1,27	0,70–1,45	0,69–1,48	0,85–1,80	0,74–1,52	0,84–1,21	0,98–1,32
Placebo	2,4	5,5	5,4	4,9	4,6	5,5	5,2	4,4
4. Krebsmortalität								
Clofibrat	1,9	3,2	2,9	2,1	3,2	1,5	2,6	2,4
	1,03 – 2,42	0,56–1,41	0,62–1,69	0,48–1,48	0,78–2,16	0,33–1,14	0,73–1,22	0,81–1,23
Placebo	1,2	3,6	2,8	2,5	2,5	2,5	2,4	2,4

[a] 95 %-Vertrauensintervalle des relativen Risikos (*RR*). Das RR ist statistisch signifikant (*unterstrichen*), falls das ganze Intervall entweder über oder unter 1,0 liegt.

Mißerfolg der Cholesterinsenkung in bezug auf die Gesamtsterblichkeit sowie auf die auffällige statistisch signifikante Häufung gewaltsamer Todesfälle in den Behandlungsgruppen und auf mögliche psychologische und neurologische Erklärungen hingewiesen worden [25]. Solche möglichen unerwünschten Mortalitätseffekte sind gering, aber offensichtlich nicht kleiner als die geringe Wirkung der Cholesterinsenkung auf die Infarktmortalität.

So kann heute aufgrund des inzwischen umfangreichen Datenmaterials festgestellt werden, daß die Behandlung einer asymptomatischen Hypercholesterinämie die Todesrate nicht vermindert, sondern nur die Todesart verändert. Obwohl die Lipidtheorie z.Z. sicher genauer untersucht ist als mögliche Wirkungsmechanismen solcher Nebenwirkungen, sind letztere konsistent zu beobachten. Das gängige Argument der Screeningprotagonisten, der Wirkungsmechanismus solcher Nebenwirkungen sei unklar und die Nebenwirkungen deshalb bedeutungslos, ist wenig überzeugend. Vom Standpunkt eines entweder an einem Infarkt oder an Nebenwirkungen gestorbenen Patienten dürfte es ziemlich unwichtig sein, ob die Medizin den genauen Mechanismus seines Sterbens erklären kann oder nicht.

Direkte, besondere gastrointestinale Nebenwirkungen treten unter allen Lipidsenkern (v.a. bei Behandlungsbeginn) häufig auf, verlieren sich aber oft im Verlauf der Behandlung [4, 9, 19]. Die Fibrate führten in den Langzeitstudien zu einer Verdoppelung der Cholezystektomierate (gepoolte Analyse: $p < 0,01$); diese Zunahme betrug 1 Fall pro 1000 Behandlungsjahre.

Zahlenmäßig bedeutsamer sind möglicherweise unerwünschte Wirkungen und Befindlichkeitsstörungen durch das Screening selbst. Vom Hypertoniescreening ist bekannt, daß allein schon die neue Patientenrolle als Risikofaktorenträger zu einer Verdoppelung des Absentismus führen kann. Bei bis zu 20% der nun in eine Krankheitsrolle geratenen Risikopatienten traten vermehrt Depression und eine diffuse Befindlichkeitsstörung auf [2, 13, 20]. Einem praktischen Arzt sind solche Auswirkungen des Screenings als nicht allzu selten bekannt. Solche „intangible" Auswirkungen des Cholesterinscreenings sind bisher jedoch kaum untersucht worden. Lediglich eine Studie ist dieser Frage nachgegangen mit dem Ergebnis, daß das betreffende Cholesterinscreeningprogramm zu keinen solchen negativen Auswirkungen führte [11]. Bedeutsam schien dabei allerdings zu sein, daß das Screening von einer Beratung durch psychologisch geschulte Fachleute begleitet war. Daß beispielsweise Übergewichtige einer fachgerechten Beratung bedürfen, ist jedoch unabhängig vom Cholesterinspiegel. Ob ein Screening in der Arztpraxis oder auf dem Marktplatz ohne diese aufwendige Beratung die Befindlichkeit beeinträchtigt, muß mangels Studien offen bleiben.

Schlußfolgerungen und Thesen

Kein Screening der asymptomatischen Hypercholesterinämie

- Eine cholesterinsenkende Behandlung bei symptomloser Hypercholesterinämie verändert lediglich die Krankheits- und Todesart, ohne die Gesamtrate senken zu können.

- Im Screening der asymptomatischen Hypercholesterinämie ist die individuelle Risikoklassifizierung aus Gründen der geringen Spezifität des Cholesterinspiegels und der großen intraindividuellen Schwankungen sowie aus Gründen von Fehlklassifizierungen durch Laborungenauigkeiten praktisch unmöglich.
- Damit führt ein Cholesterinscreening in der gesunden asymptomatischen Bevölkerung lediglich zu einer fehlerhaften Risikostigmatisierung ohne nützliche Konsequenzen.
- Ein Cholesterinscreening in der gesamten unselektionierten Bevölkerung ist demnach wertlos und hat eher unerwünschte Auswirkungen. Ein ungezieltes Screening ist deshalb weder auf dem Marktplatz (Massenscreening) noch in der Arztpraxis („case-finding") von Vorteil.

Behandlung nur bei hohem Risiko

- Screening ist per definitionen eine individuelle und keine bevölkerungsweite Prävention. Dabei sollen das individuelle Risiko bestimmt und individuelle Maßnahmen ergriffen werden. Entscheidende Beurteilungsparameter im Screening sind deshalb erwünschte und unerwünschte Wirkungen in *absoluten* Risiken (Rate verhinderter Infarkte pro 1000 Behandlungsjahre). Studienergebnisse in relativen Risiken ausgedrückt (Prozent Senkung der Infarktrate) sind für die Nutzensbeurteilung wertlos und irreführend.
- Theoretisch nimmt der absolute Nutzen bei steigendem individuellen Risiko zu; die Nebenwirkungen einer Behandlung bleiben theoretisch pro Individuum gleich. Damit ist eine Verbesserung des Nutzen-Risiko-Verhältnisses einer Behandlung bei Hypercholesterinämikern mit manifester koronarer Herzkrankheit oder anderweitigen gleichzeitigen Risikofaktoren anzunehmen. Wenn das durch Nebenwirkungen bedingte Mortalitätsrisiko einer Lipidsenkerbehandlung rund 0,5 Todesfälle in 1000 Behandlungsjahren beträgt (gemäß Beobachtung aus bisherigen Studien), so kann die Gesamtmortalität theoretisch positiv beeinflußt werden, wenn das Infarkttodesrisiko bei über 2,5 pro 1000 jährlich liegt. (Eine 20 %ige Senkung entspräche ebenfalls einem Mortalitätsunterschied von 0,5 pro 1000 jährlich).
- Diese theoretischen Überlegungen sind jedoch bisher in Langzeitstudien nicht bestätigt worden. Es liegt lediglich eine ältere, methodisch recht mangelhafte Studie vor: Diese weist jedoch darauf hin, daß das Behandlungsergebnis in einer Hochrisikogruppe mit großenteils vorbestehender koronarer Herzkrankheit günstiger sein könnte.
- Cholesterinbestimmungen in Hochrisikogruppen (v. a. Männer mittleren Alters mit koronarer Herzkrankheit oder mit weiteren Risikofaktoren und einer positiven Familienanamnese) sind sehr wahrscheinlich von Nutzen, weil auch die Senkung eines nur grenzwertigen Cholesterins in dieser Gruppe einen relativ großen absoluten Nutzen erzeugen könnte, der die Nebenwirkungen ziemlich sicher überwiegt.

Ein „case-finding" in der Arztpraxis ist deshalb sinnvoll, wenn solcherart selektionierte Cholesterinbetimmungen vorgenommen werden.

- Die Erarbeitung von Screening- bzw. Case-finding-Strategien nach Kriterien von absoluten Risiken (und damit des positiven Vorhersagewertes eines Cholesterinspiegels) sollte die heute empfohlene undifferenzierte „Hypercholesterinämie"bestimmerei und -behandlerei ersetzen. Weitere entsprechende Langzeitstudien sind erforderlich.

Lipidsenker sind nicht harmlos

- Lipidsenker können ein erhebliches Nebenwirkungspotential aufweisen, das zumindest bei asymptomatischer Hypercholesterinämie die Gesamtmortalität erhöhen kann. Deshalb sind Substanzen, die nicht in kontrollierten Langzeitstudien erprobt wurden, von unsicherem Nutzen und potentiell gefährlich.
- Bisher zeigten sich nur Colestyramin und Gemfibrozil in Langzeitstudien als einigermaßen sicher: Sie erhöhten zwar die Nichtinfarktmortalität genauso wie sie die Infarktmortalität senkten, führten jedoch immerhin zu keiner Zunahme der Gesamtsterblichkeit.

  Gemfibrozil ist v. a. für die Hypertriglyzeridämie Typ IIb geeignet, für Typ IIa kommen in erster Linie Ionenaustauschharze in Frage.
- Andere „unsichere" Fibrate und Reduktasehemmer sollten nicht oder nur mit größter Zurückhaltung verwendet werden.

Diät ist eine wenig wirksame Alternative

- So schön die Idee einer nebenwirkungsfreien Diät als Ersatz für die medikamentöse Cholesterinsenkung wäre, so sicher wissen wir heute, daß eine cholesterinsenkende Diät als Prophylaxe wirkungslos ist. Nur für Hochrisikogruppen mit manifester kardiovaskulärer Erkrankung besteht wahrscheinlich ein schwacher Nutzen der Diät.
- Der Cholesteringehalt der Nahrung ist ein weitgehend wertloser Parameter. Früher wegen ihres geringen Cholesteringehalts als „präventiv" erklärte Nahrungsmittel (Margarine) sind nach neuen Erkenntnissen ungünstig zusammengesetzt. Biochemische Spekulationen können epidemiologische Langzeitstudien über Nutzen und unerwünschte Auswirkungen von Diätveränderungen nicht ersetzen. Was für das Herz gut sein soll, könnte zudem für andere Organe nachteilig sein.
- Eine Cholesterinbestimmung als Grundlage und Kontrollinstrument von Diätempfehlungen ist nicht rational. Gewisse allgemeine Diätempfehlungen (kalorisch angepaßt, faserreich) müssen nicht von einer Cholesterinspiegelbestimmung abhängig gemacht werden.

Literatur

1. American Heart Association (1973) Coronary risk. Handbook
2. Bloom JR, Monterossa S (1981) Hypertensive labelling and sense of well-being. Am J Public Helth 71 : 1228–1232
3. Broughton PM, Bullock DG, Cramb R (1990) Improving the quality of plasma cholesterol measurements in primary case. Scand J Clin Lab Invest [Suppl] 198 : 43–48
4. Committee of Principal Investigators (1984) WHO trial on primary prevention of IHD with clofibrat to lower serum cholesterol: Final mortality follow-up. Lancet II: 600–604
5. Coronary Drug Project Research Group (1975) Clofibrate and niacin in CHD. JAMA 231 : 360–381
6. Dorr AE, Gundersen K, Schneider Jr JC, Spencer TW, Martin WB (1978) Colestipol hydrochloride in hypercholesterolemic patients – effect on serum cholesterol and mortality. J Chronic Dis 31 : 5–14
7. Fletcher RH, Fletcher SW, Wagner EH (1982) Clinical epidemiology: the essentials. Williams & Wilkins, Baltimore London
8. Frantz ID, Daxson EA, Ashman PL et al. (1989) Test of effect or lipid-lowering by diet of cardiovascular risk. The Minnesota Coronary Survey. Arteriosclerosis 9 : 129–135
9. Frick MH, Elo O, Haapa K et al. (1987) Helsinki Heart Study: primary-prevention trial with gemfibrozil in middle-aged men with dyslipidemia. Safety of treatment, changes in risk factors, and incidence of coronary heart disease. N Engl J Med 317 : 1237–1245
10. Gordon T, Kagan A, Garcia Palmiori M et al. (1981) Diet and its relation to CHD and deaths in three populations. Circulation 63 : 500–515
11. Havas S, Reisman J, Hsu L, Koumjian L (1991) Does cholesterol screening result in negative labelling effects? Arch Intern Med 151 : 113–119
12. Haynes RB, Sackett DL, Tylor DW, Gibson ES, Johnson AL (1978) Increased absenteeism from work after detection and labelling of hypertensive patients. N Engl J Med 1978; 299:741–744
13. Hegsted DM, Nicolosi RJ (1987) Individual variation in serum cholesterol levels. Proc Natl Acad Sci 84 : 6259–6261
14. Isles CG, Hole DJ, Gillis CR et al. (1989) Plasma cholesterol, coronary heart disease, and cancer in the Renfrew and Paisley survey. Br Med J 298 : 920–924
15. Kannel WB, Castelli WP, Gordon T (1979) Cholesterol in the prediction of arteriosclerotic heart disease. New perspectives based on the Framingham Study. Ann Intern Med 90 : 1985–1991
16. Keys A, Aravanis C, Blackburn H et al. (1972) Probability of middle-aged men developing coronary heart disease in five years. Circulation 45 : 815–828
17. Kromhout D, Bosschieter EB, de Lezenne CC (1982) Dietary fibre and 10-year mortality from CHD, cancer, and all causes. Lancet II: 518–522
18. Kromhout D, Bosschieter EB, de Lezenne CC (1985) The inverse relation between fish consumption and 20-year mortality from CHD. N Eng J Med 312 : 1205–1209
19. The Lipid Research Clinics Coronary Primary Prevention (1984) Trial results: I. Reduction in incidence of coronary heart disease. JAMA 251 : 351–364
20. Macdonald LA, Sackett DL, Haynes RB et al. (1984) Labelling in hypertension: a review of the behavioural and psychological consequences. J Dis 37 : 933–942
21. Mensink RP, Katan MB (1990) Effect of dietary trans fatty acids on high-density and low-density lipoprotein cholesterol levels in healthy subjects. N Engl J Med 323 : 439–445
22. Miettinen TA, Huttunen JK, Nankkarinen V et al. (1985) Multifactorial primary prevention of cardiovascular disease in middle-aged men: Risk factor changes, incidence, and mortality. JAMA 254 : 2097–2102
23. Mogadam M, Ahmed SW, Mensch AH, Godwin ID (1990) Within-person fluctuations of serum cholesterol and lipoproteins. Arch Intern Med 150 : 1645–1648
24. Morris JN (1977) Diet and heart: A postscript. Br Med J II: 1307–1314

25. Muldoon MF, Manuck JB, Matthews KA (1990) Lowering cholesterol concentrations and mortality: a quantitative review of primary prevention trials. Br Med J 301 : 309–314
26. Sackett DL, Haynes RB, Tugwell P (1985) Clinical epidemiology: a basic science for clinical medicine. Little, Brown & Company, Boston Toronto
27. Schmidt J (1987) Risiko und Nutzen einer Behandlung: das Beispiel Clofibrat. Schweiz Med Wochenschr 117 : 773–776
28. Schmidt JG (1990) Wie sinnvoll ist ein Cholesterin-Screening? Z Allg Med 66 : 789–794
29. Stamler J (1987) Lifestyle, major risk factors, proof and public policy. Circulation 58 : 3–19
30. Thompson SG, Pocock SJ (1990) The variability of serum cholesterol measurements: implications for screening and monitoring. J Clin Epidemiol 43 : 783–789
31. The Toronto Working Group on Cholesterol Policy (1990) Asymptomatic hypercholesterolemia: a clinical policy review. J Clin Epidemiol 43 : 1028–1121

Hypercholesterinämie und kardiovaskuläre Risikofaktoren

Thomas Eisenhauer

Einleitung

Erhöhte Cholesterinspiegel stellen einen der Hauptrisikofaktoren für die Entwicklung einer vorzeitigen Atherosklerose dar. Neben tierexperimentellen Studien ist inzwischen in zahlreichen großangelegten, epidemiologischen Studien eindeutig belegt, daß eine strenge und unabhängige Beziehung zwischen der Höhe des Cholesterinspiegels und der Inzidenz einer koronaren Herzerkrankung besteht [1, 5, 8].

Obwohl diese Beziehung seit über 10 Jahren übereinstimmend anerkannt wird, ist die Evidenz, daß eine Verringerung der Cholesterinspiegel zu einer Verminderung des koronaren Risikos führt, nicht so klar. Deshalb ist der klinische Nutzen von therapeutischen Interventionen zur Senkung des Cholesterinspiegels bisher Gegenstand erheblicher öffentlicher Kontroversen.

Kardiovaskuläre Komplikationen einer vorzeitigen Atherosklerose stellen die Haupttodesursache in westlichen Ländern dar. Dies hat dazu geführt, daß das Thema in den verschiedenen Medien vor einem breiten Publikum diskutiert wurde und aufwendige nationale und internationale Programme zur Cholesterinsenkung ausgearbeitet worden sind. Diese Programme sind jedoch nicht ohne Kritik geblieben. Die Empfehlung, einer großen Zahl gesunder Menschen mit Hypercholesterinämie eine strenge cholesterinarme Diät oder sogar cholesterinsenkende Medikamente zu geben, hat erhebliche wirtschaftliche Folgen. Obwohl natürlich einige gut definierte Patientengruppen mit einem hohen Atheroskleroserisiko von dieser Therapie profitieren, trifft dies nicht für alle Menschen mit hohen Cholesterinwerten zu. Der potentielle Nutzen einer Behandlung großer Bevölkerungszahlen muß sorgfältig gegen die möglichen Risiken der Einnahme von Medikamenten und der Probleme und Kosten von Änderungen der Diät abgewogen werden.

Zur Senkung erhöhter Cholesterinwerte sind 2 verschiedene Strategien angewendet worden [11]:

1. Der patientenorientierte Weg: Er hat zum Ziel, Individuen mit hohem Risiko zu identifizieren, bei denen eine intensive Intervention von Nutzen ist. Für diese Patienten müssen klare Kriterien herausgearbeitet werden, um die Gruppe zu definieren, die von einer medikamentösen Intervention profitieren kann. Außerdem müssen genaue Richtlinien vorgegeben werden, wie diese Patienten zu behandeln und zu überwachen sind.
2. Eine Bevölkerungsstrategie: Sie hat zum Ziel, die Verteilung der Cholesterinwerte in der gesamten Bevölkerung auf ein niedrigeres Niveau zu verschieben.

Rationale Pharmakotherapie in der Allgemeinpraxis
Rational Pharmacotherapy in General Practice
M. M. Kochen (Hrsg.)

Dies geschieht durch Erziehung und Veränderung der Ernährungsgewohnheiten.

Es ist gezeigt worden [9], daß allein die Messung des Cholesterinwertes im Blut und eine kurze Aufklärung über die Ernährungsgewohnheiten zu einer positiven Veränderung der Eßgewohnheiten und zu einer Absenkung des Cholesterinspiegels führen kann.

Wen screenen?

Nach den Empfehlungen des National Cholesterol Education Program [11] sollte der Gesamtcholesterinspiegel im Serum bei allen Erwachsenen über 20 Jahre wenigstens alle 5 Jahre kontrolliert werden.

Spiegel unter 200 mg/dl gelten als normal, während Spiegel über 240 mg/dl als erhöht eingestuft werden. Cholesterinkonzentrationen zwischen 200–240 mg/dl werden als grenzwertig betrachtet.

Ein Stellenwert von 240 mg/dl für die Definition eines erhöhten Cholesterinspiegels wurde deshalb ausgewählt, weil in mehreren Studien gezeigt werden konnte, daß das Risiko für das Auftreten einer koronaren Herzerkrankung abrupt ansteigt, wenn dieser Wert überschritten wird.

Gleichfalls wird empfohlen, bei allen Patienten weitere Risikofaktoren für die Entwicklung einer koronaren Herzerkrankung zu erfassen. Diese Risikofaktoren sind: Zigarettenrauchen, Hochdruck, Diabets mellitus, Übergewicht und eine fämiliäre Belastung mit koronarer Herzerkrankung.

Eine Lipoproteinanalyse sollte sowohl bei allen Patienten mit erhöhtem Gesamtcholesterin (> 240 mg/dl) als auch bei den Patienten mit grenzwertigem Cholesterin (200–240 mg/dl) durchgeführt werden, die zusätzlich ein hohes kardiovaskuläres Risiko aufweisen. Dieses wird definiert als eine schon vorbestehende koronare Herzerkrankung oder das Vorliegen von mindestens 2 weiteren Risikofaktoren. Die Patienten der Gruppe mit grenzwertigen Cholesterinwerten, die keine weiteren kardiovaskulären Risikofaktoren aufweisen, sollten eine Diätempfehlung erhalten und nach einem Jahr kontrolliert werden.

Die Behandlungsindikation von Patienten mit erhöhten Cholesterinwerten sollte sich an den LDL-Cholesterinspiegeln orientieren. Diese werden übereinstimmend als Schlüsselparameter in der Therapieentscheidung benutzt. LDL-Cholesterinwerte über 160 mg/dl werden als „Hochrisiko"-LDL-Cholesterinwerte betachtet, LDL-Spiegel zwischen 130–159 mg/dl als *grenzwertig* „Hochrisiko"-LDL-Cholesterin. Bei den *„Hochrisiko"*patienten und den Patienten mit *„grenzwertigen"* LDL-Werten, die zusätzlich 2 oder mehr kardiovaskuläre Risikofaktoren aufweisen, sollte nach einer vollständigen klinischen Untersuchung mit der cholesterinsenkenden Behandlung begonnen werden.

Wen behandeln?

Es ist geschätzt worden, daß bei Verwendung der Richtlinien des National Cholesterol Education Programs etwa 36 % aller amerikanischen Erwachsenen zwischen 20–74 Jahren entweder als Patienten für eine Diätberatung oder sogar für eine cholesterinsenkende Behandlung in Frage kämen [13]. Dies würde, wenn man die Bevölkerungsdaten der USA von 1986 zugrunde legt, etwa 70 Mio. Amerikaner betreffen und einen enormen personellen und wirtschaftlichen Aufwand erfordern [7]. Deshalb sind diese Richtlinien von verschiedenen Autoren kritisiert worden [4, 14]. Zum Beispiel ist bisher nicht gezeigt worden, ob die Beziehung zwischen Cholesterinspiegeln und koronarer Herzkrankheit bei über 60jährigen weiterbesteht [4]. Des weiteren ist berichtet worden, daß diese Beziehung für Frauen erheblich geringer ist [14].

Kardiovaskuläre Erkrankungen sind für fast die Hälfte aller Todesfälle in den USA verantwortlich, und die als sehr hoch geschätzten Kosten einer lebenslangen medikamentösen Therapie gelten als wichtiges Argument gegen die weit verbreitete prospektive Anwendung von cholesterinsenkenden Medikamenten [10].

Die Grundlage der Therapie der Hypercholesterinämie stellt eine cholesterinarme Diät dar. Die von der American Heart Association [6] empfohlene Diät besteht aus einer Verringerung des Nahrungsfettes auf 30 % der Gesamtkalorien oder weniger. Wobei die Erziehung des Patienten, insbesondere die Korrektur seiner Eßgewohnheiten, das Anstreben einer Gewichtsreduktion bei übergewichtigen Patienten und die Verringerung der Aufnahme von saturierten Fettsäuren bei Begrenzung der Gesamtkalorien von größter Wichtigkeit ist. Die Cholesterinaufnahme sollte wenigerals 300 mg/24 h betragen.

Ziel der Diättherapie ist die Reduktion der LDL-Cholesterinwerte unter 160 mg/dl bei Patienten ohne weitere Risikofaktoren und ohne koronare Herzerkrankung.

Bei Patienten, die mehr als 2 zusätzliche kardiovaskuläre Risikofaktoren aufweisen oder bei Patienten mit Sekundärprävention, (aufgrund dokumentierter vorbestehender koronarer Herzerkrankung) ist eine stärkere LDL-Absenkung anzustreben. Für diese Patienten wird von dem National Cholesterol Program ein Zielwert des LDL-Cholesterins von < 130 mg/dl vorgeschlagen.

Eine medikamentöse Therapie sollte nach sorgfältiger Analyse jedes individuellen Patienten erfolgen, da cholesterinsenkende Medikamente über lange Zeit und oft sogar lebenslang gegeben werden müssen. Der Nutzen einer medikamentösen Senkung der Cholesterinspiegel für eine Verringerung der kardiovaskulären Mortalität ist bei der primären Prävention noch nicht eindeutig belegt. Es gibt jedoch neue und sehr überzeugende Studien, die klar erwiesen haben, daß bei Patienten mit bekannter koronarer Herzerkrankung und Hypercholesterinämie die Reduktion der Cholesterinspiegel das Risiko eines zweiten Herzinfarktes und die Mortalität signifikant senkt [2, 3].

Fazit einer zusammenfassenden Analyse von mehreren großen epidemiologischen Studien ist die Feststellung von Rossouw et al. [12]:

In den Studien zur Sekundärprävention ist erwiesen worden, daß eine 10%ige Cholesterinreduktion eine Reduktion der Inzidenz von nichttödlichen Reinfarkten um 19% und von tödlichen Infarkten um 12% erwarten läßt (S. 1117).

Ungeachtet der Tatsache, daß zwei Drittel aller Patienten mit koronarer Herzerkrankung Cholesterinwerte über 200 mg/dl aufweisen, ist der Behandlung der erhöhten Cholesterinwerte bei diesen Patienten bisher sehr wenig Aufmerksamkeit entgegengebracht worden.

Unter Berücksichtigung dieser neuen Erkenntnisse wird deshalb empfohlen, die medikamentöse cholesterinsenkende Therapie gezielt zur Sekundärprävention der koronaren Herzerkrankung einzusetzen. Eine solche Therapie sollte bei der primären Prävention der koronaren Herzerkrankung auf individuelle Patienten mit besonders schwerer Hypercholesterinämie, die ein deutlich erhöhtes Risiko für die Entstehung einer koronaren Herzerkrankung aufweisen, begrenzt werden.

Abschließend sollte darauf hingewiesen werden, daß es bisher nicht möglich ist, das Vorhandensein einer atherosklerotischen Veränderung vor seiner klinischen Manifestation zu diagnostizieren. Es gibt leider keinen einfachen, nichtinvasiven Test, um die Patienten mit erhöhten Cholesterinwerten zu identifizieren, die später eine koronare Herzerkrankung entwickeln werden.

Literatur

1. Blankenhorn DH, Nessum SA, Johnson RL, Sanmarco ME, Azen SP, Cashin-Hemphill L (1987) Beneficial effects of combined colestipolniacin therapy on coronary atherosclerosis and coronary venous bypass graft. JAMA 257:3233–3240
2. Brown G, Albers JJ, Fisher LD et al. (1990) Regression of coronary artery disease as a result of intensive lipid-lowering therapy in men with high levels of apolipoprotein B. N Engl J Med 323:1289–1298
3. Buchwald H, Varko LL, Matts PJ et al. (1990) Effect of partial ileal bypass surgery on mortality and morbidity from coronary heart disease in patients with hypercholesterolemia: Report of the Program on the Surgical Control of the Hyperlipidemias (POSCH). N Engl J Med 323:946–955
4. Castelli WP, Garrison RJ, Wilson PW, Abbott RD, Kalousdian S, Kannel WB (1986) Incidence of coronary heart disease and lipoprotein cholesterol levels: The Framingham Study. JAMA 256:2835–2838
5. Frick MH, Elo O, Haapa K et al. (1987) Helsinki Heart Study: Primary prevention trial with gemifibrozil in middle-aged men with dyslipidemia. N Engl J Med 317:1237–1245
6. Gotto A Jr, Bierman EL, Connor WE et al. (1984) Recommendations for treatment of hyperlipidemia in adults: A joint statement of the Nutrition Committee and the Council on Arteriosclerosis. Circulation 69:1065A–1090A
7. Leaf A (1989) Management of hypercholesterolemia. Are preventive interventions advisable? N Engl J Med 321/10:680–684
8. Lipid Research Clinics Program (1984) The Lipid Research Clinics Coronary Primary Prevention Trial results. JAMA 251:351–364
9. Murray DM, Luepker RV, Pirie PL, Grimm RH, Bloom E, Davis MA, Blackburn H (1986) Systematic risk factor screening and education: a community-wide approach to prevention of coronary heart disease. Prev Med 1:661–672

10. Oster G, Epstein AM (1987) Costeffectiveness of antihyperlipidemic therapy in the prevention of coronary heart disease: The case of cholestyramine. JAMA 258 : 2381–2387
11. Report of the National Cholesterol Education Program Expert Panel (1988) On detection, evaluation, and treatment of high blood cholesterol in adults. Arch Intern Med 148 : 36–69
12. Rossouw JE, Lewis B, Rifkind BM (1990) The value of lowering cholesterol after myocardial infarction. N Engl J Med 18 : 1112–1119
13. Sempos C, Fulwood R, Hains C et al. (1989) The prevalence of high blood cholesterol levels among adults in the United States. JAMA 262 : 45–52
14. Wilson PW, Christiansen JC, Anderson KM, Kannel WB (1989) Impact of national guidelines for cholesterol risk factor screening: The Framingham Offspring Study. JAMA 262 : 41–44

Hypercholesterinämie und Myokardinfarktrisiko: Ergebnisse der GRIPS-Studie

Rainer Muche, Olaf Gefeller, Dorothea Nagel und Peter Cremer

Einleitung

Krankheiten des Herz-Kreislauf-Systems sind weiterhin die häufigste Todesursache in den industrialisierten Ländern. Laut offizieller Statistik verzeichnete die Bundesrepublik Deutschland im Jahre 1988 insgesamt 341 428 Todesfälle (Männer: 147 339, Frauen: 194 089) infolge dieser Erkrankungen. Damit entfällt die Hälfte aller Todesfälle (Männer: 46 %, Frauen: 53 %) auf diese Krankheitssparte. Während bei Frauen diese Erkrankung erst im höheren Alter als Todesursache in den Vordergrund treten, sind sie bei Männern bereits in den mittleren Lebensjahren (45–65 Jahre) mit 27 219 Fällen (= 36 %) die dominierende Todesursache.

Die Bemühungen um eine wirksame Verhütung dieser Krankheit basieren auf dem sog. Risikofaktorkonzept [13]. Grundsätzlich kann man in dem Prozeß atherosklerotischer Veränderungen einen chronischen, allmählich progredienten Vorgang sehen, der bis zu einem gewissen Grad altersphysiologisch erscheint. Durch ungünstige Einflüsse kann die Progredienz jedoch derart beschleunigt werden, daß es frühzeitig zu klinischen Folgen kommt. Dabei sind Risikofaktoren Merkmale, die mit einem forcierten Ablauf atherosklerotischer Gefäßveränderungen und einer damit verbundenen Erhöhung der Erkrankungswahrscheinlichkeit einhergehen. In einer Vielzahl epidemiologischer Studien in den letzten Jahrzehnten [16, 18, 19] sind potentielle Risikofaktoren für spezielle Herz-Kreislauf-Erkrankungen, insbesondere für den Myokardinfarkt, untersucht worden. Dabei konnten u. a. Hypertonie, Diabetes mellitus, Zigarettenrauchen und bestimmte Fettstoffwechselstörungen (speziell erhöhter Serumcholesterinspiegel) als wesentliche Risikofaktoren identifiziert werden.

In der GRIPS-Studie (*G*öttinger *R*isiko-, *I*nzidenz- und *P*rävalenz*s*tudie) [9] soll speziell der Einfluß des Lipidstoffwechsels auf die Myokardinfarktinzidenz mit Hilfe einer differenzierten Analytik detailliert untersucht werden. Alle Lipide befinden sich im Plasma ausschließlich als Bestandteile komplexer Transportpartikel, der sog. Lipoproteine. Aufgrund unterschiedlicher, physikochemischer Eigenschaften lassen sich die Lipoproteine nach ihrer Dichte in 3 reguläre Hauptlipoproteinfraktionen unterteilen: HDL („high density lipoproteins"), LDL („low density lipoproteins") und VLDL („very low density lipoproteins"). Der Stellenwert dieser Fraktionen hinsichtlich ihres atherogenen Risikopotentials wird kontrovers diskutiert. In der LRC-Studie (Lipid Research Clinics Coronary Primary Prevention

Rationale Pharmakotherapie in der Allgemeinpraxis
Rational Pharmacotherapy in General Practice
M. M. Kochen (Hrsg.)

Trial) [15] wird die gefäßschädigende Rolle der LDL-Komponente in den Vordergrund gestellt, während andere Studien (z. B. PROCAM, Prospektive Cardiovascular Münster-Studie) [1, 17], Framingham [4] die gefäßprotektive Bedeutung der HDL-Komponente betonen.

Ein Manko vieler Studien liegt jedoch darin, daß nicht alle der 3 Komponenten *direkt* gemessen wurden. Häufig kam die Friedewald-Formel zum Einsatz, die aus HDL-Cholesterin, Serumcholesterin und Triglyzeridkonzentration den LDL-Cholesterinwert approximiert. Diese Vorgehensweise ist aber mit z. T. gravierenden Fehlern behaftet [5]. Mit der quantitativen Lipoproteinelektropherese stand der GRIPS-Studie eine valide, direkte Meßtechnik zur Quantifizierung aller Fraktionen zur Verfügung [5]. Somit ist GRIPS die erste prospektive Großstudie, in der auch LDL-Cholesterin direkt gemessen wurde. Sie ist daher besonders geeignet, den prognostischen und diagnostischen Stellenwert der verschiedenen Lipoproteinfraktionen zu untersuchen.

Studienziele

Die Ziele der Studie waren:
- Erfassung der Myokardinfarktinzidenz in dieser klar definierten Population,
- Bestimmung des Einflusses verschiedener Lipoproteinfraktionen auf die Entstehung eines Myokardinfarkts,
- Analyse der dadurch möglichen Verbesserung der individuellen Prädiktion.

Dabei sollten weitere kardiovaskuläre Risikofaktoren simultan Berücksichtigung finden. Unter Myokardinfarkt wurden dabei folgende Zielereignisse zusammengefaßt:
- gesicherter nichttödlicher Herzinfarkt,
- gesicherter tödlicher Myokardinfarkt,
- akuter Herztod.

Die Sicherung dieser Zielereignisse erfolgte nach definierten Kriterien [9] angelehnt an Richtlinien der LRC [15].

Material und Methoden

Studiendesign und -kollektiv der GRIPS-Studie

Die GRIPS-Studie [6, 9] ist eine prospektive Kohortenstudie an 40–60jährigen männlichen Beschäftigten eines Industrieunternehmens. Die Erhebung der Basisdaten begann im Frühjahr 1982. Neben einer umfassenden klinischen, laborchemischen und anamnestischen Erfassung der potentiellen Risikofaktoren und typischen Folgekrankheiten der Atherosklerose erfolgte die Bestimmung des differenzierten Lipoproteinstatus. Nach 3 bzw. 5 Jahren erfolgten Follow-up-Untersuchungen. Dabei wurden die Zielereignisse (Myokardinfarkt, koronare Herzkrankheit, Schlaganfall, periphere arterielle Verschlußkrankheit) gesichert und erfaßt [7, 9]. Die Zusammensetzung des Studienkollektivs sowie die erzielte Beteiligung am 5-Jahres-Follow-up sind Tabelle 1 zu entnehmen.

Tabelle 1. Studienkollektiv der GRIPS-Studie

	n
Grundgesamtheit der 40- bis 60jährigen männlichen deutschen Beschäftigten eines Industrieunternehmens	7430
Beteiligung an der Basisuntersuchung	6029 (81,1 %)
– davon koronargesund	5738
Teilnahme am 5-Jahres-Follow-Up	5467 (95,3 %)
Myokardinfarkte	107
– davon tödlich	27
Konkurrierende Zielereignisse	228

Erhebung der Studienvariablen

Die Basisdaten der GRIPS-Studie wurden zwischen Januar und April 1982 direkt in dem Industrieunternehmen erhoben. Dabei wurde zuerst bei den Probanden eine umfangreiche Anamnese durch ein persönliches Interview erhoben. Anschließend erfolgte die Gewichts- und Größenbestimmung sowie die Blutdruckmessung unter standardisierten Bedingungen.

Die Blutabnahme bei der Basiserhebung erfolgte frühestens 5–6 h nach der letzten Nahrungsaufnahme. In Pilotuntersuchungen wurde gezeigt, daß bei der in der GRIPS-Studie eingesetzten Lipoproteinelektropherese die Ergebnisse der Lipoproteinquantifizierung vom Nüchternzustand des Patienten nicht beeinflußt werden [12]. Darüber hinaus erlaubt dieses Analyseverfahren unter der Annahme eines konstanten Cholesterin- und Triglyzeridanteils in den Lipoproteinfraktionen die Bestimmung eines Triglyzeridwertes, der sehr gut mit tatsächlichen Nüchternspiegeln übereinstimmt [12]. Die Blutproben wurden gekühlt und jeweils am selben Tag im Zentrallabor des Universitätsklinikums Göttingen analysiert. Ergänzend dazu wurden Serum- und Plasmaproben von jedem Studienteilnehmer eingefroren. Potentielle Risikofaktoren, die bei Studienbeginn noch nicht bekannt waren, können so nachträglich berücksichtigt werden.

Für die Variable „Zigarettenrauchen" wurden die differenzierteren Informationen aus der ersten Nachbefragung für die Analyse benutzt. So ließen sich 3 Ausprägungen definieren: Nichtraucher, Exraucher, Raucher.

Die Analyse berücksichtigte bekannte Risikofaktoren aus früheren epidemiologischen Studien. Weitere mögliche Einflußfaktoren wurden durch unifaktorielle Auswertungen der GRIPS-Daten identifiziert [8]. Tabelle 2 gibt eine Übersicht über die bei der Modellierung einbezogenen Variablen und ihre Kategorisierungen.

Tabelle 2. Potentielle Einflußfaktoren und ihre Kategorisierungen (*MI* Myokardinfarkt)

Einflußfaktor	Kategorien
Alter	< 50 Jahre; ≥ 50 Jahre
Triglyzeride	< 200 mg/dl; ≥ 200 mg/dl
Blutzucker	< 120 mg/dl; 120 – 150 mg/dl; ≥ 150 mg/dl
Body Mass Index	< 25 kg/m^2; 25 – 30 kg/m^2; ≥ 30 kg/m^2
Familiäre Disposition	0 Verwandte MI; ≥ 1 Verwandte MI
Zigarettenrauchen	nie; früher; jetzt
Blutdruck	WHO-Definition: normoton, grenzwertig, hyperton
Alkoholkonsum	nie; unregelmäßig + regelmäßig
Sportliche Aktivität	selten; gelegentlich + regelmäßig

Statistische Methodik

Die mathematische Modellierung der dichotomen Variable „Myokardinfarkt“ erfolgte durch das logistische Regressionsmodell [14]. Dabei konnten alle potentiellen Risikofaktoren und deren Wechselwirkungen simultan auf ihren Einfluß geprüft werden. Dadurch sind die Ergebnisse für den interessierenden Risikofaktor adjustiert für die weiteren im Modell befindlichen Einflußfaktoren. In der vorliegenden Auswertung kam eine spezielle Auswertungsstrategie zur Anwendung, die unter Beachtung des Hierarchieprinzips [3] ein geeignetes Selektionsverfahren unter den potentiellen Einflußfaktoren durchführte, um nur diejenigen Einflußfaktoren zu berücksichtigen, welche die Beziehung zwischen den Lipoproteinfraktionen und dem Myokardinfarkt im vorliegenden Datenmaterial beeinflußten.

Die berechneten Modellparameter erlauben anschließend direkt eine inhaltliche Interpretation als relative Veränderung des Myokardinfarktrisikos. Ergänzend dazu wurden zur Einschätzung der Veränderung des absoluten individuellen Risikos durch das Vorliegen eines Risikofaktors auf der Grundlage des Modells absolute Risikodifferenzen für verschiedene Risikofaktorprofile berechnet [2].

Ergebnisse

Der Modellbildungsprozeß führte nach mehreren Zwischenschritten zu dem in Tabelle 3 abgebildeten Endmodell. Neben dem p-Wert des Likelihood-Ratio-Tests auf Signifikanz der entsprechenden Einflußvariable sind der adjustierte Schätzer für die relative Risikoveränderung (Odds Ratio) und dessen 95 %-Konfidenzintervall aufgeführt.

Es zeigte sich, daß sowohl unter den Lipoproteinen, als auch insgesamt LDL-Cholesterin die stärkste Beziehung zum Myokardinfarktrisiko aufweist. Zur Darstellung des Risikopotentials wurden für diesen stetigen Parameter zwei international diskutierte Grenzwerte (160 mg/dl bzw. 190 mg/dl) ausgewählt [1,10,11].

Tabelle 3. Endmodell nach Einflußvariablenselektion in der GRIPS-Studie. *OR* Odds Ratio; *CI* Konfidenzintervall; *MI* Myokardinfarkt

		p	OR	95%-CI
LDL-Cholesterin[a]	(stetig)	<0,0001		
	≥ 190 mg/dl		5,547	3,526; 8,726
	≥ 160 mg/dl		4,853	3,051; 7,721
HDL-Cholesterin	≥ 35 mg/dl	0,0045	0,482	0,292; 0,797
VLDL-Cholesterin	≥ 30 mg/dl	0,1936	1,349	0,859; 2,120
Familiäre Disposition	≥ 1 Verwandter MI	<0,0001	3,714	2,280; 6,136
Blutzucker	≥ 150 mg/dl	0,0013	3,522	1,632; 7,602
Zigarettenrauchen	jetzt	0,0015	2,054	1,319; 3,198
Alter	≥ 50 Jahre	0,0012	2,041	1,326; 3,140
Alkoholkonsum	gelegentlich + regelmäßig	0,0257	0,552	0,328; 0,931
Blutdruck	hyperton	0,0290	1,703	1,056; 2,745

[a] Zur Illustration des Risikopotentials sind 2 spezielle Grenzwerte verwendet worden. Ansonsten wurde LDL-Cholesterin als stetige Variable in das Modell einbezogen.

Gegenüber einer 5- bis 5,5fachen Risikosteigerung bei erhöhtem LDL-Cholesterinspiegel ergab sich bei normaler vs. verminderter Konzentration des HDL-Cholesterins eine Halbierung des Myokardinfarktrisikos. VLDL-Cholesterin zeigte keinen signifikanten Einfluß im Endmodell, das Odds Ratio von 1,35 deutete eine Tendenz zur Risikosteigerung an.

Die weiteren wesentlichen Einflußfaktoren in der Beziehung der Lipoproteine zum Myokardinfarktrisiko mit relativen Risikoerhöhungen um 3,5 waren *familiäre Disposition* und stark erhöhter *Blutzuckerspiegel*. Allerdings nur 9 bzw. 3 % der Studienteilnehmer waren davon betroffen. Bei den weiteren Risikofaktoren wurden jeweils die höchsten Ausprägungsstufen in das Endmodell aufgenommen. Speziell beim Blutdruck und Zigarettenrauchen entfiel dadurch die ursprüngliche Unterteilung in 3 Klassen.

Anschließend wurde die Auswirkung der weiteren Einflußfaktoren im Modell auf die Beziehung des LDL-Cholesterins zum Myokardinfarktrisiko untersucht. Unter Verwendung der geschätzten Koeffizienten des Endmodells ist für verschiedene Risikofaktorprofile die Wahrscheinlichkeit für einen Myokardinfarkt innerhalb von 5 Jahren in Abhängigkeit vom Ausgangswert des LDL-Cholesterins berechnet worden. In Abb. 1 sind die Resultate für 3 spezielle Risikofaktorprofile dargestellt. Dabei ist neben den Kurven der beiden „Extremprofile" (gänzlich unbelastet mit weiteren Risikofaktoren, alle identifizierten Risikofaktoren vertreten) die Kurve des durchschnittlichen Risikofaktorprofils in der GRIPS-Studie abgebildet.

Die Abb. 1 weist darauf hin, daß die Bedeutung des LDL-Cholesterins als Risikofaktor für den Myokardinfarkt durch die Existenz weiterer Risikofaktoren entscheidend beeinflußt wird. Während bei extrem Hochrisikobelasteten der Anstieg des LDL-Cholesterins selbst im unteren Bereich mit einem deutlichen Wahrschein-

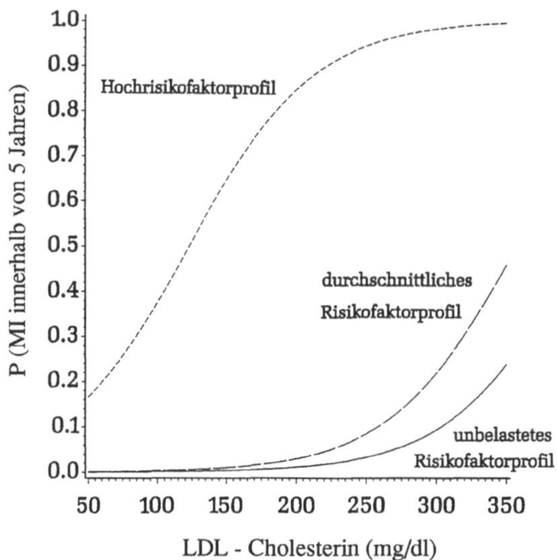

Abb. 1 Geschätzte Myokardinfarktwahrscheinlichkeit in Abhängigkeit vom LDL-Cholesterin bei verschiedenen Risikofaktorprofilen (*MI* Myokardinfarkt)

lichkeitszuwachs für den Myokardinfarkt einherging, verlief beim Fehlen weiterer Riskofaktoren die Kurve bis ca. 190 mg/dl LDL-Cholesterin sehr flach, um erst dann deutlich anzusteigen.

Tabelle 4 beinhaltet die auf Grundlage des Endmodells berechneten absoluten Risikodifferenzen für die beschriebenen Risikofaktorprofile. Dabei ist für die jeweilige Situation die Differenz der Myokardinfarktwahrscheinlichkeiten mit und ohne Störung im Lipoproteinbefund (LDL- und VLDL-Erhöhung, HDL-Verminderung) angegeben. Diese Risikodifferenzen ermöglichen die Beurteilung des absoluten Zuwachses der Myokardinfarktgefährdung eines exponierten Individuums.

LDL-Cholesterin zeigt – wie schon bei den relativen – auch bei den absoluten Risikodifferenzen einen stärkeren Einfluß auf das individuelle Myokardinfarktri-

Tabelle 4. Risikodifferenzen [%] für verschiedene Risikofaktorprofile

Lipoprotein	Risikofaktorprofil		
[mg/dl]	niedrig	durchschnittlich	hoch
LDL <> 160	0,76	2,12	31,44
LDL <> 190	1,41	3,80	27,52
HDL <> 35	0,21	0,92	8,23
VLDL <> 30	0,09	0,39	3,78

siko als HDL-Cholesterin und VLDL-Cholesterin. Jedoch sind die absoluten Risikodifferenzen beim durchschnittlichen Risikofaktorprofil mit 3,8 bzw. 2,1 % je nach Entscheidungsgrenze für LDL-Cholesterin gering. Nur bei ansonsten extrem risikobelasteten Personen erhält man absolute Steigerungen des Myokardinfarktrisikos von 27,5 bzw. 31,4 %.

Diskussion

Die hier vorgestellten Auswertungen im multifaktoriellen Modell bestätigen die vorläufigen Ergebnisse zum Stellenwert der verschiedenen Variablen für die Prädiktion des Myokardinfarktrisikos [8]. LDL-Cholesterin konnte als dominierender Risikofaktor identifiziert werden. Der Einfluß auf das Myokardinfarktrisiko war wesentlich stärker als der des HDL-Cholesterin. Jedoch zeigte HDL-Cholesterin auch in dieser Studie eine signifikante inverse Beziehung zum Myokardinfarktrisiko. VLDL-Cholesterin spielte eine untergeordnete Rolle. Es konnte nicht als Risikofaktor nachgewiesen werden.

Aus diesen Ergebnissen, speziell den gegenläufigen Wirkmechanismen des LDL- und HDL-Cholesterins, folgt, daß statt der Messung des Gesamtcholesterins eine differenzierte Lipoproteinanalytik zur diagnostischen Bewertung des Koronarrisikos unverzichtbar ist. Speziell dem LDL-Cholesterinwert sollte besondere Aufmerksamkeit gewidmet werden. Allerdings ist der Einfluß des LDL-Cholesterins auf die Wahrscheinlichkeit eines Myokardinfarkts stark abhängig von der Existenz zusätzlicher Risikofaktoren.

Weitere identifizierte Risikofaktoren für den Myokardinfarkt sind: familiäre Disposition, erhöhter Blutzuckerspiegel, Zigarettenrauchen, Alter und Bluthochdruck. Als inverse Einflußgröße auf das Myokardinfarktrisiko fand sich neben HDL-Cholesterin auch regelmäßiger und unregelmäßiger Alkoholkonsum. Beim Vorliegen weiterer Risikofaktoren sind bereits Anstiege des LDL-Cholesterins im unteren Wertbereich mit einer deutlichen Steigerung des Myokardinfarktrisikos verbunden, während bei unbelasteten Personen erst mit höherem LDL-Spiegel eine spürbare Zunahme des Myokardinfarktrisikos zu beobachten ist.

Die absoluten Risikodifferenzen bei verschiedenen Risikoprofilen zeigen allerdings, daß eine Reduktion des Myokardinfarktrisikos durch eine LDL-Cholesterinabsenkung unter 160 bzw. 190 mg/dl nur bei Vorliegen extremer Risikosituationen einen substantiellen Beitrag zur Verminderung der individuellen Gefährdung erbringen kann. Schwellenwertangaben bzw. Diagnoseempfehlungen allein auf der Grundlage von Lipoproteinwerten ohne Berücksichtigung der weiteren Risikofaktoren sind daher nicht adäquat.

In der Literatur sind viele Screeningvorschläge veröffentlicht, die auf der Grundlage der obigen Risikofaktoren versuchen, „Hochrisikopatienten" zu identifizieren und einer Therpie zuzuführen. Die hier vorgestellten Ergebnisse, speziell die absoluten Risikodifferenzen, lassen vermuten, daß dies kein vielversprechender Weg ist. In einer weiteren Arbeit in diesem Band sollen diese Screening-Vorschläge anhand des GRIPS-Datenmaterials auf ihre Eignung hinsichtlich einer individuellen Myokardinfarktprädiktion geprüft werden (s. folgenden Beitrag: Gefeller et al.).

Literatur

1. Assmann G, Schriewer H (1986) Verbesserte Hyperlipidämie-Diagnostik unter Einbeziehung von HDL-Cholesterin. Lebensversich Med 2: 47–51
2. Berkson J (1958) Smoking and lung cancer. Some observations on two recent reports. J Am Statist Assoc 53: 28–38
3. Bishop YMM, Fienberg SE, Holland PW (1975) Discrete multivariate analysis: theory and practice. MIT Press, Cambridge
4. Castelli W, Garrison RJ, Wilson PWF et al. (1986) Incidence of coronary heart disease and lipoprotein cholesterol levels – The Framingham Study. JAMA 256: 2835–2838
5. Cremer P, Seidel D, Wieland H (1985) Quantitative Lipoproteinelektropherese: Ihre routinemäßige Anwendung im Vergleich mit anderen Verfahren zur differenzierten Untersuchung des Fettstoffwechsels. Lab Med 9: 39–51
6. Cremer P, Wieland H, Seidel D (1988) Göttinger Risiko-, Inzidenz- und Prävalenzstudie (GRIPS): Aufbau und bisherige Ergebnisse. MMW 130: 268–274
7. Cremer P, Elster H, Labrot B et al. (1988) Incidence rates of fatal and nonfatal myocardial infarction in relation to the lipoprotein profile: first prospective results from the Göttingen Risk, Incidence and Prevalence Study (GRIPS). Klin Wochenschr [Suppl XI] 66: 42–49
8. Cremer P, Muche R, Kruse-Lösler B et al. (1989) Myokardinfarktrisiko bei 40- bis 60jährigen Männern in Abhängigkeit von potentiellen Risikofaktoren der Atherosklerose – Zwischenauswertungen der Göttinger Risiko-, Inzidenz- und Prävalenzstudie (GRIPS) nach einem 5-jährigen Beobachtungszeitraum. Versicherungsmed 41: 154–162
9. Cremer P, Nagel D, Labrot B et al. (1991) Göttinger Risiko-, Inzidenz- und Prävalenzstudie (GRIPS) Springer, Berlin Heidelberg New York Tokyo
10. Consensus Conference (1985) Lowering blood cholesterol to prevent heart disease. JAMA 253: 2080–2086
11. The Expert Panel (1988) Report of the National Cholesterol Education Program Expert Panel on detection, evaluation, and treatment of high blood cholesterol in adults. Arch Intern Med 148: 36–51
12. Herbst M (1987) Möglichkeiten der Lipid-, Lipoprotein- und Apoproteinanalytik im Postprandialstadium. Med Dissertation, Universität Göttingen
13. Kannel WB, Schatzkin A (1984) Risk factor analysis. Prog Cardiovasc Dis 26: 309–332
14. Kleinbaum DG, Kupper LL, Chambless LE (1982) Logistic regression analysis of epidemiologic data: theory and praxis. Comm Statist Theor Meth 11: 485–547
15. The Lipid Research Clinics Program (1984) The lipid research clinics coronary primary prevention trial results. JAMA 251: 351–374
16. MRFIT Research Group (1982) Multiple Risk Factor Intervention Trial – Risk factor changes and mortality results. JAMA 248: 1465–1477
17. Schulte H, Assmann G (1988) Ergebnisse der Prospective Cardiovascular Münster (PROCAM) Studie. Soz Präv Med 33: 32–36
18. Shaper AG, Pocock SJ (1987) Risk factors for ischaemic heart disease in British men. Br Heart J 57: 11–16
19. Truett J, Cornfield J, Kannel W (1967) A multivariate analysis of the risk of coronary heart disease in Framingham. J Chronic Dis 20: 511–524

Cholesterinscreening: Vergleich verschiedener Strategien anhand der Daten der GRIPS-Studie

Olaf Gefeller, Rainer Muche, Dorothea Nagel und Peter Cremer

Einleitung

Diagnostische Konzepte zur Früherkennung Koronargefährdeter, basierend auf Cholesterinmessungen und Erfassung weiterer kardiovaskulärer Risikofaktoren, sind unter dem Begriff „Cholesterinscreening" in vielen Varianten vorgeschlagen worden [3–6, 9, 15, 16, 18]. In der Bundesrepublik Deutschland hat eine kontroverse Diskussion dieses Themas eingesetzt, nachdem im April 1990 ein 13köpfiges Expertengremium unter dem Titel *Nationale Cholesterin-Initiative* ein „Strategiepapier zur Erkennung und Behandlung von Hyperlipidämien" im *Deutschen Ärzteblatt* publizierte [16]. In diesem Artikel werden bevölkerungsweite Screeninguntersuchungen propagiert. Weiteren Zündstoff für eine öffentliche Diskussion des Themas lieferte im November 1990 die Titelgeschichte „Mythos Cholesterin" des in einer Auflage von 1 Mio. Exemplaren verbreiteten, führenden deutschen Nachrichtenmagazins „Der Spiegel" [2]. Die z. T. emotional geführte Kontroverse soll in diesem Beitrag nicht aufgearbeitet und kommentiert werden. Vielmehr ist es unser Ziel, auf der Basis des umfangreichen Datenmaterials einer prospektiven Studie, der Göttinger Risiko-, Inzidenz- und Prävalenz-Studie (GRIPS), die verschiedenen Cholesterinscreeningstrategien hinsichtlich ihrer Eignung als Früherkennungsmaßnahme für den Myokardinfarkt zu untersuchen. Dabei ist die Evaluation auf die Güte des Instruments „Cholesterinscreening" als diagnostisches Verfahren zur Vorhersage des Myokardinfarkts beschränkt. Die unverzichtbare Diskussion weiterer Aspekte, die bei der Etablierung und Evaluation von Screeningmaßnahmen zu prüfen sind, wird hier nicht geführt [14]. Um die verschiedenen Dimensionen einer sorgfältigen Prüfung von Screeningmaßnahmen wenigstens anzudeuten, ist in Anlehnung an eine WHO-Schrift von Wilson u. Jungner [20] ein 10-Punkte-Katalog aufgelistet (s. unten), der die notwendigen Kriterien für die Einführung eines Screeningprogramms zusammenstellt (eine ähnliche Liste findet sich in [19]). In der Terminologie dieser Liste ausgedrückt, beschäftigt sich diese Arbeit ausschließlich mit der Analyse des Cholesterinscreenings hinsichtlich der Erfüllung des Punktes 5.

Rationale Pharmakotherapie in der Allgemeinpraxis
Rational Pharmacotherapy in General Practice
M. M. Kochen (Hrsg.)

Anforderungen an Screeninguntersuchungen. (Nach Wilson u. Jungner [20])

1. Die zu entdeckende Krankheit sollte ein wichtiges Gesundheitsproblem für den einzelnen wie für die Gesellschaft darstellen.
2. Es sollte ein allgemein anerkanntes Therapieverfahren für die diagnostizierten Erkrankungen bestehen.
3. Im medizinischen Versorgungssystem sollten Kapazitäten für die weitere diagnostische Abklärung und die evtl. notwendigen Behandlung vorhanden sein.
4. Es muß ein erkennbares Frühstadium der betreffenden Krankheit geben.
5. Es muß ein geeigneter Test zur Verfügung stehen, der zur Früherkennung eingesetzt werden kann.
6. Der Test muß für die Zielgruppe akzeptabel sein.
7. Der natürliche Verlauf der Erkrankung, einschließlich der Entwicklung von einem latenten zu einem manifesten Stadium, sollte hinreichend bekannt sein.
8. Es muß Übereinstimmung bestehen, wer als Patient behandelt werden soll.
9. Die Kosten für das Screening einschließlich der aus dem Screening resultierenden Ausgaben für weitere diagnostische Abklärung und Behandlung der Patienten sollten in Relation zu den gesamten Gesundheitsausgaben abgewogen werden.
10. Screeninguntersuchungen sollten einen kontinuierlichen Prozeß und keine „Einmal-und-nicht-wieder"-Aktion darstellen.

Material und Methoden

Screeningstrategien

Im Rahmen des Vergleichs werden die folgenden Screeningstrategien betrachtet:

- Richtlinien des „Expert Panels" des amerikanischen National Cholesterol Education Programs (NCEP; [15]);
- Empfehlungen der European Atherosclerosis Society (EAS; [9]);
- Strategiepapier der Nationalen Cholesterin-Initiative (NatCI, [16]).

Die Beschränkung auf die 3 genannten Strategien erfolgte unter dem Gesichtspunkt, daß diese Vorschläge – insbesondere das NCEP- und EAS-Konzept – Vorbildcharakter für andere Screeningstrategien zu diesem Thema besitzen, die häufig nur kleine Modifikationen dieser Grundtypen beinhalten. Zudem basieren die beiden erstgenannten Konzepte auf den Resultaten spezieller Konsensuskonferenzen der jeweiligen Fachgesellschaften im amerikanischen und europäischen Raum. Der Vorschlag der Nationalen Cholesterin-Initiative wurde aufgrund seiner Bedeutung in der Bundesrepublik Deutschland hinzugenommen. Die Umsetzung der Empfehlungen der EAS und der NatCI in folgende Ablaufschemata wird durch eine wenig konkrete Endpunktdefinition in den Veröffentlichungen sehr erschwert. In den Empfehlungen der EAS und der NatCI findet sich neben der eigentlichen Screeningstrategie zusätzlich eine Einteilung in 5 Risikogruppen A–E. Der darauf basierende gemeinsame Screeningvorschlag beider Institutionen (EAS und NatCI) wird in Abb. 4 gezeigt.

In den Abb. 1–4 sind die Screeningstrategien als Flußdiagramme graphisch dargestellt. Die darin enthaltenen Grenzwerte für Gesamt- und LDL-Cholesterin variieren sehr. Zur Identifizierung koronargefährdeter Personen wird in allen Screeningvorschlägen zusätzlich Information über weitere kardiovaskuläre Risikofaktoren herangezogen, wobei diese gleichrangig und nur in dichotomisierter Form einfließt. Weitere, in dieser Untersuchung aufgrund des GRIPS-Studiendesigns nicht in die Screeningstrategien einfließende Risikofaktoren (jugendliches Alter, männliches Geschlecht und orale Antikonzeptiva) sind aus Gründen der Übersichtlichkeit weg-

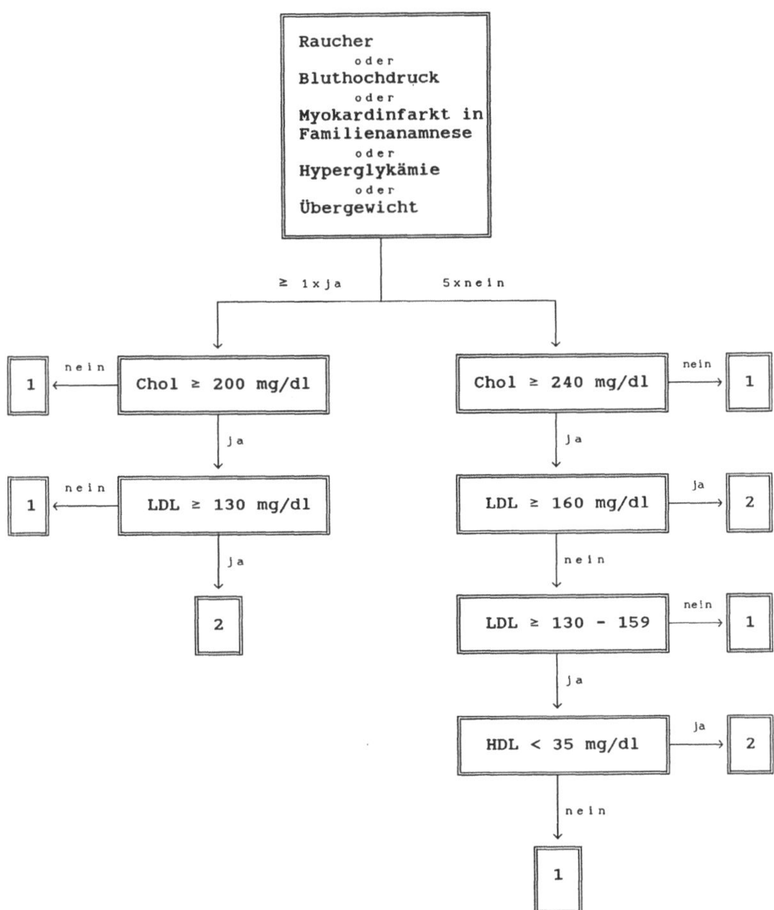

Abb. 1. Screeningstrategie: Expert Panel des NCEP (*1* nicht koronargefährdet, *2* koronargefährdet

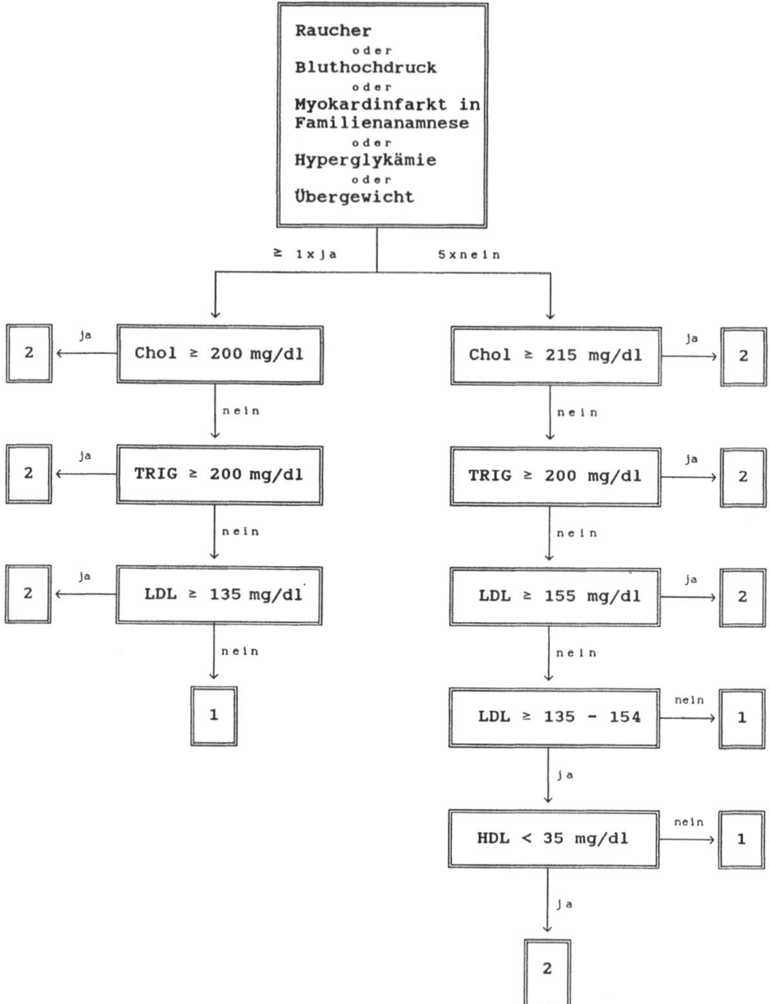

Abb. 2. Screeningstrategie: European Atherosclerosis Society (EAS; *1* nicht koronargefährdet, *2* koronargefährdet)

gelassen worden. Die Darstellung des Vorgehens in den Strategien erfolgt in der an die Praxis angelehnten Reihenfolge: erst allgemeine Untersuchungen, anschließend Lipidanalyse und ggf. Lipoproteinanalyse. (Auf eine detaillierte Erläuterung muß aus Platzgründen verzichtet werden, wir verweisen dazu auf die ausführliche Originalliteratur [9, 15, 16]).

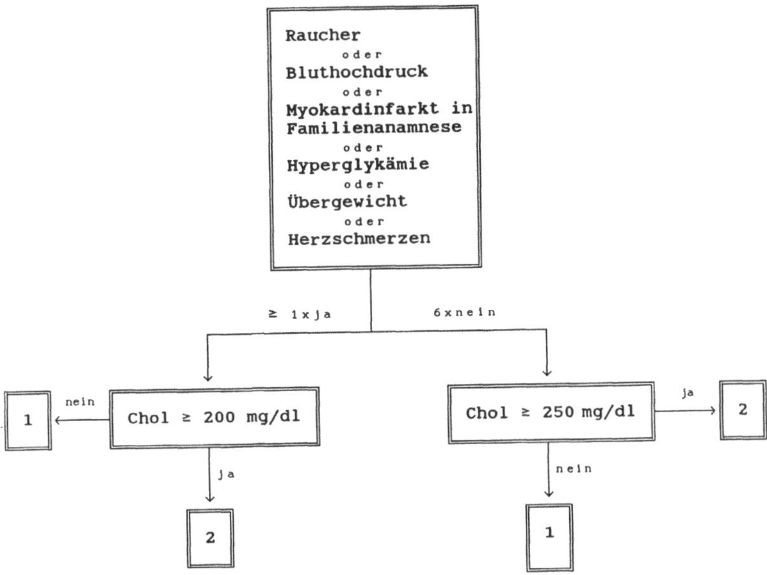

Abb. 3. Screeningstrategie: Nationale Cholesterin-Initiative (NatCI; *1* nicht koronargefährdet, *2* koronargefährdet)

Methodisches Vorgehen

Auf der Grundlage der Daten des 5-Jahres-Follow-up der GRIPS-Studie, einer prospektiven Kohortenstudie an 6029 männlichen Beschäftigten eines Industrieunternehmens der Altersgruppe 40–60 Jahre (ausführliche Darstellung der Studie s. vorheriger Beitrag in diesem Band sowie in [7, 8]), werden für alle Screeningstrategien Sensitivität, Spezifität und prädiktive Werte bei der Vorhersage der späteren Myokardinfarktfälle mit Hilfe der in der Baseline-Untersuchung erhobenen Merkmale berechnet. Dabei werden „Risikofälle" (Ausgang 2 in den Abb. 1–4) von „Nichtrisikofällen" (Ausgang 1) getrennt. Risikofälle sind dabei solche Personen, die als interventionsbedürftig eingestuft werden. Es erfolgt in dieser Arbeit keine Unterscheidung hinsichtlich der Form der Intervention (diätetische und/oder medikamentöse Therapie).

Mit den Ergebnissen kann die Effektivität eines hypothetischen Screenings der GRIPS-Kohorte zu Studienbeginn beurteilt werden. Die GRIPS-Studie beinhaltet keine Intervention bei den Studienteilnehmern, sie ist als reine Beobachtungsstudie angelegt. Dadurch sind keine Verzerrungen bei der Berechnung von Sensitivität, Spezifität und prädiktiven Werten zu erwarten. Mit *Sensitivität* wird dabei der Anteil der im Screening als koronargefährdet eingestuften Personen unter allen späteren Myokardinfarktfällen des Kollektivs bezeichnet, während die *Spezifität* den Anteil der im Screening als nicht koronargefährdet eingestuften Personen unter allen nach 5 Jahren (noch) keinen Myokardinfarkt aufweisenden Personen

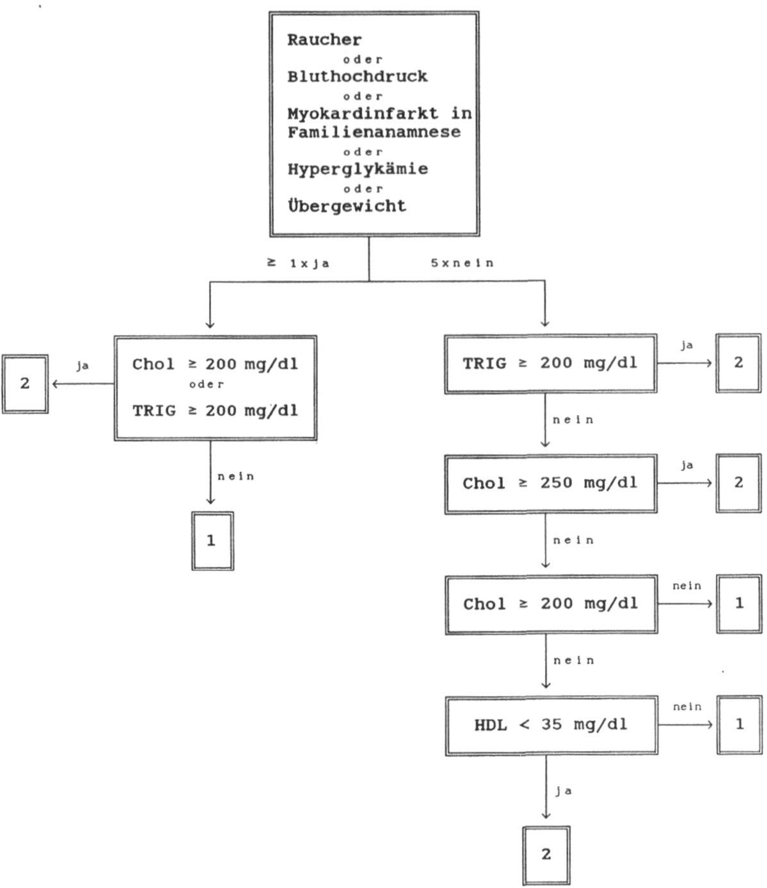

Abb. 4. Screeningstrategie: European Atherosclerotic Society und Nationale Cholesterin-Initiative (EAS & NatCI; *1* nicht koronargefährdet, *2* koronargefährdet)

des Kollektivs angibt. Beide Größen lassen Aussagen über die Güte der Screeninguntersuchung in der Entdeckung bzw. dem Ausschluß des interessierenden Zielkriteriums, hier des Myokardinfarkts, zu. Ihre alleinige Kenntnis reicht jedoch zur Entscheidung über die Einsetzbarkeit der Screeninguntersuchung nicht aus. Die *prädiktiven Werte* bestimmen entscheidend die klinische Brauchbarkeit der Screeningmaßnahme. Dabei ist hier unter dem *positiven prädiktiven Wert* (häufig auch: positive Korrektheit) der Anteil der Myokardinfarktfälle unter allen als koronargefährdet eingestuften Personen des Kollektivs zu verstehen, während der *negative prädiktive Wert* (häufig auch: negative Korrektheit) den Anteil der nach 5 Jahren (noch) gesunden Personen unter allen als nicht koronargefährdet eingestuften Personen des Kollektivs bezeichnet. Beide Werte sind von der Krankheitshäufigkeit in dem untersuchten Kollektiv ebenso abhängig wie von der Güte des Screeningtests. Der gleiche Screeningtest hat in einem Kollektiv mit einer höheren Krankheitshäufigkeit einen größeren positiven prädiktiven Wert als in einem Kollektiv mit niedriger Krankheitshäufigkeit.

Ergebnisse

Die Sensitivitäten, Spezifitäten und prädiktiven Werte der verschiedenen Screeningstrategien für die Prädiktion des Myokardinfarkts innerhalb von 5 Jahren sind in Tabelle 1 zusammengestellt.

Tabelle 1. Kennwerte verschiedener Cholesterinscreeningstrategien auf der Basis der GRIPS-Kohorte (*pW* prädiktiver Wert)

Strategie	Sensitivität [%]	Spezifität [%]	Positiver pW [%]	Negativer pW [%]
NCEP	80,4	55,9	3,7	99,3
EAS	93,5	30,8	2,7	99,6
NatCI	83,2	53,0	3,6	99,3
EAS und NatCI	86,0	48,6	3,4	99,4

Das EAS-Konzept erzielte mit 93,5 % die höchste Sensitivität bei der Prädiktion des Myokardinfarkts, wies jedoch gleichzeitig die mit 30,8 % niedrigste Spezifität auf. Umgekehrt verhielt es sich mit dem Vorschlag des NCEP. Der niedrigsten Sensitivität unter allen Screeningstrategien von 80 % stand die höchste Spezifität von knapp 56 % gegenüber. Die positiven prädiktiven Werte lagen bei allen Screeningmodellen unter 4 %. Sie müssen in Relation zur Myokardinfarktinzidenz im GRIPS-Kollektiv von 1,9 % betrachtet werden. Somit führen die Screeningstrategien zu einer absoluten Verbesserung der Prädiktion des Myokardinfarkts von nur 0,8–1,8 %. Auch die hohen negativen prädiktiven Werte müssen im Zusammenhang mit der Wahrscheinlichkeit von 98,1 %, innerhalb von 5 Jahren keinen Myokardinfarkt zu erleiden, gesehen werden. Ihnen kommt bei der Bewertung der Screeningstrategien ohnehin nur eine untergeordnete Rolle zu.

Diskussion

Die Beurteilung des Cholesterinscreenings als Früherkennungsmaßnahme für den Myokardinfarkt auf Bevölkerungsebene bedarf einer umfangreichen Abwägung unter Einbeziehung vielfältiger Überlegungen (z. B. Kosten-Nutzen-Analysen). In der vorliegenden Arbeit ist einzig die Brauchbarkeit verschiedener Screeningstrategien als valides diagnostisches Verfahren zur Prädiktion des Myokardinfarkts untersucht worden. Die erzielten Ergebnisse sind nicht direkt auf ein bevölkerungsweites Screening in der Bundesrepublik Deutschland übertragbar. Die GRIPS-

Kohorte als Datengrundlage der Berechnungen umfaßt nur Männer der Altersgruppe 40–60 Jahre und stellt damit ein selektiertes Kollektiv dar. Die Auswirkungen einer Ausdehnung auf die Gesamtbevölkerung hinsichtlich der Veränderung des positiven prädiktiven Wertes sind jedoch vorhersehbar: er wird weiter sinken, da die Myokardinfarktinzidenz in der Gesamtbevölkerung niedriger als in der GRIPS-Kohorte ist. Erfahrungen aus dem Bereich des Krebsscreenings lassen vermuten, daß sich auch die testspezifischen Gütekriterien, Sensitivität und Spezifität, beim Übergang von einem selektierten zu einem umfassenderen Kollektiv verändern werden [11]. Somit dürfen die hier berichteten Werte zur Sensitivität, Spezifität und positiven bzw. negativen Korrektheit der verschiedenen Screeningmaßnahmen nicht im Sinne einer Prognose für die bei einem bevölkerungsweiten Screening zu erzielenden Prozentsätze mißverstanden werden. Dennoch liefern die vorgelegten Zahlen wertvolle Information zur kritischen Beurteilung der vorgeschlagenen Screeningkonzepte. Einer durchaus akzeptablen Sensitivität von 80–94 % steht eine deutlich niedrigere Spezifität von nur 31–56 % gegenüber. Durch diese geringe Spezifität wird bei einer bevölkerungsweiten Einführung der Screeningstrategien ein erheblicher Teil der Bundesbürger unberechtigterweise zu Hochrisikofällen erklärt und möglicherweise belastenden, präventiven Therapien zugeführt. Nur für eine Minderheit von unter 4 % der durch das Screening zu Patienten erklärten Personen besteht überhaupt die potentielle Möglichkeit, Nutzen im Sinne der Vermeidung eines Myokardinfarkts innerhalb der nächsten 5 Jahre aus dem Screening zu ziehen. Auf die kontroverse Diskussion, ob dieser Nutzen durch eine medikamentöse oder diätetische Behandlung der Hypercholesterinämie tatsächlich zu erzielen ist, soll in diesem Beitrag nicht eingegangen werden [1, 10, 12, 13, 17].

Eine vergleichende Bewertung der Screeningstrategien ist entscheidend davon abhängig, ob einer Maximierung der Sensitivität oder der Spezifität der Vorrang eingeräumt wird, da die „beste"Strategie hinsichtlich einer maximalen Sensitivität die „schlechteste" im Hinblick auf die Spezifität ist und umgekehrt. Keines der analysierten Screeningmodelle erweist sich bei einer simultanen Betrachtung von Sensitivität und Spezifität im Vergleich als spürbar überlegen. Einzig die Aussage erscheint gerechtfertigt, daß das EAS-Konzept im Streben nach einer hohen Sensitivität des Verfahrens die Spezifität völlig aus den Augen verliert und daher bei einer gleichzeitigen Würdigung beider Gütekriterien den anderen Screeningstrategien unterlegen ist. Dies dokumentiert sich auch in dem mit 2,7 % niedrigsten positiven prädiktiven Wert. Die Ursache dafür liegt in offensichtlich zu niedrig angesetzten Grenzwerten für Gesamtcholesterin (200 mg/dl bzw. 215 mg/dl) und LDL-Cholesterin (135 mg/dl bzw. 155 mg/dl).

Probleme bei der Interpretation dieser Zahlen bereitet die kurze Follow-up-Dauer von 5 Jahren. Eine Verbesserung sowohl der Spezifität als auch der prädiktiven Qualität des Screenings könnte bei einer Verlängerung der Beobachtungsdauer eintreten. Atherosklerotische Gefäßveränderungen stellen einen allmählich progredienten Prozeß dar, der nicht unbedingt innerhalb einer Fünfjahresspanne zu klinisch manifesten Folgeerkrankungen wie Myokardinfarkt führt. Über das Ausmaß einer evtl. durch ein verlängertes Follow-up zu erzielenden Erhöhung von

Spezifität und positivem prädiktivem Wert läßt sich bislang allerdings nur spekulieren. Weitere Aufschlüsse zu diesem Aspekt wird die im Herbst 1991 durchzuführende 3. Follow-up-Untersuchung im Rahmen der GRIPS-Studie liefern. Damit stehen dann die Daten eines 9-Jahres-Follow-up-Zeitraums zur Verfügung, die eine erneute Beurteilung der Screeningstrategien hinsichtlich ihrer langfristigen Prädiktion eines Myokardinfarkts ermöglichen.

Insgesamt betrachtet, führen alle untersuchten Screeningstrategien bei Ausrichtung auf eine akzeptable Sensitivität zu unbefriedigenden Ergebnissen hinsichtlich der Spezifität und des positiven prädiktiven Wertes. Dies zeigt, daß zusätzliche Anstrengungen zur Identifikation weiterer Risikofaktoren notwendig sind. Auf der Grundlagen der heutigen Kenntnisse läßt sich somit kein Vorschlag zum Bevölkerungsscreening auf Myokardinfarkt empfehlen. Die notwendige Verbesserung der Güteeigenschaften dieser Strategien ist möglicherweise bei verlängerter Beobachtungsdauer sowie durch Einbeziehung zusätzlicher Variablen zu erzielen.

Literatur

1. Ahrens EH (1985) The diet-heart question in 1985: Has it really been settled?
2. Anonymus (1990) Mythos Cholesterin. Der Spiegel 44/45 : 256–272
3. Arbeitsgruppe Lipide der Schweizerischen Stiftung für Kardiologie (1989) Lipide und die Prävention der koronaren Herzkrankheit: Diagnostik und Maßnahmen. Schweiz Ärzteztg 7 : 1279–1292
4. Assmann G, Gleichmann U (1989) Stufenmodell zur Erkennung von Hochrisikopatienten für den Myokardinfarkt. Dtsch Ärztebl 86 : 1885–1886
5. Assmann G, Schulte H, Wahrburg U (1988) Konzepte zur Atherosklerose-Prävention. MMW 130 : 260–267
6. Cremer P, Muche R (1990) Göttinger- Risiko-, Inzidenz- und Prävalenz-Studie (GRIPS): Empfehlungen zur Prävention der koronaren Herzkrankheit. Ther Umsch 47 : 482–491
7. Cremer P, Elster M, Labrot B et al. (1988) Incidence rates of fatal and nonfatal myocardial infarction in relation to the lipoprotein profile: first prospective results from the Göttingen Risk-, Incidence-, and Prevalence-Study (GRIPS). Klin Wochenschr 66 : 42–49
8. Cremer P, Nagel D, Labrot B et al. (1991) Göttinger Risiko-, Inzidenz- und Prävalenzstudie (GRIPS). Springer, Berlin Heidelberg New York Tokyo
9. European Atherosclerosis Society Study Group (1988) The recognition and management of hyperlipidemia in adults: a policy statement of the European Atherosclerosis Society. Eur Heart J 9 : 571–600
10. Frick MH, Elo O, Haapa K et al. (1987) Helsinki Heart Study: Primary prevention trial with gemfibrozil in middle-aged men with dyslipidemia: safety of treatment, changes in risk factors and incidence of coronary heart disease. N Engl J Med 317 : 1237–1245
11. Köbberling J, Trampisch HJ, Windeler J (Hrsg) (1989) Memorandum zur Evaluierung diagnostischer Maßnahmen. (Schriftenreihe der Deutschen Gesellschaft für Medizinische Dokumentation, Informatik und Statistik, Heft 10). Schattauer, Stuttgart
12. Kronmal RA (1985) Commentary on the published results of the Lipid Research Clinics Coronary Primary Prevention Trial. JAMA 253 : 2091–2093
13. Lipid Research Clinics Program (1984) The Lipid Research Clinics Program Trial Results: I. Reduction in incidence of coronary heart disease. JAMA 251 : 351–364
14. Morrison AS (1985) Screening in chronic disease. Oxford Univ Press, New York

15. National Cholesterol Education Program Expert Panel (1988) Report of the National Cholesterol Education Program Expert Panel on detection, evaluation and treatment of high blood cholesterol in adults. Arch Int Med 148 : 36–63
16. Nationale Cholesterin-Initiative (1990) Strategie-Papier zur Erkennung und Behandlung von Hyperlipidämien. Dtsch Ärztebl 87 : 1358–1382
17. Schmidt J (1990) Wie sinnvoll ist ein Cholesterin-Screening? Z Allg Med 66 : 789–794
18. Weiss K, Egger S, Hirmann P, Widhalm K, Sinzinger H (1990) Risikofaktoren für Atherosklerose und Risikobewußtsein bei Mitarbeitern einer Wiener Versicherung. Wien Klin Wochenschr 140 : 513–519
19. Whitby LG (1974) Screening for disease. Definitions and criteria. Lancet II : 819–822
20. Wilson JMG, Jungner G (1968) Principles and practive of screening for disease. WHO, Genf (WHO Public Health Papers, No 34)

Schmerztherapie bei unheilbar Kranken

Analgesia in Terminal Care

Tumorschmerztherapie

Gerd-Gunnar Hanekop, Dirk-Bodo Eggebrecht, Ingrid Gutberlet
und Jan Hildebrandt

Epidemiologie des Tumorschmerzes

Weltweit sterben jährlich ca. 5–6 Mio. Menschen an den Folgen eines Tumorleidens. Es existieren zwar ausgiebige Morbiditäts- und Mortalitätsstatistiken bei weitgehender Differenzierung nach Tumorarten, es gibt aber vergleichsweise wenige Daten über Umfang und Intensität von Tumorschmerzen aufgegliedert nach Geschlecht, Alter, Tumorart und Stadium der Erkrankung sowie evtl. durchgeführter Therapien.

Kaye [18] gibt eine Tumorschmerzprävalenz von 71 % an. Diese Häufigkeit liegt im Bereich der Angaben, die andere Autoren berichten [2, 8, 12–15, 21, 28], und die sich zwischen minimal 10 und maximal 96 % (Mittelwert 51 % [8]) für alle Tumorstadien bewegen. Die beträchtliche Streuung dieser Prävalenzangaben beruht sowohl auf der häufig sehr kleinen Zahl als auch auf der Inhomogenität

Tabelle 1. Anteil der Patienten mit Schmerzen, aufgegliedert nach Stadium der Tumorerkrankung

Tumorart und Stadium	Patienten ohne Schmerz [%]	Patienten mit Schmerz [%]	Anzahl der Patienten n
Mammakarzinom			
– metastasiert	36	64	196
– nicht metastasiert	60	40	93
Prostatakarzinom			
– metastasiert	24	76	38
– nicht metastasiert	70	30	10
Kolorektales Karzinom			
– metastasiert	53	47	107
– nicht metastasiert	60	40	20
Zervixkarzinom			
– metastasiert	100	0	6
– nicht metastasiert	65	35	85
Korpuskarzinom			
– metastasiert	60	40	5
– nicht metastasiert	86	14	22
Ovarialkarzinom			
– metastasiert	41	59	29
– nicht metastasiert	61	39	56

Rationale Pharmakotherapie in der Allgemeinpraxis
Rational Pharmacotherapy in General Practice
M. M. Kochen (Hrsg.)

der untersuchten Patientenkollektive in bezug auf die Tumorart oder den Metastasierungsgrad. Für die beiden letztgenannten Faktoren liegen Untersuchungen vor, die einen Zusammenhang mit der Häufigkeit von Tumorschmerzen belegen. Daut u. Cleeland [12] verglichen die Inzidenz von Tumorschmerzen bei 6 ausgewählten Tumorarten unter Einbeziehung des Tumorstadiums. Unterscheidungskriterium war das Vorhandensein von Metastasen. Bei fast allen Tumorarten berichteten Patienten mit fortgeschrittenem Tumorleiden und Metastasen über stärkere Schmerzen als Patienten mit Tumoren ohne Metastasenbildung. Für die Patienten mit Mamma- und Prostatakarzinom waren die Unterschiede signifikant ($p < 0,005$; Tabelle 1).

Bonica [7] schätzte die Häufigkeit von Tumorschmerzen bei unterschiedlichen Tumorarten anhand einer Metaanalyse von diversen Studien zum Krebsschmerz (Tabelle 2). Dieses Verfahren war notwendig, da nirgendwo auf nationaler Ebene verläßliche epidemiologische Daten über die Prävalenz von Schmerzen im Verlauf einer Tumorerkrankung verfügbar waren.

Tabelle 2. Prävalenz von Tumorschmerzen bei fortgeschrittenem Leiden

Tumorart bzw. Lokalisation	Patienten mit Schmerzen Bereich [%]	Mittelwert [%]
Oro-Pharynx	54– 80	66
Ösophagus	80– 93	87
Magen	67– 93	78
Kolorektal	47– 95	70
Pankreas	72–100	81
Leber/Galle	65–100	79
Lunge	57– 88	73
Knochen (primär)	70– 85	80
Knochen (Metastase)	55– 96	83
Mamma	56–100	74
Gebärmutter	40–100	75
Ovar	49–100	72
Prostata	55–100	72
Niere/Harnwege	62–100	69
ZNS	55– 83	70
Weichteile	50– 82	60
Lymphome	20– 69	58
Leukämie	5– 76	54
Sarkome	75– 89	85

Weder für die Bundesrepublik Deutschland noch für die ehemalige DDR liegen aussagekräftige epidemiologische Studien über die Inzidenz und Prävalenz von Tumorschmerzen vor, so daß die oben beschriebenen Anhaltszahlen auch für uns gelten können. Viele deutschsprachige Autoren legen deshalb diese Angaben ihren Untersuchungen zugrunde [19,23].

Die Schmerzen bei Tumorpatienten sind nicht immer durch den Tumor selbst bedingt. Adler [1] zeigte, daß 78 % der Schmerzen durch das Tumorleiden, 19 % durch die Tumortherapie und 3 % durch andere, vom Tumor unabhängige Erkrankungen bedingt waren. Viele Tumorpatienten klagen über mehr als einen Schmerz [8, 13, 26]; den einzelnen Schmerzlokalisationen liegen in der Regel auch unterschiedliche Entstehungsmechanismen zugrunde.

Diverse Vorschläge zur Behandlung von Tumorschmerzen wurden in den zurückliegenden Jahren veröffentlicht. Die größte Bedeutung hat der *Stufenplan der WHO* [31] erlangt, an dem sich viele andere Vorschläge orientieren. Die Therapierichtlinie der WHO wurde so konzipiert, daß sie in jedem Land der Erde durchgeführt werden kann. Ausschlaggebend für die Entwicklung dieses Stufenplans war die Erkenntnis, daß auch in den Industrieländern 50–80 % der Tumorschmerzpatienten keine ausreichende Linderung ihrer Schmerzen erfuhren [7]. Die Ursachen für diesen Umstand sind vielfältig:

1. Die Drogengesetzgebung behindert die Verschreibung von Opioiden.
2. Die Kenntnisse der behandelnden Ärzte in bezug auf die Pharmakokinetik und -dynamik der benutzten Analgetika sind unzureichend.
3. Dem Schmerz per se wird kein großer Stellenwert beigemessen.

Weitere Gründe sind in der folgenden Übersicht genannt:

Ursachen für eine ungenügende oder fehlende Schmerztherapie

Nicht angepaßte Verordnung von Analgetika:

- Gabe nach „Bedarf" anstelle der Gabe nach der „Uhr",
- Verordnung eines der Schmerzursache nicht angepaßten Medikamentes,
- Nichtanwendung des Stufenplanes,
- Unterdosierung eines wirksamen Analgetikums,
- häufiger Wechsel zwischen Medikamenten der gleichen Stufe,
- keine Anwendung von Opioiden der 3. Stufe, speziell Morphium,
- keine prophylaktische Behandlung von Nebenwirkungen,
- keine Anwendung adjuvanter Medikamente,
- Kombination von Opioidagonisten und -antagonisten.

Keine Kenntnis über weitere Behandlungsmöglichkeiten von Schmerzzuständen:

- palliative Strahlentherapie, z. B. bei Knochenmetastasen,
- chirurgische Intervention, z. B. bei drohenden Frakturen,
- psychologische Maßnahmen, z. B. zur Aufarbeitung von Angst, Unsicherheit, Einsamkeit, Depression und Hilflosigkeit,
- Neurolysen, z. B. bei Pankreaskarzinom.

Furcht vor Abhängigkeit und Sucht bei Verschreibung von Betäubungsmitteln

---

Über die Effektivität einer medikamentösen Schmerztherapie liegen diverse Studien vor. Schug et al. [23] konnten bei 90 % ihrer Patienten mittels medikamentöser Therapie eine weitgehende Schmerzbefreiung erreichen. Ein ähnliches Ergebnis erzielten Ventafridda et al. ([28]; 71 % Schmerzfreiheit), ebenso auch Takeda [25], der 87 % seiner Patienten analgetisch erfolgreich behandeln konnte. In allen genannten Untersuchungen wurde das Stufenschema der WHO [31] angewendet.

Psychosoziale Faktoren und Tumorschmerz

Obwohl die Effektivität des Stufenplans der WHO unbestritten ist, gibt es doch Kritik wegen der unzureichenden Berücksichtigung psychosozialer Faktoren [10, 16]. Würden psychologische und psychotherapeutische Methoden häufiger bei Krebspatienten eingesetzt, ließe sich eine weitere Verbesserung der Schmerzsituation erreichen. Diese Annahme wird gestützt durch Untersuchungsergebnisse von Bond [4–6]. Er stellt fest, daß die durch Tumorschmerz bedingten emotionalen Belastungen um ein Vielfaches höher sind als solche, die durch andere chronische Schmerzsyndrome nichtmaligner Genese entstehen.

Dalton u. Feuerstein [1] weisen darauf hin, daß jede Schmerzwahrnehmung auf 3 wesentlichen Dimensionen beruht:

1. sensorisch-diskriminative Komponente,
2. motivational-affektive Komponente,
3. kognitiv-evaluative Komponente.

Diese 3 Anteile beeinflussen die Schmerzantwort und -wahrnehmung. Die erste Komponente ist der pharmakologischen Therapie zugänglich; bei den beiden anderen ist die medikamentöse Behandlung in ihrer Wirksamkeit limitiert, hier sind psychologische Verfahren besser geeignet. Wie weitreichend das Spektrum der Einflußfaktoren auf den Schmerz ist, zeigt Abb. 1.

Um eine umfassende Therapie des als Gesamtschmerz bezeichneten Geschehens bei Krebspatienten zu ermöglichen, ist ein interdisziplinärer Ansatz notwendig.

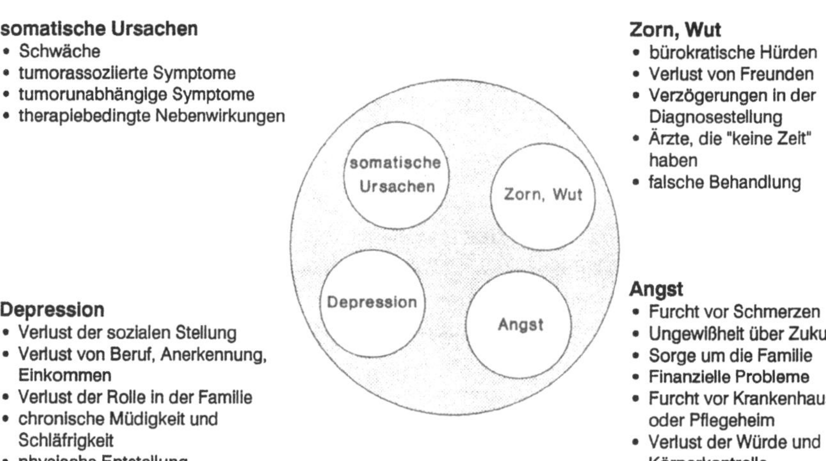

Abb. 1. Einflußfaktoren auf die Schmerzwahrnehmung. (Mod. nach Twycross [27], eigener Entwurf)

Anatomie und Physiologie des Tumorschmerzes

Die bei Krebspatienten auftretenden akuten wie auch chronischen Schmerzen lassen sich grob in 3 Grundformen einteilen:

- somatischer Schmerz,
- viszeraler Schmerz,
- Deafferentierungsschmerz.

Somatischer und viszeraler Schmerz werden durch Nozizeptorerregung ausgelöst. Der Deafferentierungsschmerz resultiert aus einer Störung des peripheren und zentralen Nervensystems. Die einzelnen pathophysiologischen Vorgänge bei der jeweiligen Schmerzart sind komplex und nicht bis in alle Einzelheiten geklärt. Über grundlegende Charakteristika der 3 Schmerzarten informiert Tabelle 3.

Nach Wall [29] wird Schmerz nicht nur durch das Vorhandensein einer peripheren Verletzung wahrgenommen, sondern auch durch die Modulation parallel ablaufender Veränderungen im peripheren (z. B. Änderungen der Muskelspannung über spinale Reflexkreise) und im zentralen Nervensystem (absteigende inhibitorische Bahnen vom Hirnstamm: Locus coeruleus, Raphekerne, Formatio reticularis; [33]). Diese Hemmsysteme eröffnen therapeutische Möglichkeiten bei der Behandlung von Tumorschmerzen.

Schmerzerfassung und Schmerzanalyse

Voraussetzung für eine sinnvolle Anwendung und Kombination schmerztherapeutischer Maßnahmen ist eine gezielte *klinische Schmerzanalyse*. Der Untersuchungsgang bei einem Patienten mit Krebserkrankung sollte folgende Teile enthalten:

Schmerzanamnese:
- allgemeine Anamnese,
- spezielle Tumorschmerzanamnese,
- psychosoziale Anamnese.

Körperliche Untersuchung:
- allgemeine körperliche Untersuchung,
- spezieller neurologischer Status,
- spezieller orthopädischer Status.

Bei der *speziellen Tumorschmerzanamnese* geht es v. a. um die örtliche, qualitative, quantitative und zeitliche Erfassung der Schmerzwahrnehmung. Wichtigste Beurteilungskriterien sind:

Wo tut es weh?

Ist der Schmerz unilokulär, multilokulär oder diffus, ein- oder beidseitig; radikulär, pseudoradikulär oder segmental? Die vom Patienten erhaltenen Aussagen sollten in ein Körperschema eingetragen werden.

Tabelle 3. Schmerzarten und ihre Charakteristika

Art	Charakter	Mechanismus	Beispiel	Therapie
Somatisch	Dauerschmerz, gut lokalisiert, nagend, drückend,	Nozizeptor-aktivierung	Knochen-metastasen	antineoplastische Therapie (z. B. Radiatio), Analgetika (opioide und nichtopioide Analgetika), Nervenblockaden
Viszeral	Dauerschmerz, schlecht lokalisiert, drückend, ziehend oft übertragen in Dermatome	Nozizeptor-aktivierung	Leber-/Lungenmeta-stasen (projizieren in die Schulter via N. phrenicus)	antineoplastische Therapie, Analgetika (opioide und nichtopioide Analgetika), Nervenblockaden
Neuropathisch	einschießende Paroxysmen/ brennender Dauerschmerz	spontane, paroxysmale Entladungen im PNS + ZNS	brachiale und lumbosakrale Plexopathien	Antikonvulsiva, Antidepressiva, TENS Sympathikusblockaden, Analgetika

Wann tut es weh?

Zu welcher Tages- oder Nachtzeit, sind die Schmerzen konstant oder intermittierend, gibt es spezielle Auslöser; gibt es neben einem Dauerschmerz auch gelegentlich Schmerzspitzen? Wurden schon Analgetika eingenommen oder andere Therapieverfahren angewendet? Welchen Effekt haben diese Maßnahmen auf den Schmerz gehabt?

Wie tut es weh?

Hier geht es um den Schmerzcharakter, der jedoch nicht immer einen Rückschluß auf die Schmerzursache gestattet. Gebräuchliche Deskriptoren sind: brennend, drückend, dumpf, einschießend, krampf- oder kolikartig, scharf, stechend, ziehend etc.

Wie stark ist der Schmerz?

Da Schmerz etwas Subjektives und nicht ausreichend kommunizierbar ist, sollte er für jeden Patienten quantitativ erfaßt werden. Für diesen Zweck gibt es diskrete oder stetige Skalen. Beispiel für eine diskrete Skala wäre eine Erfassung über die Kategorien: schwach, mittel oder stark. Eine stetige Quantifizierung ist über numerische oder visuelle Analogskalen möglich. Bei der visuellen Analogskala (VAS) handelt es sich um eine Linie von 100 mm Länge, mit Extrempunkten: links 0 = kein Schmerz und rechts 100 = stärkster vorstellbarer Schmerz. Der Patient gibt auf dieser Skala den Wert an, der seinem aktuellen Schmerzniveau relativ zu den beiden Extrempunkten entspricht [22].

Die Quantifizierung des Schmerzes ist eine wesentliche Voraussetzung für die Bewußtwerdung des Schmerzproblems bei Tumorpatienten und ein wichtiges Hilfsmittel zur Überprüfung des Effektes schmerztherapeutischer Interventionen.

Therapieverfahren bei Tumorschmerzen

Ziel einer adäquaten analgetischen Therapie bei Krebskranken ist es, das Auftreten von Schmerzen zu verhindern (antizipatorische Therapie). Um dieses Ziel zu erreichen, ist es in der Regel notwendig, medizinische und psychologische Verfahren zu kombinieren.

Therapeutische Interventionen:

- Pharmakotherapie (kontinuierlich: per os, rektal, intravenös, subkutan)
- neurostimulatorische Verfahren (transkutane elektrische Nervenstimulation TENS, Akupunktur etc.),
- Nervenblockaden (reversible Unterbrechung der Schmerzleitung mittels Lokalanästhetika),
- Psychologische Verfahren (Gesprächstherapie, AT, Progressive Muskelrelaxation)
- invasive neuroablative Methoden (Chordotomie, perkutane Rhizotomie, perkutane Ganglion-coeliacum-Blockade mit Neurolytika etc.),
- peridurale, intrathekale und intraventrikuläre Medikamentengabe,
- physikalische Therapie.

Hervorzuheben bleibt, daß alle genannten Maßnahmen nicht als Alternativen zu verstehen sind, sondern komplementär eingesetzt werden. Gerade in der Initialphase eines Tumorleidens (in vielen Fällen ist der Schmerz das erste Symptom) sollte eine suffiziente analgetische Versorgung erfolgen, um dem Patienten die Schmerzen während der Diagnostik zu ersparen. Ist nach Abschluß der Untersuchungen eine kurative Therapie möglich, kann die eingeleitete Schmerztherapie nach erfolgter Behandlung und wiedererlangter Schmerzfreiheit beendet werden.

Der Schwerpunkt der symptomatischen Schmerzbehandlung liegt eindeutig bei der systemischen oralen Pharmakotherapie [30]. Mit ihren Methoden ist es möglich, bei 85–90 % der Patienten eine befriedigende Schmerzkontrolle zu erreichen [3].

Bei der medikamentösen Einstellung von Tumorpatienten sind folgende Behandlungsprinzipien zu beachten:

- individuelle Dosisfindung,
- Bevorzugung einer oralen Medikation,
- Gabe nach Plan, d. h. zu festen Zeiten,
- konsequente Behandlung von Nebenwirkungen,
- gezielter Einsatz von Koanalgetika,
- Behandlung der Schlaflosigkeit,
- sorgfältige Überprüfung des Therapieeffekts.

Wurde der Patient schon zuvor mit Schmerzmedikamenten behandelt, so ist unter folgenden Aspekten zu prüfen, ob die Medikation den Schmerzen angemessen war:

- adäquat in bezug auf die Ursache,
- ausreichend dosiert,
- regelmäßig verordnet.

Stufenplan der WHO

Ist eine der Forderungen nicht erfüllt, so gilt es, die Therapie entsprechend umzustellen und den Erfolg nach 1–2 Tagen zu kontrollieren. Wurde bislang keine analgetisch medikamentöse Behandlung durchgeführt, so ist diese z. B. gemäß dem *WHO-Stufenplan* einzuleiten (vgl. Abb. 2 und Tabelle 4):

Starke Opioide
+ nichtopioidhaltige Analgetika
+/- Koanalgetika
Stufe 3
Schwache Opioide
+ nichtopioidhaltige Analgetika
+/- Koanalgetika
Stufe 2
Nichtopioidhaltige Analgetika
+/- Koanalgetika
Stufe 1

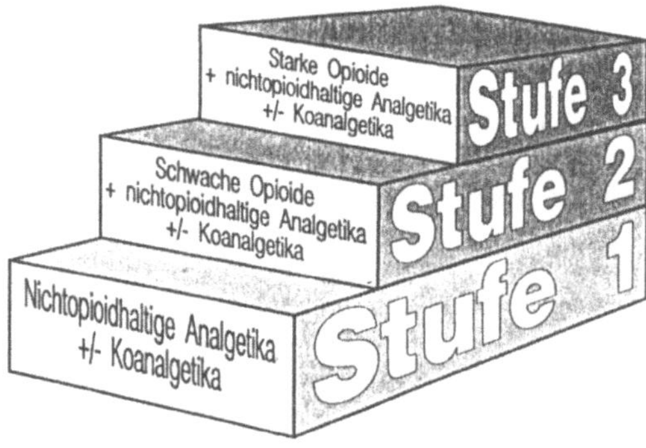

Abb. 2. Stufenplan der WHO. (Mod. nach [31])

Tabelle 4. Therapie nach dem WHO-Stufenplan

Arzneistoffe und Präparate	Dosierung	Nebenwirkungen
Stufe 1		
Acetylsalicylsäure (Aspirin, Generika)	250–1000 mg alle 4 h	gastrointestinale Störungen erhöhte Blutungsneigung
Diclofenac (Voltaren, Generika)	50–100 mg alle 6–8 h	gastrointestinale Störungen
Ibuprofen (Brufen, Generika)	400-800 mg alle 6–8 h	gastrointestinale Störungen
Paracetamol (Ben-u-ron, Generika)	500–1000 mg alle 4 h	Lebertoxizität bei Dosen > 10 g
Metamizol (Novalgin, Generika)	500–1000 mg alle 4 h	Agranulozytose Allergie
Stufe 2		
Codein (z. B. Tricodein)	30–100 mg alle 4 h 60 mg Retardform alle 8–12 h	Obstipation Übelkeit, Erbrechen
Tramadol (Tramal)	50–100 mg alle 2–4 h	Übelkeit, Erbrechen Obstipation
Tilidin + Naloxon (Valoron N)	50–100 mg alle 2–4 h	Übelkeit, Erbrechen Obstipation
Dextropropoxyphen (nur in Retardform verfügbar)	100–150 mg alle 6–8 h	Übelkeit, Erbrechen Verwirrtheit
Stufe 3		
Morphium (MST)	10–30–60–100 mg Retardtabletten alle 8–12 h Lösung (1–4 %) alle 4 h	Obstipation, Übelkeit Erbrechen, Müdigkeit
Methadon (L-Polamidon)	Beginn: 2,5–5 mg alle 6–12 h cave: Kumulation!	Obstipation, Übelkeit, Erbrechen
Buprenorphin (Temgesic)	Beginn: 0,2–0,4 mg alle 6–8 h	Obstipation, Übelkeit, Erbrechen
	ab ca. 4 mg „Ceiling“-Effekt, d. h. keine Steigerung der Analgesie, jedoch Zunahme der Nebenwirkungen bei höherer Dosierung	

In der *1. Stufe* kommen nichtopioide Analgetika ± adjuvante Behandlung zum Einsatz.

In der *2. Stufe* werden, bei nicht ausreichender Wirksamkeit der 1. Stufe zusätzlich schwach wirksame Opioide verordnet. Für die Bundesrepublik Deutschland bedeutet dies, daß Präparate angewendet werden, die nicht unter die BtM-VV fallen.

In der *3. Stufe* werden die schwach wirksamen Opioide durch stark wirksame ersetzt.

Bei der Anwendung von Opioiden der 2. Stufe sollte daran gedacht werden, daß die verfügbaren Präparate häufig nicht länger als 2–4 h wirken. Einzig die retardierten Präparationen zeigen längere Wirkungszeiten.

Die analgetische Potenz aller Substanzen der 2. Stufe im Verhältnis zu Morphium liegt zwischen 1:5 bis 1:10 [20]. Diese als Äquipotenzdosen bezeichneten Relationen gestatten es, einen Patienten, der bisher mit einem Opioid der 2. Stufe ungenügend eingestellt war, relativ problemlos auf ein solches der Stufe 3 umzustellen. Die gewählte Dosis des Opioids der 3. Stufe sollte dabei deutlich (20–50 %) über der Äquipotenzdosis des ersetzten Opioids der 2. Stufe liegen, um eine bessere Wirksamkeit zu gewährleisten.

Bei einem gleichbleibenden Dauerschmerz ist es sinnvoll, die Patienten in der 3. Stufe mit einem Retardpräparat zu versorgen. Kommen zusätzlich neben den konstanten Schmerzen auch Schmerzspitzen vor, zeigt der Tumorschmerz einen wellenförmigen oder unregelmäßigen Verlauf, so ist neben der Verordnung eines retardierten Medikaments auch die Verschreibung von Morphintropfen indiziert. Die Logik für die Kombination von Tropflösungen mit einem Retardopioid liegt in der verzögerten Wirkung der Retardpräparation, die bei plötzlich und unvorhergesehenen Schmerzen nicht rechtzeitig eintreten kann. Das retardierte Morphium hat sein Wirkungsmaximum erst nach ca. 5 h, bei Morphiumtropfen ist jedoch schon 30–40 min nach der Einnahme ein Wirkspiegel vorhanden [17].

Vorsichtig dosiert werden sollten alle starkwirksamen Opioide bei Patienten in reduziertem Allgemeinzustand, mit hohem Lebensalter, eingeschränktem Sensorium, erhöhtem intrakraniellem Druck, eingeschränkter Leber- und Nierenfunktion, obstruktiven Ventilationsstörungen sowie erschwerter Blasenentleerung.

Die Wirksamkeit einer Schmerztherapie bei Tumorpatienten nach dem Stufenschema der WHO überprüfte Ventafridda [2]. Initial wurden alle in die Studie aufgenommenen Patienten (n = 292) mit Medikamenten der Stufe 1 behandelt. Nach 4 Wochen waren 9 % der Patienten gestorben, 17 % wurden noch nach Stufe 1, 49 % nach Stufe 2 und 25 % nach Stufe 3 therapiert. In der 9. Woche waren 20 % der aufgenommenen Patienten gestorben. Medikamente der Stufe 1 erhielten noch 6 %, 18 % nahmen Pharmaka der Stufe 2 und 56 % der Stufe 3. Die Patienten wurden durchschnittlich 19 Tage nach Stufe 1, 28 Tage nach Stufe 2 und 47 Tage nach Stufe 3 behandelt.

Neben den Analgetika kommen in der Schmerztherapie des Tumorpatienten Medikamente zum Einsatz, die nicht zu den eigentlichen Schmerzmitteln zählen, aber in bestimmten Situationen eine Schmerzreduktion bewirken. Diese als Koanalgetika bezeichneten Substanzen wirken entweder selbst analgetisch (z. B. durch Membranstabilisierung bei neuropathischen Schmerzen oder durch eventuelle Aktivierung absteigender noradrenerger bzw. serotoninerger Bahnen) oder lindern Begleitsymptome, die zu einer Schmerzverstärkung beitragen (Tabelle 5).

Tabelle 5. Koanalgetika

Medikamentengruppe	1. Wahl	Alternative
1. Antikonvulsiva (bei Schmerzparoxysmen)	Carbamazepin (z. B. Tegretal, Timonil)	Clonazepam (Rivotril)
2. Antidepressiva (bei Dysästhesien)	Amitryptilin (Saroten, Generika)	Mianserin (Tolvin)
3. Kortikoide (bei Hirndruck, Nervenkompression, Leberkapselschmerz)	Prednisolon (Decortin H, Generika)	Dexamethason (Decadron, Generika)
4. Neuroleptika (bei Übelkeit und Erbrechen)	Haloperidol (Haldol, Generika)	Chlorpromazin (Megaphen) (Neurocil, Generika)

Die als Begleitmedikamente bezeichneten Substanzgruppen und Pharmaka dienen der symptomatischen Behandlung hauptsächlich analgetikabedingter Nebenwirkungen. Da es sich bei der Tumorschmerztherapie in der Regel um eine Dauertherapie handelt, einige der potentiellen Nebenwirkungen, wie z. B. die Obstipation unter Opioidgabe, nahezu immer auftreten, muß auch die Verordnung von Begleitmedikamenten entsprechend der Analgetikaverschreibung erfolgen (Tabelle 6).

Sinnvolle und in der Praxis erprobte Dosierungsschritte bei der oralen Morphintherapie wären für wäßrige Morphinlösungen (mögliche Konzentrationen 0,1–4 %): 10, 15, 20, 30, 40, 60, 90, 120 ... mg/h [32].

Bei der Verordnung eines Retardpräparats nach vorangegangener Opioidtherapie mit einem Medikament der Stufe 2 erfolgt die Umrechnung anhand der Äquipotenzdosis. Bei Neueinstellung auf ein Opioid, Beginn mit 2mal 10 mg MST oder 3mal 10 mg MST/Tag. Bei notwendig werdender Dosiserhöhung haben sich bei uns folgende Steigerungsstufen bewährt:
2mal 10 mg, 3mal 10mg, 2mal 20 mg, 2mal 30 mg, 3mal 30 mg, 2mal 60 mg, 3mal 60 mg, 2mal 100 mg, 3mal 100 mg ... Die Dosis sollte in 24-h-Intervallen solange erhöht werden, bis eine ausreichende Schmerzreduktion erreicht worden ist. Zur Beurteilung des Effekts einer Dosiserhöhung haben sich die Instrumente der quantitativen Schmerzmessung, verbale Ratingskalen bzw. visuelle oder nominelle Analogskalen, als sehr hilfreich erwiesen.

Medikamente, die der Betäubungsmittelgesetzgebung unterliegen

Für die Verordnung von Betäubungsmitteln (BTM) ist die Verwendung des amtlichen dreiteiligen Formblatts vorgeschrieben. Welche Medikamente Betäubungsmittel sind, ist im Betäubungsmittelgesetz (BtMG) festgelegt; ihre Verschreibung wird in der Betäubungsmittel-Verschreibungs-Verordnung (BtMVV) geregelt. Die Rezeptvordrucke können von jedem approbierten Arzt unter folgender Adresse kostenlos angefordert werden:

Bundesopiumstelle, Institut für Arzneimittel, Bundesgesundheitsamt, Gentiner Straße 38, W-1000 Berlin 30, Bundesrepublik Deutschland.

Dazu sind ein formloser Antrag sowie eine beglaubigte Kopie der Approbationsurkunde an die Bundesopiumstelle zu senden.

Tabelle 6. Begleitmedikamente zur Symptomkontrolle (keine Koanalgetika!)

Indikation und Wirksamkeit	Arzneistoffe und Präparate
Laxanzien	
Prophylaktische Gabe bei Tumorpatienten angeraten, die ein Opioid erhalten, um der auftretenden Obstipation entgegenzuwirken:[a]	Lactulose (Bifiteral, Generika) Sennoside (z. B. Agiolax) paraffinhaltige Mittel (z. B. Obstinol) Stimulantien (z. B. Natriumpicosulfat/ z. B. Laxoberal) Förderung der Darmperistaltik (z. B. Bisacodyl/Dulcolax, Generika)
Antiemetika[b]	
Zentral wirksam	Haloperidol (Haldol, Generika)
motilitätssteigernd	Metoclopramid (Paspertin, Generika)
(v. a. bei dyspeptischen Beschwerden)	Domperidon (Motilium, Generika)
serotoninantagonistisch	Ondansetron (Zofran)
Arzneimittel zur Ulkusprophylaxe	
H_2-Rezeptorenblocker	Cimetidin (Tagamet, Generika) Ranitidin, (Sostril, Zantic)
Anticholinergika	Pirenzepin (Gastrozepin, Generika)
Antazida	Sucralfat (Ulcogant, Generika) Aluminium und Magnesiumsalze (z. B. Gelusil, Maaloxan, Solugastril)

[a] Hinweis: Alle Tumorpatienten, die ein Opioid rezeptiert bekommen, sollten auf die Notwendigkeit der regelmäßigen Stuhlentleerung (alle 2–3 Tage) hingewiesen werden. Dazu ist in der Regel die prophylaktische Verordnung eines Relaxans empfehlenswert. Sollte es trotz der Anwendung von Laxanzien zu einer Stuhlverhaltung kommen, ist die Durchführung von Klysmen, Einläufen und ggf. die manuelle Ausräumung indiziert.

[b] Bei Nichtansprechen von Antiemetika auch andere Ursachen für die Übelkeit und Erbrechen mit in die Überlegungen einbeziehen, z. B. Hirnmetastasen, Magenausgangsstenosen, Subileus.

Notwendige Angaben auf dem Betäubungsmittelrezept

Auf dem Betäubungsmittelrezept sind folgende Angaben vorzunehmen:

1. Name, Vorname und Anschrift des Patienten:
   Vom Arzt oder Personal handschriftlich oder maschinell auszufüllen.
2. Ausstellungsdsatum:
   Vom Arzt handschriftlich einzutragen.
3. Bezeichnung, Darreichungsform, Gewichtsmenge des enthaltenen Betäubungsmittels je Packungseinheit, bei abgeteilten Zubereitungen Angabe der abgeteilten Form; die Stückzahl, die Gewichtsmenge in Gramm oder Milligramm, die Stückzahl in arabischen Ziffern und in Worten wiederholen:
   Vom Arzt handschriftlich einzutragen.
4. Gebrauchsanweisung, mit Einzel- und Tagesgabe:
   Vom Arzt handschriftlich einzutragen.
5. Name des Arztes, seine Berufsbezeichnung, vollständige Anschrift und Telefonnummer:
   Vom Arzt oder Personal handschriftlich oder maschinell oder per Stempel anzugeben.
6. Bei Überschreiten der Tageshöchstmenge von 200 mg sind zusätzlich erforderlich der Vermerk „Menge ärztlich begründet“ und die Angabe, für wie viele Tage diese Menge verschrieben wird:
   Vom Arzt handschriftlich einzutragen.
7. Ungekürzte Unterschrift:
   Vom Arzt handschriftlich zu vollziehen.
8. Evtl. Zusatz „in Vertretung“:
   Vom Arzt eigenhändig zu vermerken.

Vom Ausstellungsdsatum des Betäubungsmittelrezeptes bis zur Vorlage bei der Apotheke dürfen nicht mehr als 7 Tage vergangen sein!

Tageshöchstmengen

Tageshöchstmengen		
Buprenorphin:	10 mg	Überschreiten bis zum 2-fachen der einfachen
Levomethadon:	60 mg	Tageshöchstmenge für den Bedarf von bis zu 7 Tagen,
Morphium	200 mg	mit Vermerk: *„Menge ärztlich begründet“* und
		„Bedarf für x Tage“ (x = maximal 7 Tage).

Bei *Morphin-retard-Tabletten* zur oralen Applikation, Überschreitung je Anwendungstag bis zum 5fachen der einfachen Tageshöchstmenge = 1000 mg/Tag.

Bei *Morphinlösungen* bis zu einem Morphingehalt von 4 % unter Zusatz von mindestens 1 %igem Carboxymethylzellulose-Natrium je Anwendungstag bis zum 10fachen der einfachen Höchstmenge = 2000 mg/Tag.

Alternativen zur oralen medikamentösen Behandlung

Diese Applikationsformen sollten zum Einsatz kommen, falls die orale Medikation nicht oder aufgrund von Nebenwirkungen nicht mehr möglich ist.

Eine Möglichkeit stellt die subkutane Bolusgabe von Morphin dar, die auch vom Patienten oder von einem Angehörigen vorgenommen werden kann. Die s.c.-Gabe muß alle 4 h erfolgen, um einen durchgehenden Wirkspiegel zu erhalten. Die parenterale Opiatgabe wird – soweit erforderlich – mit der oralen oder rektalen Gabe eines nichtopioiden Analgetikums kombiniert (Ausnahme ASS: wegen seiner keratolytischen Wirkung nicht rektal applizieren!).

Eine weitere Applikationsform stellt die kontinuierliche subkutane Gabe von Morphin mit Hilfe einer tragbaren Pumpe und über eine Butterflykanüle dar. Diese Methode hat den Vorteil, daß sie gleichmäßigere Morphinspiegel liefert, geringere Nebenwirkungen aufweist und wegen der geringeren Punktionsfrequenz eine höhere Akzeptanz hat als die Bolusgabe [9].

Bei der Umstellung einer oralen auf die parenterale Opiatgabe gilt die folgende Äquivalenzrelation:
10 mg Morphin oral = 3 mg Morphin subkutan.

Ist mit diesen, auch für den niedergelassenen Kollegen durchführbaren Therapieformen keine zufriedenstellende Analgesie zu erreichen, sollte der Patient in einer Fachabteilung oder bei einem niedergelassenen Schmerztherapeuten vorgestellt werden.

Literatur

1. Adler RH, Hürny C (1988) Differential diagnosis of pain in cancer patients. Springer, Berlin Heidelberg New York Tokyo (Recent results in cancer research, vol 108, pp 1–8)
2. Ahles TA, Ruckdeschel JC, Blanchard EB (1984) Cancer related pain. I. Prevalence in an outpatient setting as a function of stage of disease and type of cancer. J Psychosom Res 28:115–119
3. Baines MJ (1984) Cancer pain. Postgrad Med J 60:852–857
4. Bond MR (1976) Pain and personality in cancer patients. In: Bonica JJ, Albe-Fessard D (eds) Advances in pain research and therapy, vol 1. Raven, New York, pp 311–316
5. Bond MR (1979) Psychologic and psychiatric techniques for the relief of pain of advanced cancer. In: Bonica JJ, Ventafridda V (eds) Advances in pain research and therapy, vol 2. Raven, New York, pp 215–222
6. Bond MR (1985) Cancer pain: psychological substrates and therapy. In: Fields HL, Dubner R, Cervero F (eds) Advances in pain research and therapy, vol 9. Raven, New York, pp 559–567
7. Bonica JJ (1985) Treatment of cancer pain: current status and future needs. In: Fields HL et al. (eds) Advances in pain research and therapy, vol 9. Raven, New York, pp 589–615
8. Bonica JJ (1990) Cancer pain. In: Bonica JJ (ed) The management of pain. Lea & Febiger, Philadelphia, pp 400–460
9. Bruera E, Brenneis C, MacDonald RN (1987) Continuous s.c. infusion of narcotics for the treatment of cancer pain: an update. Cancer Treat Rep 71:953–958
10. Cleeland CS (1989) Pain control-public and physicians' attitudes. In: Hill CS, Field WS (eds) Advances in pain research and therapy, vol 11. Raven, New York, pp 81–89

11. Dalton JA, Feuerstein M (1988) Biobehavioral factors in cancer pain. Pain 33 : 137–147
12. Daut RL, Cleeland CS (1982) The prevalence and severity of pain in cancer. Cancer 50 : 1913–1918
13. Foley KM (1979) Pain syndroms in patients with cancer. In: Bonica JJ, Ventafridda V (eds) Advances in pain research and therapy, vol 2. Raven, New York, pp 59–75
14. Foley KM (1985) The treatment of cancer pain. N Engl J Med 313 : 84–95
15. Greenwald HP, Bonica JJ, Bergner M (1987) The prevalence of pain in four cancers. Cancer 60 : 2563–2569
16. Hildebrandt J, Pfingsten M (1990) Nachsorge als supportive Maßnahme bei palliativ operierten Patienten – Schmerztherapie. Langenbecks Arch Chir [Suppl] 2 : 255–260
17. Jage J (1991) Medikamente gegen Krebsschmerzen. Edition Medizin, Weinheim
18. Kaye P (1989) Notes on symptom control in hospice and palliative care. Hospice Education Institute, Essex CT, pp 1–3
19. Kolkmann F-W (1990) Leitfaden zur Schmerztherapie bei Tumorpatienten. Eine gemeinsame Empfehlung der Tumorzentren, der Kassenärztlichen Vereinigungen und der Landesärztekammer Baden-Württemberg
20. Lehmann KA (1990) On-demand Analgesie. In: Lehmann KA (Hrsg) Der postoperative Schmerz. Springer, Berlin Heidelberg New York Tokyo, S 237–265
21. Pannuti F, Martoni A, Rossi AP (1979) The role of endocrine therapy for the relief of pain due to advanced cancer. In: Bonica JJ (ed) Advances in pain research and therapy, vol 2. Raven, New York, pp 145–165
22. Porges P (1988) Der Karzinomschmerz. Schmerz 2 : 59–65
23. Schug SA, Zech D, Dorr U (1990) Cancer pain management according to WHO analgesic guidelines. J Pain Symptom Manage 5 : 27–32
24. Shepard DA (1977) Principles and practice of palliative care. Can Med Assoc J 116 : 522–526
25. Takeda F (1986) Results of field-testing in Japan of the WHO draft interim guideline on the relief of cancer pain. Pain Clin 1 : 83–89
26. Twycross RG, Fairfield S (1982) Pain in far advanced cancer. Pain 14 : 303–310
27. Twycross RG, Lack SA (1989) Totaler Schmerz. In: Twycross RG, Lack SA (Hrsg) Therapie bei Krebs im Endstadium. Fischer, Stuttgart New York, S 207
28. Ventafridda V, Tamburini M, Caraceni A, DeConno F, Nabli F (1987) A validation study of the WHO method for cancer pain relief. Cancer 59 : 850–856
29. Wall PD (1988) Neurological mechanisms in cancer pain. Cancer Surv 7 : 127–140
30. Walsh TD, Saunders CM (1981) Oral morphine for relief of chronic pain from cancer. N Engl J Med 305 : 1417–1418
31. WHO (1986) Cancer pain relief. WHO, Geneva
32. Zech D, Schug SA (1989) Medikamentöse Therapie. In: Hankmeier U, Bowdler J, Zech D (Hrsg) Tumorschmerztherapie. Springer, Berlin Heidelberg New York Tokyo, S 25–61
33. Zimmermann M (1990) Physiologie von Nociception und Schmerz. In: Basler HD, Franz C, Kröner-Herwig B, Rehfisch HP, Seemann H (Hrsg) Psychologische Schmerztherapie. Springer, Berlin Heidelberg New York Tokyo, S 46–88

Psychosoziale Probleme bei fortgeschrittenen Tumorerkrankungen aus der Sicht von Patienten, Angehörigen und Therapeuten

Dirk-Bodo Eggebrecht, Ingrid Gutberlet, Gerd-Gunnar Hanekop und Jan Hildebrandt

Einleitung

Die Problembereiche, die sich in der Betreuung von Tumorpatienten ergeben können, sind perspektivisch sehr divergent. Dabei erfordert die Situation des Patienten und die seiner Angehörigen von allen in die Behandlung involvierten Personen/Disziplinen über die rein körperliche Behandlung hinaus ein großes Maß an Einfühlung, und zwar ganz unabhängig vom Lebenszeitpunkt, an dem die Krebserkrankung auftritt bzw. diagnostiziert wird. Trotz einer weitgehenden verbalen Enttabuisierung des Wortes Krebs in den letzten Jahren hat es für die Betroffenen kaum etwas von seiner lähmenden Wirkung verloren. Krebs ist immer noch ein Thema, das viele Menschen schockiert und von ihnen in sehr direkter Weise mit Sterben und einem Leben unter Schmerzen und Qualen in Verbindung gebracht wird.

Aus der Sicht der Patienten

Die Konfrontation mit der Diagnose Krebs macht meist sprachlos, läßt die so Betroffenen häufig „wie vom Blitz getroffen" erstarren. Viele Menschen fühlen sich in dieser Situation entsetzlich einsam, hilflos und alleingelassen. Andere haben beinahe grenzenlose Angst und Panik. Allen gemeinsam ist sicherlich, daß sie schnelle Hilfe möchten und zunächst gar nicht die Bedeutung dessen realisieren, was ihnen da gerade mitgeteilt wurde. Sie möchten das alles nicht wahrhaben. Und doch wissen die meisten, daß eine Operation oder eine andere Behandlung in Form von Chemo- oder Strahlentherapie auf sie zukommen wird. So setzen die Patienten meist alle Energien in die Unterstützung der medizinischen Behandlung und hoffen auf den Behandlungserfolg, hoffen auf den Fortschritt der Technik und der Forschung sowie auf das Können der Ärzte. Patienten möchten ihre Hoffnung unterstützt sehen, möchten Zuversicht vermittelt bekommen. Aus ihrer Sicht bleibt jedoch oft viel zuwenig Raum für die zwischenmenschliche Begegnung, den direkten Kontakt auf der emotionalen Ebene. Viele Patienten erleben eine solche Behandlungsrealität als unzureichend.

Patienten erwarten gerade in der Phase der Diagnosemitteilung ausreichend Zeit, so daß ein Nachfragen hinsichtlich wichtiger Details möglich ist und für sie wichtige Informationen nicht „zwischen Tür und Angel" verlorengehen. Darüber hinaus

Rationale Pharmakotherapie in der Allgemeinpraxis
Rational Pharmacotherapy in General Practice
M. M. Kochen (Hrsg.)

wünschen sie sich während des gesamten Krankheitsverlaufs Offenheit und ausreichende Informationen über die jeweiligen Behandlungsmaßnahmen. Während der Behandlung und auch später erhoffen sie sich, bezogen auf ihre Lebensqualität, so wenig Einschränkungen wie möglich.

Bei einer Verschlechterung der Erkrankung stellt sich wiederholt die Frage: Wieviel Zeit habe ich noch?/Wieviel Zeit bleibt uns (Familie, Partner/in, Angehörige) noch? Hinzu kommt die Angst vor nicht oder nur noch unzureichend behandelbaren Schmerzen, so daß schon allein aufgrund dieser Anspannungen und Unsicherheiten ein Belastungszustand entsteht, der viele Patienten in ihren Aktivitäten lähmt und verzweifeln läßt. Für den Patienten ist es jetzt sehr erleichternd, wenn er diese Ängste ansprechen kann, wenn er eine Person seines Vertrauens hat, mit der er sich regelmäßig austauscht, um nicht alles allein bewältigen zu müssen. Der Wunsch nach Nähe, Wärme und emotionaler Unterstützung bleibt in unserer derzeitigen Medizinlandschaft weitgehend unberücksichtigt [1]. Hinsichtlich einer vorhandenen Schmerzangst kann man Patienten entlasten indem man sie über die heutzutage möglichen und sehr umfangreichen Schmerztherapiemaßnahmen informiert. Für die Patienten ist mit dem Verlust der Gesundheit die persönliche Zukunft in Frage gestellt, und mit jeder Verschlechterung der Krebskrankheit nimmt diese Unsicherheit zu, zeigt oftmals auch soziale Auswirkungen. Das Wissen um die akute Krise, die Bedrohung des eigenen Lebens konfrontiert die so betroffenen Menschen mit einer unlösbaren Aufgabe, mit ihren eigenen Todesängsten, mit ihrem eigenen Sterben [5].

Patienten, denen die Therapie eine Möglichkeit des Weiterlebens eröffnet hat, erleben besonders den Übergang vom „Kranksein" hin zum „Gesundsein" als sehr beschwerlich. Auch in dieser Zeit können zusätzliche über die reine Organmedizin hinausgehende Therapieangebote (Entspannung; begleitende, nichtaufdeckende Gesprächsangebote) sehr entlastend für die Patienten sein und helfen, die aktuelle Lebenssituation positiv zu verändern [6].

Aus der Sicht der Angehörigen

Traditionell ausgerichtete Gesundheitsversorgung hat sich bisher fast ausschließlich auf den Patienten konzentriert und die Belange der Angehörigen, der Familie mehr oder weniger außer Acht gelassen. Die Bedeutung der Einbindung des Patienten in sein soziales Umfeld wurde dabei oft vernachlässigt [4].

Durch eine Krebserkrankung wird jedoch nicht nur der Patient in einen Zustand der Unordnung und Unruhe gebracht, auch Angehörige sind hiervon erheblich mitbetroffen, werden sie doch oftmals zu einer Art Langzeitbetreuer der Erkrankten. Im direkten Kontakt mit den Betroffenen werden sie immer wieder mit den (Noch)Fähigkeiten des Patienten konfrontiert.

Patienten und Angehörige berichten immer wieder, daß sie sich durch eine gegenseitige Verantwortungszuschreibung im Sinne eines „Ich muß helfen!" oder „Ich darf mir nicht so viel anmerken lassen!" belastet fühlen. Ihr gemeinsamer Alltag, der häufig schon allein aufgrund der Bedrohung durch die Erkrankung negativ verändert ist, erfährt durch eine vorhandene Schmerzproblematik eine zusätzliche Belastung. In diesem Zusammenhang wünschen sie sich oftmals eine entlastende Ansprache von außen, da sie selbst sich scheuen, von sich aus die eigene Bedürftigkeit oder gar Schwäche vor Außenstehenden zuzugeben. Angehörige neigen in Zeiten der Bedrohung ihres Familiensystems zu „Alles-oder-nichts"-Reaktionen. Es ist von daher wichtig, sie von Beginn an mit in die Behandlung zu integrieren und auch für sie als Ansprechpartner dazusein bzw. solche zu vermitteln.

Aus der Sicht der Therapeuten

In seiner Tätigkeit sollte der Arzt intensiven Einblick in die gegenwärtige Situation des Patienten erhalten. Dafür benötigt er neben ausreichender Zeit auch die Motivation, sich immer wieder neu auf die Betreuung Tumorkranker einzulassen [3]. Darüber hinaus muß er sich zu Beginn einer jeden Behandlung von Krebskranken immer wieder die Frage seiner eigenen emotionalen Belastbarkeit stellen. Genau wie der Krebspatient muß sich der Arzt auf einen erst einmal nicht abzuschätzenden Zeitraum der Begleitung des Patienten einstellen. Dabei sollte der Arzt sich darüber klar werden, daß der Patient seine größte Stärke in der Therapie der beklagten körperlichen Beschwerden sieht. Dadurch besteht die Gefahr, den emotionalen Beziehungsaspekt zu vernachlässigen.

Ausgehend von einer ständig zunehmenden Zahl von Krebspatienten erscheinen kombinierte ambulant-stationäre Versorgungseinrichtungen mit einem integrativen Behandlungs- und Betreuungsansatz (bio-psycho-sozial) immer notwendiger. Die bisher bestehenden Behandlungskonzepte für akut Kranke sind nicht länger auf chronisch Kranke übertragbar.

In der Behandlung von Krebspatienten erleben viele Ärzte, daß sich ihr Handlungsbereich langfristig in Diagnostik und Therapie erschöpft. Damit unterbleibt oftmals die persönliche Auseinandersetzung mit der Diagnose Krebs. Vor dem Hintergrund einer tragfähigen Arzt-Patienten-Beziehung, die den Patienten dabei unterstützen kann, seine Lebenswürde in jeder Phase der Erkrankung aufrechtzuerhalten bzw. wiederzuerlangen, ist es jedoch notwendig, die eigenen Gefühle wahrzunehmen und zu reflektieren [2].

Ausblick

Betrachtet man den Alltag der Patienten und auch der behandelnden Ärzte, zeigt sich im ambulanten Bereich ein großes Defizit an psychosozialer Versorgung für Tumorpatienten. Viele Patienten wollen und benötigen zusätzliche Behandlungsangebote. Viele Ärzte wollen dies unterstützen, können für ihre Patienten jedoch kaum auf solche Angebote zurückgreifen. Darüber hinaus gilt für alle Beteiligten die starke Verunsicherung gerade in der terminalen Phase der Krebserkrankung. Die Patienten selbst haben Angst, in der letzten Lebensphase alleingelassen und isoliert zu werden sowie unter starken Schmerzen und Qualen sterben zu müssen.

Angehörige haben Angst, nicht genug zu tun bzw. nicht genug tun zu können. Sie erleben sich in dieser Zeit hilflos und leiden unter ihrer als eher passiv erlebten Rolle. Behandelnde Ärzte zeigen in der letzten Lebensphase oft noch einmal viele Aktivitäten, häufig auch aus dem Gefühl heraus, den Ansprüchen und Wünschen des Patienten auf Heilung nicht gerecht geworden zu sein. Unternimmt man den Versuch, die vorhandenen Problembereiche von der Metaebene her zu betrachten, ist festzuhalten, daß die gezeigte Offenheit untereinander unzureichend ist. Demzufolge läßt sich oft nur erahnen, welche Wünsche, Ängste und Erwartungen das Gegenüber (Patient, Angehöriger, Therapeut) hat. Wie will man jedoch die Behandlung von Patienten adäquat gestalten, wenn alle Beteiligten zuwenig voneinander wissen?

Literatur

1. Howe J (1982) Psychotherapie bei unheilbaren Kranken? In: Howe J (Hrsg) Therapieformen im Dialog. Kösel, München, S 145–154
2. Hürny C (1987) Das Gespräch in der Langzeitbetreuung des Krebskranken. Therapiewoche 37 : 2463–2470
3. Köhle K (1983) Ein Konzept zur Bearbeitung von psychologischen Problemen auf Schwerstkrankenstationen In: Bönisch E, Meyer JE (Hrsg) Psychosomatik in der klinischen Medizin: psychiatrisch-psychotherapeutische Erfahrungen bei schweren somatischen Krankheiten. Springer, Berlin Heidelberg New York Tokyo, S 118–139
4. Köhle K, Simons C, Kubanek B, Zenz J (1985) Zum Umgang mit unheilbar Kranken. In: Uexküll T von (Hrsg) Psychosomatische Medizin. Urban & Schwarzenberg, München, S 1203–1251
5. Leming MR, Dickenson GE (1990) Understanding, dying, death and bereavement. Holt, Rinehart & Winston, Fort Worth
6. Spiegel D, Bloom JR, Kraemer HC, Gottheil E (1989) Effects of psychological treatment on survival of patients with metastasic breast cancer. Lancet II : 888–891

Respiratorische/grippale Infekte: Verschreiben oder nur beraten?

Upper Respiratory Infections: Prescription or Just Advise?

Therapie bei „banalen“ Erkrankungen

Adalbert Keseberg

In den Herbst-, Winter- und Frühjahrsmonaten häufen sich alljährlich die Infekte der oberen Luftwege. Hierbei handelt es sich durchweg um Virusinfekte. Bakterielle Infekte treten dabei in den Hintergrund und sind meist sekundärer Natur.

Seit der letzten Gesundheitsreform werden diese Erkrankungen auch als banal apostrophiert; die Therapie der damit verbundenen Befindensstörungen wurde deshalb auch vom Gesetzgeber aus der Erstattungspflicht der sozialen Krankenversicherung herausgenommen. Man hat uns Ärzten damit den „schwarzen Peter“ in die Hand gedrückt mit dem Argument, daß wir selber entscheiden könnten, wann eine Erkrankung dieser Art nicht mehr als banal anzusehen ist.

Die sogenannte banale Erkrankung

Kein geringerer als Johann Wolfgang v. Goethe hat das Adjektiv banal in die dichterische Umgangssprache eingeführt. Als banal wird etwas Alltägliches apostrophiert. So bezeichnen wir oft eine Krankheit als banal, die der Patient jedoch keineswegs als banal empfindet, schon deshalb nicht, weil sein Allgemeinbefinden erheblich gestört wird. Dennoch zeichnen sich diese Erkrankungen durch eine hohe Selbstheilungstendenz aus. Die Frage nach sofortiger symptomatischer Therapie oder Nichtstun bzw. Beratung ist daher durchaus berechtigt. Klinisch imponieren diese Infektionen durch Katarrhe der oberen Luftwege, verbunden mit Husten, Schnupfen, Kopf- und Gliederschmerzen (Tabelle 1). In Epidemiezeiten leiden fast 60 % aller Kranken in unseren Praxen an banalen fieberhaften oder auch nicht fieberhaften Infekten der oberen Luftwege.

Tabelle 1. Symptome des banalen Virusinfektes der Atemwege. (Nach Helwig [3])

	Rhinovirus	Adenovirus	RS-Virus	Influenzavirus	Parainfluenzavirus	ECHO-Virus
Rhinitis	+	+	+	+	+	+
Laryngitis	+	+	–	+	–	+
Grippe	–	+	–	+	–	–
Krupp	–	–	–	+	+	+
Bronchitis	+	–	+	+	+	–
Bronchiolitis	–	–	+	+	+	–

Rationale Pharmakotherapie in der Allgemeinpraxis
Rational Pharmacotherapy in General Practice
M. M. Kochen (Hrsg.)

Virale Pneumotropie

Die Erreger dieser Virusinfektionen werden in primär pneumotrope und primär nichtpneumotrope Viren und Mykoplasmen eingeteilt (s. Übersicht).

Pneumotrope Viren:

Myxoviren
Influenzaviren
A, A1, A2, B, C, D
Parainfluenzaviren
Rhinoviren (30 Stämme)
Adenoviren
Coxsackieviren (30 Typen)
Reoviren (Respiratory Enteric Orphan)
Echoviren (Cytopathogenetic Human Orphan)

Primär nichtpneumotrope Viren:

Masernviren
Rubeolenviren
Varicella-zoster-Viren
mononukleose Viren
Poliomyelitisviren

Influenza, Parainfluenza, Rhinoviren, Adenoviren, Coxsackieviren und Echoviren zählen zu den pneumotropen Viren. Erkrankungen dieser Erreger manifestieren sich an den Atmungsorganen und bleiben gewöhnlich auf diese beschränkt. In seltenen Fällen kommt es zur Virämie, andere Organe wie Herzmuskel, die Meningen sowie Pleura und Herzbeutel können befallen werden. Hier sind v. a. die Coxsackieviren zu nennen.

Zu den primär nichtpneumotropen Viren gehören Masern, Rubeolen, Varizellen und Poliomyelitisviren. Erkrankungen durch diese Viren hervorgerufen, treten natürlich bei den banalen respiratorischen Infekten in den Hintergrund, man muß aber wissen, daß sie auch dort Symptome erzeugen können.

Der dritte sehr bedeutungsvolle Erreger akuter Atemwegsinfektionen ist Mykoplasma pneumoniae.

Es spielt nur eine geringe Rolle, welches Virus im einzelnen die für die Patienten so lästigen Symptome hervorruft.

Eine kausale Therapie von Virusinfektionen ist nicht oder nur in ganz beschränktem Umfang möglich.

Bleibt also die symptomatische Behandlung der Befindensstörungen. Was ist hierbei sinnvoll, was sollte besser unterbleiben?

Antipyrese ja oder nein

Der größte Teil der Patienten sucht wegen des begleitenden Fiebers einen Arzt auf. Soll man dieses Symptom unbedingt bekämpfen?

Gegen eine generelle Fiebersenkung sprechen folgende Argumente:

- Fieber ist eine Reaktion des Körpers auf verschiedene Ursachen, hier als hypothalamische Reaktion auf endogene Pyrogene. Zweck der Reaktion ist, die Krankheitserreger zu beseitigen.
- Fieber ist ein Symptom, das den Patienten zur notwendigen Inaktivität zwingt (dies ist besonders bei Kindern wichtig).

- Fieber regt die eigene Interferonproduktion an, die dem Körper hilft, mit dem Infekt fertigzuwerden.
- Eine abrupte Fiebersenkung stellt eine erhebliche Kreislaufbelastung dar.

Für eine großzügige Fieberbekämpfung sprechen nur zwei, allerdings wichtige Argumente:

1. Fiebersenkung führt zu einer Verbesserung des Allgemeinbefindens.
2. Beim Säugling und Kleinkind lassen sich durch eine großzügige Antipyrese Fieberkrämpfe verhindern.

Von der Pharmaindustrie werden eine Menge Fertigarzneimittel zur Therapie banaler Infekte angeboten, mit Mehrfachkombinationen der verschiedensten Substanzen.

Wirkstoffe sog. Grippemittel sind häufig:

1. Antipyretika bzw. Analgetika,
2. Antihistaminika,
3. kreislaufaktive Substanzen,
4. allgemeinreduzierende bzw. hustenstillende Substanzen.

Nach der OTC-Studie von 1983 [6] wurden im Rahmen der Selbstmedikation fast ausschließlich Kombinationspräparate mit den in Tabelle 2 genannten Wirkstoffen abgegeben.

Tabelle 2. In den Kombinationspräparaten enthaltene Arzneistoffe

Arzneistoff	Wirksamkeit
Acetylsalicylsäure	+
Chinin	–
Ethenzamid	+
Natriumsalicylat	+
Paracetamol	+
Phenazon	+
Propyphenazon	+
Salicylamid	<+>

Die häufigsten Substanzen sind Antihistaminika, Coffein, Antitussiva, Vitamin C und pflanzliche Ingredienzien.

Mit diesen Kombinationen soll offensichtlich eine ganze Reihe verschiedenster Symptome, gleichsam als „Mehrzweckwaffe“, behandelt werden. Da aber in der Regel nicht alle Symptome einer banalen Erkältung bzw. Grippe gleichzeitig auftreten und auch nicht alle Symptome gleich schnell abklingen, ist der therapeutische Wert dieser fixen Arzneimittelkombinationen zur Behandlung banaler Infekte von vornherein mehr als fraglich, zumal diese banalen Erkrankungen auch eine hohe Selbstheilungstendenz aufweisen.

Zur antipyretischen Therapie sind deshalb nur Monopräparate sinnvoll.

Bewertung von Kombinationen:

Sinnvoll sind: ASS/Paracetamol + Codein (30–50 mg).
Nicht sinnvoll sind: 1. Analgetika untereinander,
2. Analgetika + zentral wirksame Substanzen,
3. Analgetika + Vitamine.

Relativ ungefährlich bei zu beachtenden bekannten Nebenwirkungen und Kontraindikationen sind Paracetamol oder die Acetylsalicylsäure. Vergessen darf man auch nicht, daß mit physikalischen Maßnahmen wie Wadenwickel ebenfalls eine gute Antipyrese erreicht werden kann.

Schnupfensymptome lassen sich am besten mit lokal applizierten Sympathikomimetika, z. B. Xylometazolin, therapieren. Ihre Anwendung sollte möglichst nur abends zur Gewährleistung der Nachtruhe erfolgen. Der Gebrauch sollte auch zeitlich auf 4–5 Tage begrenzt bleiben wegen der Gefahr der Rhinitis medicamentosa.

Bei trockenem Reizhusten ist die kurzfristige Gabe von Codeinmonopräparaten durchaus sinnvoll. Zur Förderung der Expektoration ist reichlich Flüssigkeitszufuhr erforderlich.

Die Therapie mit Kombinationspräparaten, die gleichzeitig Hustenstopper wie Codein und Expektoranzien bzw. Mukolytika enthalten, ist nicht sinnvoll.

Zur Linderung unangenehmer Schluckbeschwerden kann die Gabe von lokalanästhetikahaltigen Lutschtabletten versucht werden. Antibiotikahaltige Lutschtabletten sind wegen der Gefahr der Allergisierung und der Bildung von resistenten Keimen gefährlich.

Eine bakterielle Superinfektion tritt meist unter dem Erscheinungsbild einer purulenten Tracheobronchitis oder sinusitis auf. Das Antibiotikum derWahl ist das Tetrazyklin bzw. Doxyzyklin. Zum einen werden hierbei die bronchopathogenen Keime erfaßt, zum anderen auch möglicherweise zugrundeliegende Mykoplasmen. Bei Kindern und in der Schwangerschaft empfiehlt sich die Behandlung mit Amoxycillin oder – bei nachgewiesener Penicillinallergie – Eryhtromycin (Tabelle 3).

Tabelle 3. Abgestufte Therapie der banalen Infekte. (Nach Ferlinz [1])

Infekt	Therapie
Therapie des banalen Tracheobronchialinfekts:	
Leichte Formen	keine Therapie
Höheres Fieber, Schmerzen	Antipyrese
Starker initialer Reizhusten	Antitussiva
PurulenterAuswurf mit Fieber	Tetrazykline, Amoxycillin, Co-Trimoxazol
Therapie bei Kenntnis der Erreger:	
Mycoplasma pneumoniae Ornithose Rickettsia Burneti	1. Wahl: Tetrazyklin Erythromycin Alternative: Amoxycillin

Literatur

1. Ferlinz R (1979) Die banalen Virusinfektionen des Atemtraktes beim Erwachsenen. III. Interdisziplinäres Forum der Bundesärztekammer. Deutscher Ärzte-Verlag, Köln, S 93–98
2. Füllgraff M, Palm D (Hrsg) (1989) Pharmakotherapie – Klinische Pharmakologie, 7. Aufl., Fischer, Stuttgart
3. Helwig H (1979) Der banale Virusinfekt der Atemwege bei Indern. Fortschritt und Fortbildung in der Medizin. III. Interdisziplinäres Forum der Bundesärztekammer. Deutscher Ärzte-Verlag, Köln, S 99–107
4. Keseberg A (1981) Welchen therapeutischen Wert haben sogenannte Grippemittel? Z Allg Med 57: 1854–1858
5. Keseberg A (1990) Fehldiagnosen durch falsche Beurteilung des Therapieeffektes. In: Schrömbgens HH (Hrsg) Die Fehldiagnose in der Praxis. Hippokrates, Stuttgart, S 125–134
6. OTC-Studie (1983) Selbstmedikation in der Bevölkerung der Bundesrepublik Deutschland

Die Behandlung chronisch-obstruktiver Lungenerkrankungen in der Allgemeinpraxis

Chris van Weel, Constant van Schayck, Edward Dompeling, Hans Folgering, Cees van Herwaarden und Pierre van Grunsven

Einleitung

Die chronische Bronchitis gehört ebenso wie das Asthma bronchiale zu den häufigsten chronischen Erkrankungen in der Bevölkerung [4, 8, 13]. Die meisten der betroffenen Patienten werden – jedenfalls in den Niederlanden und Großbritannien – in der Allgemeinpraxis behandelt.

Asthma und chronische Bronchitis verlaufen in schubweisen Episoden, wobei Phasen mit starken Beschwerden von Perioden gefolgt sind, in denen die Patienten entweder beschwerdefrei sind (Asthma) bzw. der Grad der Behinderung wesentlich geringer ist (chronische Bronchitis) [1, 17].

Ziel der Behandlung ist es, das Auftreten von Symptomen zu verhindern, um damit die Leistungsfähigkeit der Patienten zu verbessern. Damit soll auch langfristig die Entwicklung der Erkrankung beeinflußt werden. Es ist bekannt, daß im Laufe des Lebens die pulmonale Kapazität geringer wird, eine physiologische Entwicklung die – *zumindest hypothetisch* – durch die genannten Erkrankungen verstärkt werden könnte [6]. Vor diesem Hintergrund ist es erstaunlich, daß empirische Daten des Langzeitverlaufs von Asthma und chronischer Bronchitis weitgehend fehlen [11].

In der Praxis werden Asthma und chronische Bronchitis mit sehr unterschiedlichen Strategien behandelt. Dabei kommen symptomorientierte Therapieregimes (Intervention lediglich bei entsprechenden Beschwerden, auch „On-demand"-Therapie genannt) als auch präventionsorientiertes Vorgehen (kontinuierliche Intervention zur Verhinderung manifester Beschwerden bzw. zur Vermeidung einer pulmonalen Kapazitätsreduktion) zum Zuge. Für den praktizierenden Arzt stehen viele Arzneimittel zur Verfügung, wobei die Bronchodilatantien vom Typ β-Sympatomimetika, z. B. Salbutamol und Ipratropiumbromid, am häufigsten verordnet werden.

Ziel dieser Studie war die Dokumentation

- des Langzeitverlaufs von Asthma und chronischer Bronchitis;
- der Wirksamkeit einer Monotherapie mit inhalierten Bronchodilatanzien wobei ein Vergleich zwischen Salbutamol und Ipratropiumbromid erfolgte;
- der Wirksamkeit zusätzlicher Kortikosteroidinhalationen bei Patienten mit einer sich verschlechternden pulmonalen Kapazität.

Rationale Pharmakotherapie in der Allgemeinpraxis
Rational Pharmacotherapy in General Practice
M. M. Kochen (Hrsg.)

Methoden

Die Studie verlief in 2 Phasen, von denen jede 2 Jahre dauerte.

Die 1. Phase stellte eine randomisierte, einfachblinde (Therapeut) Studie dar, bei der *Dauerbehandlung* vs. *symptomorientierte Behandlung* mit Bronchodilatantien verglichen wurde. Innerhalb der Behandlungsstrategien war nach einem Jahr ein „cross-over" zwischen Salbutamol und Ipratropiumbromid vorgesehen.

Die 2. Phase beschränkte sich auf Patienten mit einem beschleunigten Rückgang der pulmonalen Kapazität in den ersten 2 Jahren der Untersuchung. Hier wurde die Therapie mit Bronchodilatantien durch eine Dauerbehandlung mit inhalierbaren Kortikosteroiden ergänzt. Der Verlauf der 2. Phase wurde mit dem der 1. Phase verglichen, wobei jeder Patient als eigene Kontrolle diente.

Patienten

Patienten mit einem Mindestalter von 30 Jahren wurden für die Studie durch 29 Allgemeinärzte rekrutiert. Von diesen Kranken wurden diejenigen in der 1. Phase der Studie aufgenommen, die

- nur eine geringe Atemwegsobstruktion zeigten ($FEV_1 \leq$ Vorhersagewerte [12] minus 2 Standarddeviationen, aber $FEV_1 \geq 50\,\%$ Vorhersagewert) und/oder eine

Tabelle 1. Patientencharakteristika zu Beginn der Studie. Für dichcotome Variablen wurde ein χ^2-Test durchgeführt, für die übrigen Variablen ein t-Test (student's, ungepaart)

Variable	Asthma	Chronische Bronchitis	Gesamt
Zahl (n)	60	100	160
Alter (Jahre)	49 (12)	52 (13)	51 (13)
Sex (m./f.)	28/31	61/40	89/71
Raucher (±)	25/34*	63/38	88/72
Pack Jahre	13 (15)*	18 (17)	16 (16)
Allergie (±)	23/35**	17/82	40/117
FEV_1^a	73(21)	79 (18)	77 (19)
FEV_1/IVC^b	59 (17)*	65 (12)	63 (14)
$BDR\text{-}FEV_1^c$	16 (12)***	7 (7)	10 (10)
PC_{20} [mg/ml][d]	2,4 (1,7)***	13,6 (1,9)	7,6 (2,5)

*$p < 0,05$.
**$p < 0,01$.
***$p < 0,001$.
[a] FEV_1; Liter, % Vorhersagewert.
[b] FEV_1/VIC: Liter.
[c] BDR = Bronchodilationsreaktion („bronchodilatory reaction") der FEV_1, als % der Vorhersagewert.
[d] PC_{20} – Histamine.

bronchiale Hyperreaktivität aufwiesen (PC_{20}– Histamine ≤ mg/ml; [2]);
- nicht von (oralen) Kortikosteroiden abhängig waren,
- an keiner anderen (lebensbedrohlichen) Erkrankung litten.

Patienten wurden auf der Basis einer Standardanamnese [9] den Diagnosen Asthma bzw. chronische Bronchitis zugeteilt [1].

Insgesamt nahmen 160 Patienten teil, 100 mit chronischer Bronchitis und 60 mit Asthma (Tabelle 1).

Messungen

Patienten registrierten wöchentlich ihre Symptome [3] sowie potentielle Nebenwirkungen der Therapie (mit Hilfe eines Tagebuchs) und zur selben Zeit auch den Peak Expiratory Flow (PEF). Zusätzlich wurden alle 6 Monate FEV_1 und PC_{20} gemessen, wobei vor dieser Messung alle Medikamente für mindestens 8 h abgesetzt worden waren. Am Anfang sowie nach 12 und 24 Monaten wurden alle Messungen *doppelt* ausgeführt. Die Messungen erfolgten mit Microspiro-pHI-298 (Chest inc., Japan) und Assess Peakflow Meter (Healthscan Corporation, USA) [15].

Verstärkter Rückgang der pulmonalen Kapazität

Der verstärkte Rückgang der pulmonalen Kapazität wurde definiert als eine Reduktion der FEV_1 von mehr als 80 ml/Jahr während mindestens 2 Jahren. Der Berechnung lagen 7 vorhandene Messungen zugrunde.

Therapeutische Ordnung

Alle Medikamte bis auf die Studienmedikation wurden zu Beginn der Studie abgesetzt (Tabelle 2).

Tabelle 2. Die medikamentöse Behandlung während der Studie

Phase	Therapie	Dosierung
1	*Entweder:*	
	Dauerbehandlung	Salbutamol 4mal 400 μg trockenes Pulver pro Tag *oder*: Ipratropiumbromid 4mal 40 μg/Tag
	oder	trockenes Pulver pro Tag
	Symptomorientierte Therapie:	Salbutamol 0–4mal 400 μg trockenes Pulver pro Tag *oder*: Ipratropiumbromid 0–4mal 40 μg trockenes Pulver pro Tag
2		(a) Beclomethason 200 μg/Tag (b) Salbutamol oder Ipratropiumbromid, wie im zweiten Jahr der ersten Phase

Für den Fall einer Krankheitsexazerbation konnte der betreuende Allgemeinarzt 10 Tage Prednison und (falls erforderlich) ein Antibiotikum verordnen.

Analyse

Die Entwicklung von FEV_1 und PC_{20} wurde zu den initialen Patientencharakteristika und zur medikamentösen Intervention ins Verhältnis gesetzt. Da die Randomisierung nicht vollständig gelang (Tabelle 1), sind die Ergebnisse jeweils für Alter, Geschlecht, Rauchgewohnheiten, Lungenfunktion (zu Beginn der Studie) und die entsprechende Diagnose korrigiert.

Ergebnisse

Von den 223 Patienten beendeten 63 die Studie vorzeitig: 23 aus nichtmedizinischen Gründen, 40 wegen Zunahme ihrer Beschwerden. Davon waren 27 Patienten in Dauerbehandlung; 16 Patienten vollendeten zwar die Studie, verweigerten jedoch eine Änderung der Medikation nach einem Jahr.

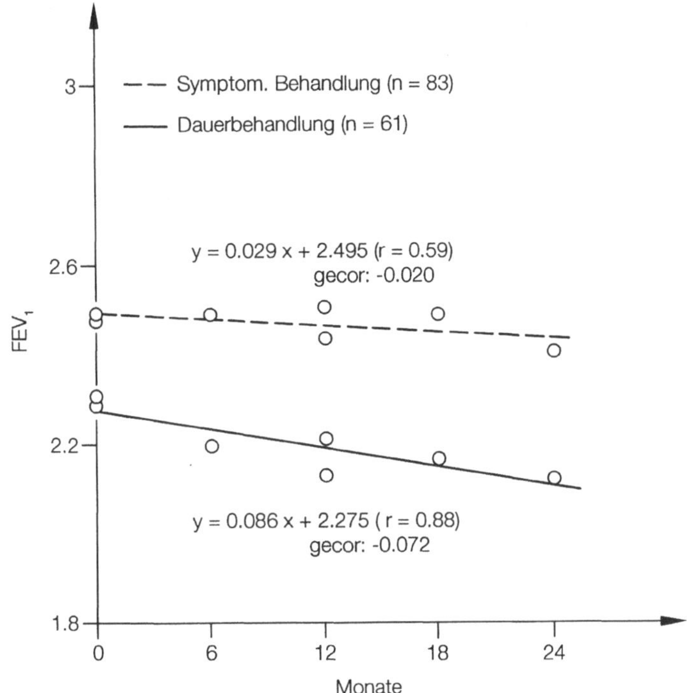

Abb. 1. Entwicklung der pulmonalen Kapazität während der 1. Phase der Studie – für Dauerbehandlung und symptomorientierte Therapie getrennt (n = 144). *gecor*: Nach Korrektur von beeinflussenden Faktoren

Abbildung 1 zeigt das Nachlassen der FEV_1: die Reduktion ist signifikant ($p < 0,05$) größer bei den dauerbehandelten Patienten ($-72,10^{-3}$L/Jahr) als bei den symptomatisch behandelten Patienten (0–20,10 $^{-3}$L/Jahr). Die Wahl des Arzneimittels (Salbutamol oder Ipratropiumbromid) zeigte keinen Effekt. Auch bezüglich des Rückgangs der FEV_1 waren keine Unterschiede zwischen Patienten mit Asthma und Patienten mit chronischer Bronchitis erkennbar.

Die bronchiale Hyperreaktivität (PC_{20}) zeigte während der Studie konstante Ausmaße, ohne wesentliche Unterschiede bei Patienten mit Asthma (Abb. 2a) oder Patienten mit chronischer Bronchitis (Abb. 2b). Überraschenderweise konnte kein Einfluß von Zigarettenrauchen auf den Verlauf der FEV_1 oder die PC_{20} festgestellt werden.

Weder die gewählte Therapieform noch die Wahl der Medikation zeigte einen Zusammenhang mit den auftretenden Beschwerden. Etwa ein Viertel der Patienten berichtete über unerwünschte Wirkungen (24 % bei Salbutamol, 25 % bei Ipratropiumbromid). Die Patienten gaben Salbutamol den Vorzug vor Ipratropiumbromid, jedoch nur dann, wenn eine symptomorientierte Behandlung erfolgte.

Bei 54 Patienten wurde eine verstärkte Reduktion der pulmonalen Kapazität festgestellt. Es war jedoch nicht möglich, den Verlauf auf der Grundlage der initialen Patientencharakteristika wie Alter, Erkrankungsdauer, Diagnose, FEV_1, PC_{20}, vorauszusagen. Abbildung 3 zeigt den Verlauf der PEF vor und nach einem Jahr Kortikosteroidinhalation. Sowohl PEF und FEV_1 (Daten nicht dargestellt) verbesserten sich auf das Niveau des Studienanfangs. Die PC_{20} war weiterhin beständig.

Diskussion

Asthma und chronische Bronchitis stellen chronische Erkrankungen dar, die einen eindeutigen Einfluß auf die Lebensqualität der betroffenen Patienten haben [7, 16].

Ein wichtiger und interessanter Aspekt dieser Erkrankungen stellt der *Langzeitverlauf* mit wechselnden Episoden von *akuten Symptomen* dar. Hier zeigt sich ein wesentlicher Unterschied im Vergleich z. B. zur arteriellen Hypertonie oder zum Altersdiabetes (Typ II). Hier richtet sich das medizinische Interesse vorwiegend nach dem Langzeitverlauf und der Vorbeugung chronischer Komplikationen.

Die Behandlung von Asthma und chronischer Bronchitis wird im wesentlichen durch das akute Beschwerdebild bestimmt. Namentlich in der Allgemeinmedizin – wo die Mehrheit aller Patienten mit diesen Erkrankungen versorgt wird – läßt sich die Verordnung von symptomatisch wirksamen Arzneimitteln [5] bzw. die Anwendung einer symptomorientierten Strategie [14] nachweisen. Die Daten unserer Untersuchung bestätigen, daß die Patienten die Wirkung der symptomatischen Therapie sowohl im Sinne der unerwünschten Wirkungen als auch als subjektive Stimulation erfahren. Dies ist wohl auch der Grund dafür, daß Salbutamol dem Ipratropiumbromid vorgezogen wird. Dennoch gibt es keinen eindeutigen Hinweis, daß Salbutamol den Krankheitsverlauf stärker beeinflußt als Ipratropiumbromid.

Über den Langzeitverlauf von Asthma und chronischer Bronchitis sind nur wenige Untersuchungen publiziert. Allerdings ist gerade für Patienten mit ei-

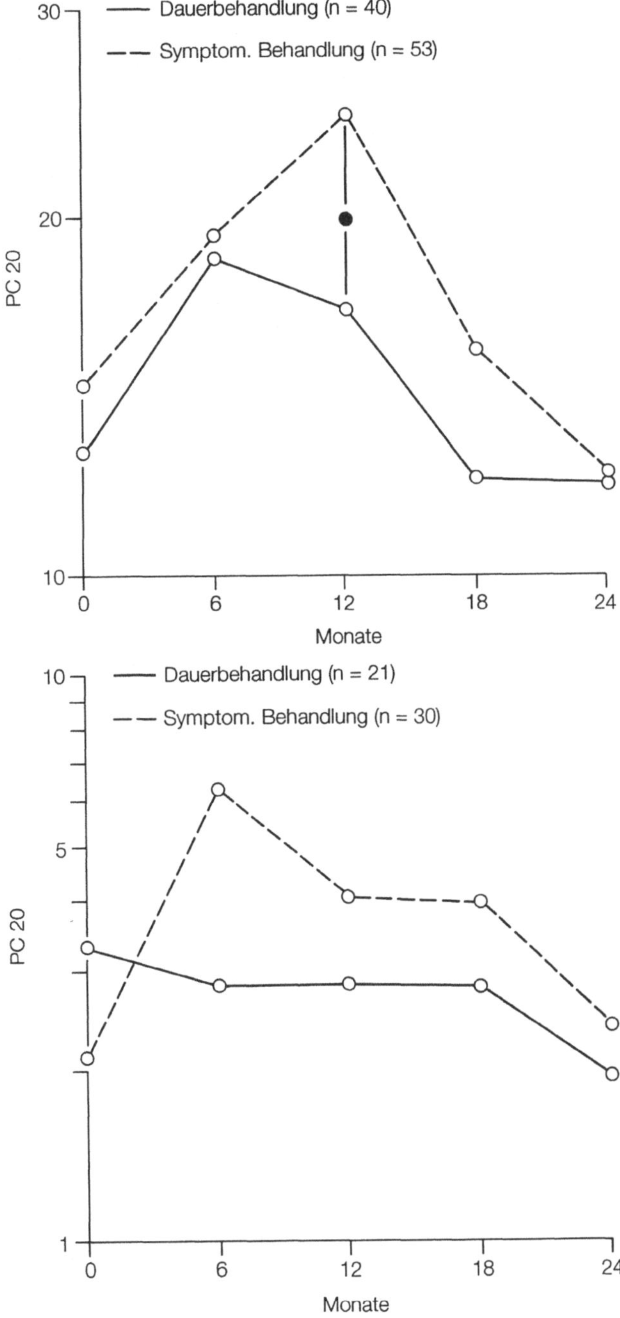

Abb. 2. Entwicklung der bronchialen Hyperaktivität: **a** bei Patienten mit Asthma während der 1. Phase der Studie (getrennt nach Dauerbehandlung und symptomorientierter Therapie; n = 51); **b** bei Patienten mit chronischer Bronchitis während der 1. Phase der Studie (getrennt nach Dauerbehandlung und symptomorientierter Therapie; n = 93)

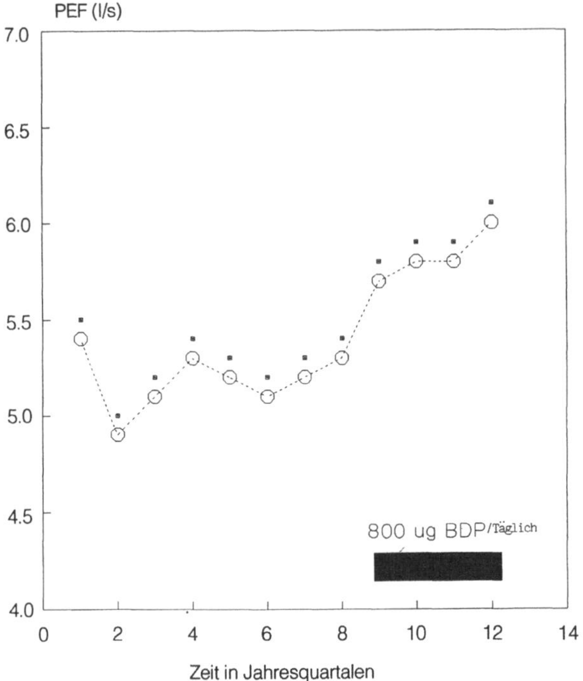

Abb. 3. Entwicklung des PEF („peak expiratory flow") während der 1. und 2. Phase der Studie (n = 54)

ner schweren Atemwegsobstruktion eine ungünstige Prognose dokumentiert. Diese Prognose scheint durch die Behandlung mit oralen Kortikosteroiden [10] verbessert zu werden. Unsere Studie weist darauf hin, daß bei Patienten mit Bronchialobstruktion im Verlauf der Untersuchung eine Verschlechterung eintritt: ca. 30 % der Patienten wiesen eine Reduktion der Lungenkapazität von mehr als 80 ml in 2 Jahren auf. Diese Entwicklung war allerdings aufgrund der klinischen Daten kaum vorhersagbar. Lediglich systematische und periodische Beobachtungen ermöglichen es, die Verschlechterung der Lungenfunktion rechtzeitig zu erkennen. Diese Beobachtungen sollten allerdings unabhängig vom symptomatischen Beschwerdebild des Patienten erfolgen, da die Symptome nur einen geringen Zusammenhang mit FEV_1 oder PC_{20} aufweisen.

Die Langzeitprognose wird aller Wahrscheinlichkeit nach durch eine antiinflammatorische Therapie (Kortikosteroide) begünstigt. Eine lediglich auf die Bronchialobstruktion gerichtete Behandlung hatte keinen Einfluß auf den Langzeitverlauf bzw. – bei kontinuierlicher Anwendung – eine eher ungünstige Wirkung. Nach diesen Daten sollte die bronchialerweiternde Medikation lediglich unterstützenden Charakter aufweisen, die Anwendung auf symptomatische Episoden beschränkt bleiben.

Literatur

1. American Thoracic Society (1987) Standards for diagnosis and care of patients with chronic obstructive pulmonary disease (COPD) and asthma. Am Rev Respir Dis 136 : 225–243
2. Cockcroft DW, Killian DN, Mellon JJA, Hargreave FE (1977) Bronchial reactivity to inhaled histamine; a method an a clinical survey. Clin Allergy 7 : 237–243
3. Dompeling E, Schayck CP van, Folgering H, Hoogen HJM van den, Weel C van (in press) Accuracy and precision of the protable flow-volume meter microspiro HI-298. Eur Respir J
4. Hoogen HJM van den, Huygen FJA, Schellekens JWG, Straat JM, Velden HGM van der (1985) Morbidity figures from general practive. Abteilung Allgemeinmedizin, Nijmegen
5. International Office of Medical Statistics (1986) Medische Index, The Netherlands, The Hague
6. Johnson RN, McNeill RS, Smith DH, Zegge JS, Fletcher F (1976) Chronic bronchitis measurements and observations over 10 years. Thorax 31 : 25–29
7. Kaptein AA, Dekker FW, Gill K, Waart MAC van der (1986) Undertreatment of asthma in Dutch general practice. Fam Pract 3 : 229–234
8. Lamberts H (1984) Morbidity in general practice. Huisartsenpers, Utrecht
9. Lende R van der, Orie NGM (1972) The MRC-ECSC questionnaire on respiratory symptoms (use in epidemiology). Scand J Respir Dis 53 : 218–226
10. Postma DS, Steenhuis EJ, Weele LTh van der, Sluiter HJ (1985) Severe chronic airflow obstruction; can corticosteroids slow down progression? Eur J Respir Dis 67 : 56–64
11. Postma DS, Vries K de, Koæter GH, Sluiter HJ (1986) Independent influence of reversibility of airflow obstruction and non-specific hyperreactivity on the long-term course of lung function in chronic airflow obstruction. Am Rev Respir Dis 134 : 276–280
12. Quanjer PH (1983) Standardised lung function testing. Bull Eur Physiopathol Respir [Suppl 5] 19 : 7–10
13. Royal College of General Practice, Office of population censuses and surveys, Department of Health and Social Security (1981–1982) Morbidity statistics from general practice 1981–82, 3rd National Study, series MB5 no 1. Her Majesty's Stationary Office, London
14. Schayck CP van, Weel C van, Folgering H, Verbeek ALM, Herwaarden CLA van (1989) Treatment of patients with airflow obstruction by general practitioners and chest physicians. Scand J Prim Health Care 7 : 137–142
15. Schayck CP van, Dompeling E, Weel C van, Folgering H, Hoogen HJM van den (1990) Accuracy and reproducibility of the assess peak flow meter. Eur Respir J 3 : 338–341
16. Schrier AC, Dekker FW, Kaptein AA, Dijkman JH (1990) Quality of life in elderly patients with chronic nonspecific lung disease seen in family practice. Chest 98 : 894–899
17. WONCA (1983) The International Classification of Health Problems in Primary Care (ICHPPC)-2-defined, 3rd edn. Oxford Univ Press, Oxford

Arzneimittel mit zweifelhafter Wirkung:
Venentherapeutika, Lebermittel, Geriatrika

Therapeutics of Doubtful Efficacy:
Drugs for Varicose Veins, Liver Disease, "Old Age"

Daten zur Verordnungshäufigkeit von Lebermitteln, Venenmitteln und Nootropika

Gerd Glaeske

Nachdem bereits die allgemeinen pharmakologischen und therapeutischen Grundlagen zu den 3 genannten Arzneimittelgruppen angesprochen wurden, möchte ich dieses Eingangsreferat um einige Daten aus der Praxis ergänzen. Sie sind den Arzneimitteldaten der AOK Kreis Mettmann entnommen, bei der für ein Arzneimittelberatungsprojekt eine arztbezogene Erfassung aller Verordnungen vorgenommen wird (AOK Mettmann: Ländlicher Bereich, ca. 180 000 Versicherte, 480 Ärzte). Aufgelistet sind jeweils die in einem 6-Monats-Zeitraum meistverordneten 10 Arzneimittel in jeder der angesprochenen Indikationsgruppen.

Lebermittel

(Tabelle 1)

Am meisten angewendet werden Lactulose-haltige Arzneimittel (Bifiteral, Lactulose Neda). Allerdings muß hier angemerkt werden, daß diese Arzneimittel möglicherweise auch als Laxantien verordnet werden. Abführmittel sind nämlich der Negativliste unterstellt und somit in der Kassenärztlichen Arzneimittelversorgung nicht verordnungsfähig – die Verordnung der laxierenden Lactulose-Präparate könnte als Ausweg genutzt werden. Lactulose gilt nicht als „Leberschutztherapeutikum", sondern wird als therapeutisch wirksames Prinzip bei Leberkoma und der chronischen Enzephalopathie zur Senkung der enteralen Ammoniakresorption eingesetzt.

An zweiter Stelle folgen die Silibinin-haltigen Arzneimittel (Legalon, Dura Silymarin), deren therapeutischer Nutzen bei der chronsichen Behandlung nach wie vor als nicht unumstritten gilt. Die in der Zwischenzeit angegebene Indikation: „Toxische Leberschäden; Adjuvans bei chronisch-entzündlichen Lebererkrankungen und Leberzirrhose" reflektiert diese therapeutische Unsicherheit. Die Anwendung Silibinin-haltiger Mittel ohne Absetzten der leberschädigenden Noxen, zumeist Alkohol, ist m. E. abzulehnen. Offensichtlich werden solche Arzneimittel aber nach wie vor mit der Assoziation „Leberschutzmittel" eingesetzt, die helfen sollen, Leberschäden auch bei chronischer Alkoholexposition zu vermeiden. Diese therapeutischen Hoffnungen gehen sicherlich weit an Möglichkeiten Silibinin-haltiger Arzneimittel vorbei, obwohl dies immer wieder durch Untersuchungen belegt werden soll [1]. Im Tierversuch, aber auch beim Menschen, hat die Substanz offensichtlich positive Effekte bei der Knollenblätterpilzvergiftung gezeigt [2], möglicherweise Folge einer gesteigerten Proteinbiosynthese in der Leberzelle [3].

Rationale Pharmakotherapie in der Allgemeinpraxis
Rational Pharmacotherapy in General Practice
M. M. Kochen (Hrsg.)

Daten zur Verordnungshäufigkeit von Lebermitteln, Venenmitteln und Nootropika

Gerd Glaeske

Nachdem bereits die allgemeinen pharmakologischen und therapeutischen Grundlagen zu den 3 genannten Arzneimittelgruppen angesprochen wurden, möchte ich dieses Eingangsreferat um einige Daten aus der Praxis ergänzen. Sie sind den Arzneimitteldaten der AOK Kreis Mettmann entnommen, bei der für ein Arzneimittelberatungsprojekt eine arztbezogene Erfassung aller Verordnungen vorgenommen wird (AOK Mettmann: Ländlicher Bereich, ca. 180 000 Versicherte, 480 Ärzte). Aufgelistet sind jeweils die in einem 6-Monats-Zeitraum meistverordneten 10 Arzneimittel in jeder der angesprochenen Indikationsgruppen.

Lebermittel

(Tabelle 1)

Am meisten angewendet werden Lactulose-haltige Arzneimittel (Bifiteral, Lactulose Neda). Allerdings muß hier angemerkt werden, daß diese Arzneimittel möglicherweise auch als Laxantien verordnet werden. Abführmittel sind nämlich der Negativliste unterstellt und somit in der Kassenärztlichen Arzneimittelversorgung nicht verordnungsfähig – die Verordnung der laxierenden Lactulose-Präparate könnte als Ausweg genutzt werden. Lactulose gilt nicht als „Leberschutztherapeutikum", sondern wird als therapeutisch wirksames Prinzip bei Leberkoma und der chronischen Enzephalopathie zur Senkung der enteralen Ammoniakresorption eingesetzt.

An zweiter Stelle folgen die Silibinin-haltigen Arzneimittel (Legalon, Dura Silymarin), deren therapeutischer Nutzen bei der chronsichen Behandlung nach wie vor als nicht unumstritten gilt. Die in der Zwischenzeit angegebene Indikation: „Toxische Leberschäden; Adjuvans bei chronisch-entzündlichen Lebererkrankungen und Leberzirrhose" reflektiert diese therapeutische Unsicherheit. Die Anwendung Silibinin-haltiger Mittel ohne Absetzten der leberschädigenden Noxen, zumeist Alkohol, ist m. E. abzulehnen. Offensichtlich werden solche Arzneimittel aber nach wie vor mit der Assoziation „Leberschutzmittel" eingesetzt, die helfen sollen, Leberschäden auch bei chronischer Alkoholexposition zu vermeiden. Diese therapeutischen Hoffnungen gehen sicherlich weit an Möglichkeiten Silibinin-haltiger Arzneimittel vorbei, obwohl dies immer wieder durch Untersuchungen belegt werden soll [1]. Im Tierversuch, aber auch beim Menschen, hat die Substanz offensichtlich positive Effekte bei der Knollenblätterpilzvergiftung gezeigt [2], möglicherweise Folge einer gesteigerten Proteinbiosynthese in der Leberzelle [3].

Rationale Pharmakotherapie in der Allgemeinpraxis
Rational Pharmacotherapy in General Practice
M. M. Kochen (Hrsg.)

Tabelle 2. Verordnungen von Venenmitteln bei der AOK Kreis Mettmann (Januar–Juni 1990). Das Gesamtvolumen aller ambulant verordneten Arzneimittel betrug 1 217 062 Verordnungen (= 33 534 238,96 DM)

Präparat	Gesamt-verordnungen	Gesamtkosten [DM]	Arzneistoff(e) (Anzahl)
Vetren ext.	3 679	33 912,55	Heparin natr. (1)
Heparin ratio ext.	2 760	40 810,05	Heparin natr. calcium (1)
Venostasin int./ext.	2 281	110 149,10	Roßkastanien- (2) extrakt
Thrombareduct ext.	2 138	35 114,80	Heparin natr.
Essaven int./ext.	1 926	60 787,70	Aescin, Heparin natr. (3)
Exhirud ext.	1 903	33 895,85	Hirudin (1)
Dehydro sanol tri	1 506	52 871,30	Triamteren Bemetizid (2)
Venalot ext./int.	1 337	63 189,78	Rutoside u. a. (2)
Phlebodril ext./int.	1 318	39 308,12	Mäusedornwurzel-stockextrakt u. a.
Venoruton ext./int.	1 226	85 688,98	Rutoside (1)
Gesamt	20 074	555 728,23	

Bei den oralen Venenmitteln dominieren die Inhaltsstoffe Roßkastanienextrakt (z. B. in Venostasin) oder Rutoside (z. B. in Venalot oder Venoruton). Die Arzneimittelkommission schreibt zu solchen Mitteln:

> Klinische Studien haben eine Besserung subjektiver Symptome, wie z. B. Spannungsgefühl in den Beinen und andere Mißempfindungen, beschrieben. Ebenso glaubt man, Einflüsse auf Ödembildung und raschere Abheilung von Ulcera beobachtet zu haben ([6]). Trotzdem muß die Frage offenbleiben, ob der mögliche therapeutische Nutzen die Breite der Anwendung rechtfertigt ([4] S. 348).

Im übrigen sind unerwünschte Wirkungen wie allergische Reaktionen und gastrointestinale Störungen bei der Anwendung zu beachten. Aescin kann nach perenteraler Gabe zu Nierenversagen und – bei Überdosierungen – zu Leberschäden führen [5].

Bei den hier vorgestellten Venentherapeutika enthält nur eines, nämlich dehydro sanol tri, ein Diuretikum (Bemetizid). Solche Diuretika können kurzfristig zur Ausschwemmung venös bedingter Ödeme als unterstützende Maßnahme sinnvoll sein, das hier vorliegende Kombinationspräparat eignet sich aber nicht für die Dauertherapie. Ursprünglich hatte es mit Hesperidinkomplex und Thiamin zwei weitere Wirkstoffe enthalten und war in der *Roten Liste* unter den Venenmitteln zu finden gewesen. Nach der Reduzierung der Inhaltsstoffanzahl auf Triamteren und Bemetizid ist es nun der Gruppe der Diuretika zugeordnet (z. B in der Roten Liste 1991).

Nootropika

(Tabelle 3)

Das Haupteinsatzgebiet der Nootropika ist der Indikationsbreich Hirngefäßerkrankungen (ICD 43), und dort die zerebralen Durchblutungsstörungen ohne nähere Angabe (ICD 437.9). Anwendung finden sie auch bei der Demenz. Verordnet werden v.a. Nootropika mit dem Inhaltsstoff Piracetam. Dies entspricht auch der in Tabelle 3 gezeigten Übersicht.

Tabelle 3. Nootropika (aus der Indikationsruppe der Psychopharmaka, Gruppe 70 der Roten Liste). Anzahl der Verordnungen und Kosten verschiedener Präparate bei der AOK Kreis Mettmann (Januar–Juni 1990). Das Gesamtvolumen aller ambulant verordneten Arzneimittel betrug 1 217 062 Verordnungen (= 33 534 238,96 DM)

Präparat	Gesamt-verordnungen	Gesamtkosten [DM]	Arzneistoff(e) (Anzahl)
Piracetam ratio	686	25 764,40	Piracetam (1)
Cerebroforte	610	22 001,90	Piracetam (1)
Nootrop	606	34 266,64	Piracetam (1)
Cuxabrain	372	13 831,70	Piracetam (1)
Normabrain	352	17 848,98	Piracetam (1)
Helfergin	318	22 110,65	Meclofenoxat (1)
Encephabol	189	17 125,30	Pyritinol (1)
Piracetam 800	126	4 850,83	Piracetam (1)
Piracetam Verla	28	926,90	Piracetam (1)
Gesamt	3 287	158 727,30	

Aufgrund unserer Kassendaten lassen sich für die Verordnung von Nootropika folgende Charakteristika feststellen:

64 % der Rezeptbezieher waren Frauen, 36 % Männer, fast 90 % waren älter als 60 Jahre.

Nootropika wurden vorzugsweise von Allgemein- und praktischen Ärzten sowie von Internisten verordnet (44 % bzw. 37 %), in 11 % der Fälle von Nervenärzten. Während eines 2-Jahres-Zeitraums erhielten die Nootropikabezieher im Durchschnitt 5,4 Verordnungen mit 146 Tagesdosierungen, d.h. ausreichend für einen 5-Monats-Zeitraum. Versichertenbezogene Analysen zeigten aber starke Abweichungen von diesen Durchschnittsverteilungen:

Rund 40 % der Verordnungen während des 2jährigen Beobachtungszeitraums waren ausreichend für einen 1-Monats-Zeitraum und nur 25 % für einen Zeitraum länger als 6 Monate. Diese Verlaufsdaten lassen die Interpretation zu, daß mit derartigen Nootropika häufig antherapiert wird, daß diese Mittel aber bald wieder abgesetzt oder – und dies zeigen die Daten ebenfalls – zusammen mit durchblutungsfördernden Substanzen oder zusammen mit Psychopharmaka (z. B. Eunerpan oder Dipiperon) verordnet werden.

Insgesamt spiegelt die geringe Verordnungshäufigkeit von Nootropika wahrscheinlich die Zweifel am Nutzen dieser Arzneimittelgruppe wieder, die der verordnende Arzt in seiner praktischen Anwendung bestätigt findet. Im Arzneiverordnungs-Report '90 ([7], S. 347) heißt es hierzu:

> Für einige Stoffe sind vigilanzsteigernde Wirkungen gezeigt worden, deren klinische Bedeutung jedoch nicht endültig beurteilbar ist, da es einwandfreie Studien zur Wirksamkeit von Nootropika und zur möglichen Vorhersage potentieller „Responder" und „Non-Responder" bisher nicht in ausreichender Zahl gibt. Der allgemeine Wert dieser Präparate ist somit nach wie vor zweifelhaft. Allerdings ist Piracetam im Rahmen der Aufbereitung zurückhaltend positiv bewertet worden.

Die Verordnungsrealität stimmt durchaus mit dieser Bewertung überein.

Literatur

1. Ferenci P, Dragosics B, Dittrich H et al. (1989) Randomisierte kontrollierte Studie über die Silymarin-Therapie bei Patienten mit Leberzirrhose. J Hepatol 9 : 1–12
2. Schenke M, Wiedemann G, Otte M (1987) Therapie der Knollenblätterpilzvergiftung. Internist Prax 27 : 293–296
3. Sonnenbichler J, Zetl I (1989) Silibinin vermehrt die „Nähmaschinen". Ärztl Prax 94 : 3279–3281
4. Arzneimittelkommission der deutschen Ärzteschaft (Hrsg) (1988) Arzneiverordnungen, 16. Aufl. Köln, S 349
5. Fricke U (1990) Venenmittel. In: Schwabe U Paffrath D (Hrsg) Arzneiverordnungs-Report '90. Stuttgart, New York, S 385–394
6. Hitzenberger G (1989) Die therapeutische Wirksamkeit des Roßkastaniensamenextraktes. Wien Med Wochenschr 139 : 385–389
7. Lohse MJ, Müller-Oerlingshausen B (1990) Psychopharmaka. In: Arzneiverordnungs-Report '90. Stuttgart New York S 335–350

Der therapeutische Nutzen von Lebertherapeutika, Venenmitteln und Mitteln zur Behandlung von Hirnfunktionsstörungen aus der Sicht einer Allgemeinärztin

Christa A. Ossmann

Vorbemerkung

Bewertungen von arzneitherapeutischen Strategien bei der Behandlung von Lebererkrankungen, Venenerkrankungen und Hirnleistungsstörungen im Alter sind immer Meinungsäußerungen aufgrund therapeutischer Erfahrungen, die in unterschiedlichem Ausmaß durch harte klinische Daten anhand von Studien belegt sind. Wenn entsprechende Daten fehlen oder widersprüchlich sind, erfolgt der Erkenntnisgewinn durch das Prinzip von trial and error in der Behandlungspraxis. Wenn ich also hier Arzneimittel beurteile, dann ist das meine therapeutische Meinung. Dieses ist klarzustellen, damit nachfolgende Äußerungen nicht als Tatsachenbehauptungen fehlinterpretiert werden.

„Lebertherapeutika"

Lebererkrankungen

Die häufigste, in der Allgemeinpraxis diagnostizierte Leberschädigung ist die *Fettleber*. Dabei kommt es zu einem erhöhten Fettgehalt in diesem Organ, der sich in einer histologisch nachweisbaren Ablagerung von Fetttropfen in den Leberzellen manifestiert. Diese Störung ist erst dann wesentlich, wenn größere Anteile der Leberzellen verfettet sind oder das ganze Parenchym von Fetttropfen durchsetzt wird.

Eine Fettleber findet sich in Europa bei ca. 20 % der Patienten.

Als häufigste Ursachen kommen in Frage: chronischer Alkoholkonsum, Überernährung, häufig verbunden mit einem Diabetes mellitus, Unterernährung (die bei uns nur von theoretischem Interesse ist), Hypertriglyzeridämie, verschiedene Pharmaka.

Die reine *alkoholische* Fettleber ist in der kurzen Zeit von 2–6 Wochen vollständig rückbildungsfähig, wenn es gelingt, den Alkohol auszuschalten.

Die *diabetische* Fettleber kommt v.a. bei den Typ-II-Diabetikern vor. Dabei scheint die Fettanhäufung in der Leber unabhängig von der Dauer und Schwere des Diabetes, nur vom Grad der Übergewichtigkeit bestimmt zu sein. Gewichtsreduktion führt nicht nur zu einer Normalisierung des Stoffwechsels, sondern auch zum Abbau der Fettleber. Bei der diabetischen Fettleber handelt es sich um eine Mastfettleber.

Rationale Pharmakotherapie in der Allgemeinpraxis
Rational Pharmacotherapy in General Practice
M. M. Kochen (Hrsg.)

Bei der *Hypertriglyzeridämie* Typ IV nach Fredrickson findet sich regelmäßig eine erhebliche Fettleber.

Die bekanntesten Pharmaka, die eine Leberzellverfettung hervorrufen können, sind Kortikosteroide und Tuberkulostatika.

Behandlung

Von seiten der Industrie werden seit Jahrzehnten eine Vielzahl von Präparaten angeboten, denen eine Wirkung auf Leberschädigungen zugeschrieben wird. So weist die Rote Liste 1990 unter dem Stichwort „Lebertherapeutika" rund 100 Fertigarzneimittel auf, die pflanzliche Extrakte, Vitamine, Phospholipide und Fettsäuren allein oder in Kombination enthalten.

Lebermittel gehörten zu einer relativ kleinen Indikationsgruppe mit einem Umsatz im Jahr 1989 von 108,6 Mio. DM und einem Rückgang des Umsatzes im Vergleich zum Vorjahr von 11,5% (= 14,1 Mio. DM).

Zwar wird behauptet, daß für die meisten Lebertherapeutika in tierexperimentellen Studien eine sog. „Leberschutzwirkung" zu beobachten sei. Dies ist aber ein oft mangelhaft definierter Begriff für willkürlich erhobene Beobachtungen und Meßwerte, denen kein sinnvolles therapeutisches Konzept zugrunde liegt. Sie läßt sich nicht auf die Lebererkrankungen des Menschen übertragen, eine therapeutische Wirksamkeit und klinische Relevanz ist beim Menschen bisher noch nicht nachgewiesen worden.

Ein Therapieerfolg mit diesen Präparaten ist somit nicht gesichert.

Trotz weltweiter Bemühungen, die Fettleber medikamentös zu beeinflussen, besteht eine wirksame Therapie nur darin, die verursachende Noxe auszuschalten.

Die wirksamste therapeutische Maßnahme bei der Behandlung der alkoholischen Fettleber ist die Alkoholkarenz, bei diabetischer bzw. ernährungsbedingter Fettleber eine Gewichtsreduktion. Innerhalb weniger Wochen kommt es in den meisten Fällen zu einer Rückbildung der Fettleber, selbst eine beginnende Zirrhose scheint noch partiell rückbildungsfähig bzw. kompensierbar zu sein. Eine kausale Therapie mit erwiesener Wirksamkeit steht also nicht zur Verfügung.

Der niedergelassene Arzt wird aber immer wieder vor die Frage gestellt, ob er bei alkoholischer, diabetischer und ernährungsbedingter Fettleber medikamentösen Nihilismus betreiben sollte oder ob es für den betroffenen Patienten beruhigender wäre, ein sog. Lebertherapeutikum einzunehmen.

Bei dieser Entscheidung sollte die kritische Einstellung des Arztes zur Pharmakotherapie und zur Belastbarkeit des Versichertensystems durch nutzlose Kostenfaktoren eine wesentliche Rolle spielen.

Bei der Verordnung solcher Präparate besteht die Gefahr, daß die Motivation des Patienten zur Alkoholabstinenz bzw. Gewichtsreduktion untergraben wird. Dem Patienten sollte intensiv vor Augen geführt werden, daß seine Erkrankung durch z.B. Alkohol bzw. Überernährung bedingt ist und *nur* durch Weglassen der Noxe geheilt werden kann. Jede zusätzliche Maßnahme verleitet den Patienten zu der Annahme, daß eine Heilung durch Arzneimittel möglich ist und der Verzicht auf Alkohol bei gewissenhafter Einnahme des Medikaments nicht nötig sei. Auch die

Fettleber des Altersdiabetikers bessert sich oder verschwindet nach Gewichtsreduktion; ebenso ist die Fettleber bei primärer Hypertriglyzeridämie einer diätetischen Behandlung zugänglich. Die medikamentös bedingte Fettleber schwindet nach Absetzen des sie verursachenden Arzneimittels; dabei wird man eine Fettleber bei bestimmten Patienten, die diese Mittel benötigen, in Kauf nehmen müssen.

Diese Erkenntnis scheint sich bei den niedergelassenen Ärzten langsam durchzusetzen: Die Verordnungshäufigkeit der sog. Lebermittel nahm im Jahr 1989 im Vergleich zu 1988 um 8,6 % ab, der Umsatz war um 11,5 % (rund 13 Mio. DM) geringer.

Präparate

Die meistverkauften Lebertherapeutika als Monopräparate sind z. B. Legalon (Silymarin), Hepa Merz (Ornithinaspartet) und die Lactulosepräparate Bifiteral, Lactulose Neda, Laevilac.

Legalon, ein Extrakt aus Früchten der Mariendistel, dessen aktives Prinzip als Silymarin bezeichnet wird und das hauptsächlich das Flavonoid Silibinin enthält, ist ein seit Jahrzehnten umstrittenes Präparat. Für die meisten Ärzte wohl unbemerkt, sind die Indikationsangaben eingeschränkt worden und lauten heute: toxische Leberschäden, Adjuvans bei chronisch-entzündlichen Lebererkrankungen und Leberzirrhose, während noch 1986 die akute Hepatitis, chronisch persistierende und chronisch aggressive Hepatitis, Leberzirrhose und toxisch metabolischer Leberschaden angeführt wurden. Trotz mehrerer kontrollierter Studien ist die Wirksamkeit des Präparats bei akuten und chronischen Lebererkrankungen weiterhin zweifelhaft und umstritten. Eine Studie über die Überlebensrate von Patienten mit Leberzirrhose ergab keine signifikanten Unterschiede zwischen behandelten und unbehandelten Patienten.

Für nichtessentielle Aminosäuren, z. B. Arginin oder sein Metabolit Ornithin – enthalten in Hepa Merz – oder Asparaginsäure, gibt es keine Belege für einen spezifischen Mangel oder eine therapeutische Wirksamkeit bei Lebererkrankungen.

Das gleiche gilt für die Kombinationspräparate, in erster Linie Essentiale forte, Eukalisan, Hepagrisevit Forte, Hepatofalk, Silibene u. a. Die darin enthaltenen lipotropen Substanzen Cholin und Methionin haben sich bei der Fettleberbehandlung als ebenso unwirksam erwiesen wie Leberhydrolysate, Frischleberextrakte, hochungesättigte Fettsäuren, verschiedene B-Vitamine, Orotsäure, Alpha-Liponsäure oder Vitamin E.

Als Ausnahme gilt lediglich die Folsäure, da bei Alkoholikern häufig ein nutritiver Folsäuremangel besteht. Gekennzeichnet ist dieser Mangelzustand durch das Auftreten einer megalozytären Anämie, die durch Folsäuregaben (initial 5–20 mg/Tag oral bis zur Remission) aber auch durch Normalkost mit durchschnittlichem Folsäuregehalt (0,2–0,5 mg/Tag) behoben werden kann.

Etwas anders verhält es sich mit Lactulose (*Bifiteral, Lactulose Neda, Laevilac*), die beim Leberkoma oder der chronischen Enzephalopathie zur Senkung der enteralen Ammoniakresorption eingesetzt wird. Lactulose säuert den Stuhl an und vermindert dadurch die Bildung von Ammoniak durch bakterielle Gärung im Dickdarm. Erfahrungen aus der Praxis geben zu der Vermutung Anlaß, daß Lactulose oft als Laxans verordnet wird, denn die Verordnungshäufigkeit ist stark angestiegen [1].

Venentherapeutika

Venenerkrankungen

Bei Störungen im venösen System wird unterschieden in Rückflußstörungen im oberflächlichen und im tiefen Venensystem, wobei für den venösen Rücktransport vorwiegend das tiefe System einschließlich der Perforansvenen bedeutsam sind. Störungen des venösen Rückflusses können bedingt sein durch oberflächliche oder tiefe Wandveränderungen mit Klappeninsuffizienz oder durch Stenosen bis hin zum Verschluß. Bei Erkrankungen im venösen System können je nach Lokalisation und Schweregrad venöse Rückflußstörungen auftreten, die akute oder chronische Venenerkrankungen zur Folge haben.

- *Akute Venenkrankheiten:* Hier liegt entweder eine oberflächliche, extrafasziale Thrombophlebitis oder Varikophlebitis mit den Zeichen einer Entzündung oder eine tiefe, intrafasziale Phlebothrombose vor, die asymptomatisch oder mit Ödem, Spannungsschmerzen bzw. Zyanose der betreffenden Extremität einhergehen kann.
- *Chronische Venenkrankheiten:* Sie sind in der Praxis weitaus am häufigsten. Hier liegt entweder eine primäre Varikose als Ektasie größerer Venen mit resultierender Klappeninsuffizienz oder eine durch entzündliche Veränderungen ausgelöste Insuffizienz oder Verschluß von tiefenVenen vor (postthrombotisches Syndrom). Bei der *chronischen Veneninsuffizienz* reichen die Symptome je nach Dauer und Ausmaß der venösen Rückflußstörung von Ödem und Zyanose über Petechien, Hämosiderose, Dermatosklerose und atrophischen Hautveränderungen bis hin zum Gewebsdefekt mit Ulkus.

Behandlung

Die sog. Venentherapeutika sollen zur adjuvanten Therapie bei primärer Varikose und chronischer Veneninsuffizienz eingesetzt werden. Dabei wird unterschieden in:

- *Venentonisierende Mittel*, z.B. Dihydroergotamin (DHE), Roßkastanienextrakte (Aescin) oder Flavonderivate (Rutin).
- *„Ödemprotektiva"*, z.B. Diosmin, Benzaron, Roßkastanienextrakte (Aescin) oder Flavonderivate (Rutin);
- *Mittel zur Ödemausschwemmung* (Diuretika);
- *Lokaltherapeutika.*

Die Rote Liste 1990 verzeichnet insgesamt 176 orale und topische Venenmittel. Der Umsatz lag im Jahr 1989 bei 578,2 Mio. DM mit einem Rückgang im Vergleich zum Vorjahr von 7,9 % (49,6 Mio. DM). Dabei ist zu beachten, daß sich unter den 2000 am häufigsten verordneten Arzneimitteln immerhin 46 Venenmittel befinden.

Eine Therapie mit *venentonisierenden Substanzen*, z.B. Dihydroergotamin (DHE), Roßkastanienextrakte und Rutoside, wird durchgeführt mit dem Ziel, durch eine Verengung der Venen den Blutstrom zu beschleunigen und so den venösen Rückfluß zu verbessern. Dadurch soll die für die Thrombosebildung gefährliche Stase verhindert werden.

Der therapeutische Nutzen dieser Mittel bei Venenerkrankungen muß jedoch außerordentlich kritisch bewertet werden.

DHE besitzt in hohen Dosen eine vasokonstriktorische Wirkung im venösen System. Es besteht aber die Gefahr peripherer Durchblutungsstörungen durch gleichzeitige Verengung der arteriellen Gefäße (Ergotismus). Für Roßkastanienextrakte und Rutoside ließen sich in pharmakologischen Tests zwar in einigen Tiermodellen und am Gesunden vasokonstriktorische Effekte postulieren, jedoch liegen keine zweifelsfreien Ergebnisse vor, die einen therapeutischen Nutzen der venentonisierenden Mittel bei der Behandlung oder zur Prophylaxe von Thromben am Patienten bestätigen.

Die Transparenzkommission beim BGA für das Gebiet „periphere venöse Durchblutungsstörungen" kommt daher zu der Schlußfolgerung, daß „nach den Ergebnissen klinisch-wissenschaftlicher Untersuchungen DHE und andere venentonisierende Substanzen bei alleiniger Gabe keine thromboseprophylaktische Wirksamkeit besitzen" [6].

Die aus Pflanzenauszügen gewonnenen Stoffe, z.B. Roßkastanienextrakte (Saponine, Aescin), Flavonoide (Diosmin, Leukocianidol, Rutin und Derivate) oder synthetische Analoga (Benzaron, Calciumdobesilat, Tribenosis), sollen membranabdichtende oder ödemprotektive Wirkungen ausüben. Aufgrund tierexperimenteller Untersuchungen werden für Aescin (in Venostasin u.a.), Benzaron (in Fragivix u.a.), Calciumdobesilat (Dexium u.a.), Rutenoside (Venoruton u.a.) und Tribenosid (Glyvenol u.a.) permeabilitätsvermindernde Wirkungen im Bereich der Endstrombahn geltend gemacht. Dem steht gegenüber, daß eine therapeutische Wirksamkeit bei Patienten mit chronischer Veneninsuffizienz, z.B. Verminderung der Ödeme oder beschleunigte Heilung von Ulzera, nicht gesichert ist. Eine Wiederherstellung der Klappenfunktion der Venen, das einzige sinnvolle Ziel therapeutischer Maßnahmen, oder eine klinisch relevante und dauerhafte Abnahme des Beinvolumens konnte bisher nicht belegt werden, auch wenn eine Besserung subjektiver Symptome anhand von kontrollierten Studien behauptet wird.

Dabei ist die Gabe von Ödemprotektiva nicht ohne Risiko: Aescin kann bei parenteraler Anwendung Nierenversagen auslösen, Flavonoide haben immunstimulierende Eigenschaften und können Fieberschübe, grippeähnliche Beschwerden, Leberschädigung, hämolytische Anämie, Myokarditis oder Pleuritis hervorrufen.

Durch die Erweiterung der Venen und Erhöhung des orthostatischen Drucks kommt es zu einem Flüssigkeitsübertritt aus den Venen in das umliegende Gewebe. *Diuretika* können theoretisch durch ihre elektrolyt- und wasserausschwemmende Wirkung auch venös bedingte Ödeme ausschwemmen. Dabei tritt jedoch gleichzeitig eine Hämokonzentration ein, die die Fließeigenschaften des Blutes verschlechtert und somit die Gefahr der Stase mit Thrombosebildung erhöht. Eine Therapie mit Diuretika kommt deshalb nur in Einzelfällen als unterstützende Maßnahme in Betracht, wenn eine Kompressionstherapie allein nicht ausreicht. Stark wirksame Schleifendiuretika wie Furosemid (Lasix) sollten wegen der erhöhten Gefahr der Hämokonzentration überhaupt nicht eingesetzt werden.

Lokaltherapeutika sind zumeist Salben oder Gele mit zahlreichen Inhaltsstoffen, die Heparin, Heparinoide, Ödemprotektiva, Antiphlogistika, sogar Antibiotika und Glukokortikoide enthalten. Diese Stoffe werden aber nur in geringem Umfang durch die Haut resorbiert, so daß auch bei großflächiger Anwendung keine systemischen gerinnungshemmenden Wirkungen zu erwarten sind. Eine Lokaltherapie bei Thrombophlebitis und Varikophlebitis dient der Linderung oder der beschleunigten Beseitigung von akuten Entzündungserscheinungen. Es ist offen, welcher Beitrag zu diesen lindernden Effekten den einzelnen Inhaltsstoffen zuzuordnen ist. Wahrscheinlich liegt der therapeutische Effekt darin, daß durch die mit dem Auftragen verbundene Gewebsmassage ein lindernder Einfluß auf die Beschwerden ausgeübt wird.

Allerdings ist zu bedenken, daß durch die Zahl der Inhaltsstoffe das Risiko von Allergisierung und Kontaktekzemen zunimmt, besonders bei Ulkuspatienten. Dies gilt nicht nur für die Inhaltsstoffe, sondern auch für die Salbengrundlage und Hilfsstoffe. Zwei Drittel der Patienten sollen von solchen Effekten betroffen sein. Wenn eine Lokalbehandlung notwendig ist, sollten solche Präparate bevorzugt werden, die wenige Inhaltsstoffe möglichst indifferenter Natur enthalten. Durch einen häufigen Wechsel der Medikamente kann theoretisch ebenfalls eine Sensibilisierung vermieden werden.

Schlußfolgerung

Die Therapie der Wahl bei Erkrankungen der Venen besteht in der Kompressionsbehandlung (Kompressionsverband oder -strümpfe), in operativen Maßnahmen (Stripping nach Babcock) und bei kleinen Varizen in der Sklerosierung. In der eigenen Praxis ist v. a. eine Bereitschaft jüngerer Patienten zu beobachten, operative Maßnahmen durchführen zu lassen. Umstritten und zweifelhaft ist der Nutzen der medikamentösen Therapie.

Behandlung von Hirnleistungsstörungen im Alter

Der Begriff „Geriatrika“ ist nicht einheitlich definiert. In der Roten Liste findet man rund 40 Präparate, die aus Pflanzenextrakten, besonders Knoblauch, aber auch Mistelkraut, Johanniskraut-Weizenkeimöl, Weißdorn, Ginseng u. a. zusammengesetzt sind. Dazu kommen Arzneimittel, die Procain, die gesamte Vitaminpalette, Spurenelemente, Organextrakte, Sexualhormone und Homöopathika enthalten. Diese Mittel haben keinen belegten therapeutischen Nutzen und sind nach den Bestimmungen der Negativliste nicht zu Lasten der gesetzlichen Krankenkassen verordnungsfähig. Wenn sich die Patienten diese Mittel kaufen, in dem Gedanken, natürliche Alterungsprozesse könnten hiermit verzögert werden, so ist dagegen nur einzuwenden, daß sie von den Mitteln keinen Nutzen haben, sondern nur der Hersteller und Verkäufer.

Das Thema sollte also besser heißen: *Mittel zur Behandlung von Hirnleistungsstörungen im Alter.* Es umfaßt dann die sog. Nootropika und durchblutungsfördernden Arzneimittel. Diese Substanzen werden trotz zweifelhafter und umstrittener Wirksamkeit in großem Umfang bei diesen Indikationen eingesetzt.

Pathophysiologie

Akute zerebrale Durchblutungsstörungen beruhen auf einer Mangelversorgung des Gehirns und werden durch Stenosen oder Verschlüsse der hirnversorgenden extrakraniellen oder intrakraniellen Gefäße verursacht. Einem zerebralen Insult gehen häufig und über längere Zeit flüchtige neurologische Ausfälle voraus, die als *TIA* (transitorisch ischämische Attacke) oder als *PRIND* (prolongiertes, reversibles ischämisch-neurologisches Defizit) bezeichnet werden.

Bei der TIA kommt es zu flüchtigen, Sekunden bis Minuten dauernden sensiblen und motorischen Ausfällen. Es wird angenommen, daß sie auf einer reversiblen Thrombozytenaggregation auf dem Boden arteriosklerotisch bedingter Gefäßstenosen beruhen.

Bei PRIND treten rezidivierende, länger anhaltende und variable Ausfälle zentralnervöser Funktionen auf, die einen Tag bis eine Woche nachweisbar sind, aber klinisch völlig ausheilen. Hier werden rezidivierende thromboembolische Prozesse vermutet, die durch Ablösen von wandständigen Thromben im Bereich arteriosklerotischer Gefäßprozesse hervorgerufen werden.

Beim akuten zerebralen Insult, der Apoplexie, kommt es in 70–80 % der Fälle zum plötzlichen Ausfall größerer Hirnanteile infolge eines thrombotischen Verschlusses der zuführenden Gefäße. Embolische Verschlüsse sind in 8–15 % der Fälle ursächlich und werden z. B. durch Embolien aus dem Herzen ausgelöst. In etwa zwei Drittel der Fälle kommt es auch ohne gezielte Therapie zur Spontanheilung bzw. zur weitgehenden Rückbildung. Eine schlechte Prognose hat dagegen die Hirnblutung, die aber nur bei 10–15 % der Insulte verursachend ist.

Schnelle Ermüdbarkeit, geistige Erschöpfbarkeit, Schwindel, Gangunsicherheit, Gedächtnisstörungen, Störungen des Schlaf-Wach-Rhythmus bis hin zur Verwirrtheit, psychomotorischer Erregung und psychotischen oder depressiven Reaktionen sind die Leitsymptome des mit zunehmendem Alter häufiger zu beobachtenden Hirnabbaus.

Der pathophysiologische Prozeß, der dem Abbau der Hirnleistungen zugrunde liegt, die Ätiologie des hirnorganischen Psychosyndroms ist noch unklar. Nur bei ungefähr 15 % der Fälle sind diese Symptome mit einer erniedrigten Hirndurchblutung infolge Arteriosklerose der zuführenden Gefäße korrelierbar. Bei der Mehrzahl der Fälle finden sich postmortal die Befunde einer Multiinfarktdemenz (25 %) oder einer Alzheimer Erkrankung (25 %) oder einer Mischform beider Erkrankungen (25 %). Die Multiinfarktdemenz beruht auf einer hyalinen Degeneration kleiner Hirngefäße mit Zelluntergang in dem Versorgungsgebiet. Bei der Alzheimer-Krankheit kommt es zum Untergang von cholinergen und anderen Neuronen in phylogenetisch älteren Abschnitten des ZNS. Diese Neurone scheinen eine Steuerung der Funktionen der Großhirnrinde auszuüben. Eine Mangeldurchblutung oder eine Stoffwechselstörung scheinen bei beiden Erkrankungen keine Rolle zu spielen. Deshalb hat bei dieser Erkrankung die Anwendung von Substanzen, die die Durchblutung fördern oder den Hirnstoffwechsel beeinflussen, keine rationale Grundlage. Eine kausale Therapie steht nicht zur Verfügung [3].

Präparate

Zur Behandlung von Hirnleistungsstörungen im Alter werden die sog. Nootropika und Arzneimittel, die eine zerebrale Durchblutungsstörung günstig beeinflussen sollen, empfohlen. Bedenkt man, daß der therapeutische Nutzen dieser Mittel in der Literatur zweifelhaft bis negativ bewertet wird, ist der Kostenfaktor dieser Therapieform unerträglich hoch.

In der Roten Liste 1990 werden die Nootropika unter dem Kapitel „Psychopharmaka" aufgelistet. Aus dem Arzneiverordnungs-Report '90 wird ersichtlich, daß die Nootropika im Jahr 1989 einen Umsatz von 103,6 Mio. DM aufweisen mit einem Umsatzrückgang im Vergleich zum Vorjahr von 7,0 % (= 7,9 Mio. DM).

Einen weitaus höheren finanziellen Stellenwert nehmen die durchblutungsfördernden Mittel mit 1195,3 Mio. DM ein; auch hier ist ein Umsatzrückgang im Vergleich zu 1988 von 16,5 % (= 236,3 Mio. DM) zu verzeichnen. Bei einem Gesamtumsatz der verordneten Arzneimittel im Jahr 1989 von 20,7 Mrd. DM nehmen die durchblutungsfördernden Mittel rund 6,0 % ein.

Zur Gruppe der sog. Nootropika gehören: Piracetam (Nootrop u.a.), Pyritinol (Encephabol u.a.) und Meclofenoxat (Helfergin u.a.), die pharmakologisch mehr als zentral stimulierende Substanzen imponieren und deshalb v.a. zur Behandlung altersbedingter Hirnleistungsstörungen eingesetzt werden, die mit rascher Ermüdbarkeit und Konzentrationsschwäche einhergehen.

Die therapeutische Relevanz der durch Nootropika hervorgerufenen Effekte ist allerdings noch nicht eindeutig beurteilbar. Eine generelle Wirksamkeit kann anhand der vorliegenden Daten nicht angenommen werden. Man kann z.B. nicht voraussagen, ob ein Patient durch die Behandlung mit Nootropika eine Besserung erfährt oder nicht. Nootropika zeigen auch keinen therapeutischen Effekt bei der Behandlung des akuten ischämischen Insults in Bezug auf Besserung von sekundären Schäden im Verlauf der Erkrankung. Diese kritische Wertung entspricht auch der stark eingeschränkt positiven Bewertung von z.B. Piracetam durch die zuständige Aufbereitungskommission beim BGA.

Dabei ist zu berücksichtigen, daß sich in der Gruppe der 2000 verordnungshäufigsten Präparate 7 Arzneimittel aus der Gruppe der Nootropika befinden, die in der Gruppe der Psychopharmaka zwar nur 5 % der Verordnungen, aber 11 % des Umsatzes ausmachen und damit eine besonders kostenintensive Arzneimittelgruppe sind.

Zu den Arzneistoffen mit umstrittener Wirksamkeit gehören auch die durchblutungsfördernden Mittel, die im Jahr 1989 zwar den in den Vorjahren gehaltenen

Rang 2 verloren, aber mit 1195,3 Mio. DM immer noch den 5. Rang der umsatzstärksten Arzneigruppe einnahmen. Diese Stoffe werden von der Industrie in der Regel für periphere *und* zentrale Durchblutungsstörungen empfohlen.

Seit Jahrzehnten wird erfolglos versucht, den Verlauf und die Progredienz von Hirnfunktionsstörungen im Alter durch die Gabe von durchblutungsfördernden Arzneimitteln zu bessern. Heute weiß man, daß eine Minderperfusion des Gehirns nur in den relativ seltenen Fällen einer Arteriosklerose der zuführenden Arterien pathophysiologisch von Bedeutung ist. Wirksam hat sich dabei bisher nur das Prinzip der Thrombozytenaggregationshemmung erwiesen, z. B. die Azetylsalizylsäure, die zur Rezidivprophylaxe bei der transitorisch ischämischen Attacke eingesetzt wird und das Risiko des Übergangs der arteriosklerotischen Gefäßerkrankung in einen manifesten ischämischen Insult um ein Drittel senken kann. Die große Mehrheit der anderen Substanzen ist bei den genannten Indikationen völlig wirkungslos.

Behandlungsmaßnahmen mit Vasodilatanzien, z. B. Pentoxifyllin (Trental u. a.), Xantinolnicotinat (Complamin u. a.), Naftidrofuryl (Dusodril u. a.), Benzyclan (Fludilat u. a.), Vincamin (Cetal, Pervincamin u. a.), Buflomedil (Bufedil u. a.) erscheinen bei zerebraler Minderperfusion sogar kontraindiziert, da durch diese Mittel die Autoregulation der Durchblutung in den nichtischämischen Bezirken aufgehoben und eine Blutumverteilung zu Lasten der ischämischen Bezirke (*Steal*phänomen) hervorgerufen werden kann.

Auch bei Co-dergocrin (Hydergin u. a.) wurde in 30jähriger Anwendungszeit kein endgültiger Beweis der Wirksamkeit erbracht. Eine jüngst erschienene Arbeit weist sogar auf eine Verschlechterung des Krankheitsverlaufs unter dieser Medikation hin [5].

Dies gilt auch für Gingko-biloba-Blätterextrakte, z. B. Tebonin und Rökan, die für Hirnleistungsstörungen und periphere arterielle Durchblutungsstörungen bei erhaltener Durchblutungsreserve zugelassen sind. Dabei nimmt Tebonin hinsichtlich der Arzneimittelkosten mit einem Umsatz von 218,9 Mio. DM im Jahr 1989 den Rang 1 aller Arzneimittel ein; dies ist noch ausgeprägter, wenn das Parallelprodukt Rökan mit einem Jahresumsatz von 61,5 Mio. DM hinzugerechnet wird.

Dem Substanzgemisch werden durchblutungssteigernde, viskositätssenkende und thrombozytenaggregationshemmende Eigenschaften zugeschrieben. Nach wie vor werden die Untersuchungen zum Nachweis der klinischen Wirksamkeit kontrovers diskutiert:

„Insgesamt liegen für diese Präparate aber immer noch weniger den heutigen methodischen Ansprüchen genügende Untersuchungen vor als für andere Präparate“ [2].

In einer anderen Studie wurden die vorliegenden Untersuchungen als nicht hinreichend für eine Wirksamkeitsaussage gewertet [4].

Wie sieht es aber mit der Verordnung dieser Pflanzenextrakte aus Gingkobaumblättern in der Praxis aus? Obwohl rezeptfrei erhältlich, ist der Wunsch nach Verschreibung zu Lasten der gesetzlichen Krankenkassen unverhältnismäßig hoch, ein Tatbestand, der sich auch in der Zahl von 4266 Mio. Verordnungen im Jahr 1989 niederschlägt. Dabei handelt es sich keineswegs um Patienten mit manifesten

Hirnleistungsstörungen im Sinne der Zulassung. Das Mittel wird aufgrund seiner pflanzlichen Zusammensetzung, im Rahmen der „grünen Welle" in der Medizin, vorbeugend gegen Altersbeschwerden, welcher Art auch immer, eingenommen.

Umgang mit Wunschverordnungen: Ein lösbares Problem?

„Wunschverordnungen" sind ein generelles Problem in der Praxis des niedergelassenen Arztes. Das gilt insbesondere für Alterspatienten mit den für sie fühlbaren Beschwerden der nachlassenden Gedächtnis- und Konzentrationskraft. Es steht keine wirksame Arzneimitteltherapie für diese Beschwerden zur Verfügung, aber der Patient verlangt vom Arzt Hilfe. Hier gegenzusteuern ist außerordentlich mühsam und mit viel Ärger verbunden. Dies gilt grundsätzlich für alle Präparate mit umstrittener Wirksamkeit, also Leber-, Venenmittel und Geriatrika bzw. Mittel zur Behandlung von Hirnfunktionsstörungen im Alter. Wenn man sich aber klar macht, daß auf Arzneimittelgruppen mit umstrittener Wirksamkeit im Jahr 1989 mit 5,3 Mrd. DM rund 25 % der Gesamtkosten für Arzneimittel entfallen und sie etwa 30,5 % des Verordnungsvolumens ausmachen, dann sollte in jedem Einzelfall überdacht werden, ob eine Verordnung zu Lasten der gesetzlichen Krankenkassen erfolgen soll oder nicht.

Es gibt zu denken, daß viele dieser Arzneimittel in den USA, Großbritannien und den skandinavischen Ländern nicht erhältlich bzw. zugelassen sind, ohne daß Nachteile für den Patienten beobachtet werden. Ein Arzneimittel zu verordnen ist einfach; ungleich schwieriger ist es dagegen, den Patienten zu einer Änderung seiner Lebensweise zu motivieren.

Es ist gleichermaßen notwendig, unsere ärztliche Einstellung zu den Marketingstrategien der Industrie zu überdenken. Man braucht nur die dümmliche Werbung in den Aussendungen und Fachzeitschriften zu betrachten, um zu erkennen, daß mit dem differenzierten Stoff Arzneimittel nicht anders umgegangen wird als mit Waschmitteln, um sie an den Arzt zu bringen. Dabei sind wir doch gerade im eigenen privaten Bereich sehr sensibel gegen diese Art von Werbung geworden und sträuben uns gegen jede Form der Manipulation.

Auch sollten wir daran denken, daß die Mittel der gesetzlichen Krankenversicherung nicht unerschöpflich sind. Die Kosten für Arzneimittel und zur Honorierung unserer ärztlichen Tätigkeit kommen aus dem gleichen Topf. Die Verschwendung von Mitteln für nutzlose Arzneimittel schmälert also auch die Mittel, die für die Honorierung unserer Leistungen zur Verfügung stehen.

Literatur

1. Dölle W, Schwabe U (1990) Leber und Gallenwegstherapeutika, Arzneiverordnungs-Report '90, Bd 6. Fischer, Frankfurt am Main, S 260
2. Held K, Schwabe U (1990) Durchblutungsfördernde Mittel, Arzneiverordnungs-Report '90, Bd 6. Fischer, Frankfurt am Main, S 202
3. Schönhöfer PS (1987) Behandlung von Hirnfunktionsstörungen im Alter. Kassenarzt-aktuell, Nr. 22/23: 39–43, 35–39

4. Schönhöfer PS, Schulte-Sasse H, Manhold C, Werner B (1989) Sind Extrakte aus den Blättern des Gingko-biloba-Baumes bei peripheren Durchblutungs- und Hirnleistungsstörungen im Alter wirksam? Internist Prax 29:585–601
5. Thompson TL et al. (1990) Lack of efficacy of hydergine in patients with Alzheimer's disease. N Engl J Med 323:445–448
6. Transparenzkommission (1984) Transparenzliste für das Indikationsteilgebiet periphere venöse Durchblutungsstörungen, S 16

Pharmakotherapieunterricht für Medizinstudenten – Neue Konzepte

Teaching Pharmacotherapy to Students: New Concepts

Teaching Pharmacotherapeutics: Experiences in Ghent

Luc Blondeel

The Medical Curriculum in Belgium and at the State University of Ghent

Universities are responsible for undergraduate medical training. The contents are provided for by the law and are the same for the seven medical schools: 3 years of preclinical teaching followed by 4 years of clinical training (theorethical and practical). Until 1982, after these 7 years the medical profession was freely accessible for general practitoners. For students who voted for a career as general practitioner, some medical schools offered a programme with specific training in general practice.

In 1982 this special training in general practice became mandatory. Departments of general practice were asked to organize this postgraduate training, which was no longer the responsibility of the university as such. The content and timing of this training was changed several times, in part as a consequence of the European directive 86/457. This directive provides for the vocational training of general practitioners; the deadline for compliance is 1 January 1995. The medical schools and the departments of general practice are now preparing a definitive scheme, to be implemented in the school year 1994–1995.

The current situation is still a transition to the post-1995 situation. The major challenge is to make a continuous education programme of 9 years for the general practitioners, with a *truncus communis* of 6 years. For this, specialists and general

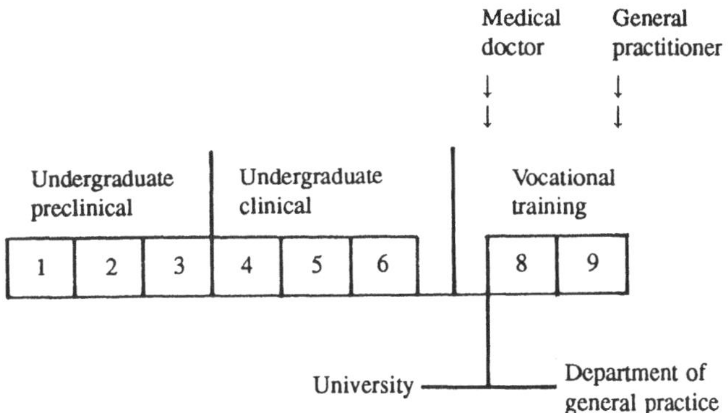

Fig. 1. Medical curriculum for medical doctors and general practitioners in terms of years of training

Rationale Pharmakotherapie in der Allgemeinpraxis
Rational Pharmacotherapy in General Practice
M. M. Kochen (Hrsg.)

practitioners have to define a common "outcome" after 6 years and to convert this into knowledge, skills and attitudes with specific educational targets.

Training in Pharmacology, Clinical Pharmacology and Therapeutics at the University in Ghent

The University of Ghent has a solid tradition in pharmacology (Heymans Institute) as well as in clinical pharmacology. The institute has neither its own ward nor its own beds whose patients could be used for teaching in the normal way. There are no formalized agreements on therapeutics between this department and the clinical entities of the university hospital.

The department of general practice was instituted in 1980 and has developed two main activities: teaching and research. There are no facilities for patient care. Patient contact can be offered to the students through an arrangement with general practitioners who collaborate on a voluntary basis.

Pharmacology, clincal pharmacology, and therapeutics are taught in a sequential way: the first two during the 4th and 5th years, the latter during the last 2 years of undergraduate training.

Pharmacology and Clinical Pharmacology: Years Four and Five

The major aim of this course is a transfer of basic knowledge about pharmacology and clinical pharmacology.

Its main characteristics are: (a) the course ist taught by a clinical pharmacologist, (b) there are lectures on specific topics, and (c) its objective is to make rational therapeutic decisions based on scientific data.

Pharmacotherapeutics: Year Six

With their knowledge of pharmacology and pathology, students are invited to go through the process of decisions about therapy. Most attention is paid to the skills. Characteristics of the course are: (a) cooperation between department of pharmacology and department of general practice for the preparation and the presentation of the discussions; (b) small-group teaching; (c) problem solving: cue identification, hypothesis generation, hypothesis testing, development of management strategies, re-evaluation of the hypothesis based on follow-up data; (d) written accounts of simulated patients with problems that can be handled at the level of general practice; (e) objective: rational prescribing on the basis of predefined therapeutic goals.

Each group (10–15 students) has eight sessions of 2 h. Subjects can change from year to year. Some topics are: fever, diarrhoea, acute otitis media, sleeping problems, chronic bronchitis, dysmenorrhoea, fever convulsions, ureteral colic, pharyngitis, anxiety, angina pectoris, peptic ulcer, peripheral vascular problems, vitamin supplements.

Special attention is paid to critical reading about pharmacotherapy. Priority is given to information derived from randomized clinical trials. Elements of prime interest are the effects of therapeutics on significant clinical outcome variables.

Pharmacotherapeutics: Year Seven

There is a specific training programme for students who choose to prepare themselves for general practice. The same sessions as in the 6th year are organised. The major difference to the forgoing year is that now students already have some experience with patient care in general practice.

The small-group teaching follows the same scheme as in the 6th year, with the difference that case histories and experiences with patient behaviour are brought in by the students themselves. Diverse aspects of the learning process are involved: (a) acquisition of new knowledge, relative to a lot of small problems encountered in general practice; (b) skills: dealing with conventional wisdom on therapeutics, handling problems for which there is no rational drug therapy, follow-up of compliance; and (c) attitudes vis-à-vis the patient: cooperation with the patient in planning and performing a therapy.

A series of whole-day discussions are organised in order to repeat and actualise the management of major health problems in general practice. General practitioners, specialists and clinical pharmacologists determine together the content of these meetings.

Vocational Training: Years Eight and Nine

Pharmacotherapy is not a separate topic in (graduate) vocational training. Lack of coordination may be responsible for very divergent messages on therapeutics during the activities that are organised in this period.

Problems and Future Developments

As a consequence of the 86/457 EEC directive, medical schools are invited to organise a program of vocational training for general practitioners. This prolongation of the medical curriculum only makes sense if a continuous programme for undergraduate and vocational training is installed. Teaching activities and contents have to be adapted for the two endpoints: medical doctor and general practitioner. This has to be translated into a logical sequence of educational objectives.

There is still a gap between training in pharmacology/clinical pharmacology and pharmacotherapeutics. There is no reason that the first could not be reoriented towards a more problem-based teaching, as has been done for pharmacotherapeutics. Integration of pharmacotherapeutics with clinical disciplines is necessary.

Evaluation of young doctors shows that they quickly adapt their (prescribing) behaviour to average daily practice medicine. This is quite different from academic medicine. Learned behaviour of patients and physicians is in part responsible for this discrepancy.

Since the practices of the colleagues who are responsible for the clinical training are important places of teaching for primary car, new contact between the university and the supervisors of vocational training is necessary. Training programs for supervisors seem to be a minimal condition in order to conserve the rationality of therapeutics.

During the first 3 years of undergraduate clinical training the major part of the training is hospital-based. Skills and attitudes are learned which are not necessarily adjusted to the work in an ambulatory setting, also with respect to pharmacothrapeutics. Inevitable re-training can be prevented by moving patient contact and specific contents of primary care to the beginning of the curriculum.

Eigenverantwortliche Qualitätsprüfung ärztlichen Verordnungsverhaltens: Wann und wie?

Medical Audit of Prescribing: When and How?

Rational Prescribing: An Exemplar of Auditing Prescribing in Updating a General Practice Formulary

David A. Gregory

Introduction

The idea of producing a general practice formulary was first suggested in 1981 [7]. Several formularies have been developed since by practices alone or in conjunction with neighbouring practices, and by groups of doctors working with university departments and local faculties of the Royal College of General Practitioners [2,3,5,6,8–10]. The aim of a formulary is to foster rational prescribing by selecting a limited number of drugs on the basis of safety, efficacy, convenience and cost [9]. Doctors involved in compiling a formulary can achieve high levels of compliance with it [4,8]. Furthermore, prescribing costs can fall following the introduction of a formulary [2,6], though the likely financial impact is difficult to predict [8].

Method

At a residential weekend course in April 1988, 23 of the 32 general practitioners who teach medical students at Newcastle University were invited to work in small groups on sections of the formulary to decide what amendments should be made. Each group was asked to report back with a list of those drugs to be included and those to be excluded in any second edition. They were invited to use the British National Formulary in particular as an authoritative resource text. A reasonable consensus was eventually achieved in plenary session. The intended changes were noted.

In July 1988 all 32 doctors were requested to record their prescribing over a 2-week period. Each was provided with prescribing tally sheets for recording patient number, presenting complaint, drugs prescribed for new conditions and drugs prescribed as repeat prescriptions. An explanatory letter and specimen tally sheet were enclosed to prevent erroneous recording. All patients consulting were to be recorded, even where no prescription was issued.

At a meeting in January 1989 the detailed analysis and anonymised individual results from the recording exercise were discussed by 25 of the doctors. Final decisions were made about the inclusion and exclusion of drugs. The method of updating (Fig. 1) was the same as that used in the original development of the formulary. The results of the own prescription recording were excluded from the analysis.

Rationale Pharmakotherapie in der Allgemeinpraxis
Rational Pharmacotherapy in General Practice
M. M. Kochen (Hrsg.)

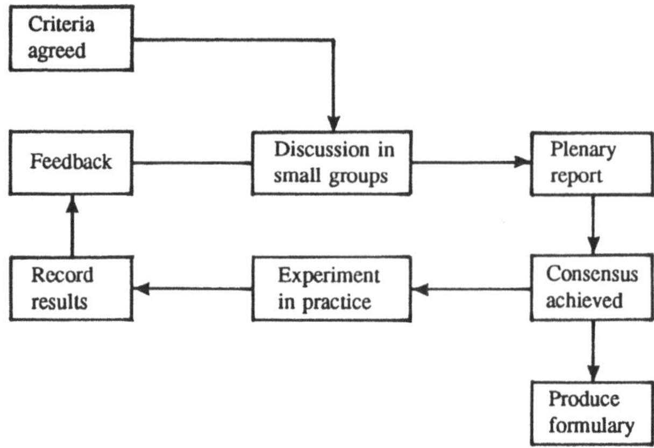

Fig. 1. Steps involved in compiling a formulary

Table 1. Amendments to existing formulary

Drugs to be added	Drugs to be omitted
Acyclovir cream	Benzhexol
Amiloride	Protryptiline
Asilone (a multi-ingredient gastro-intestinal agent)	Hydralazine
Bisacodyl suppositories	Sulphacetamide
Captopril	Trimeprazine
Chlorhexidine mouth wash	
Co-proxamol (dextropropoxyphene and paracetamol)	
Daktacort[a] (contains miconazole and corticosteroid or one of its esters)	
Enalapril	
Ephedrine nasal drops[a]	
Isosorbide mononitrate	
Loperamide	
Marvelon (hormonal contraceptive containing desogestrel and enthinyloestradiol)	
Nalidixic acid	
Oillatum[a] (paraffin and wool alcohol or arachis)	
Otosporin[a] (a multi-ingredient antibacterial agent including neomycin, polymyxin, and hydrocortisone)	
Ranitidine[b]	
Terbutaline	

Notes

[a] Added after January 1989 meeting.

[b] Included in original formulary in the appendix (drugs normally initiated by consultants).

Results

Excluding the authors, 22 of the 29 eligible doctors completed a record of their prescribing. Two doctors were on holiday and five gave no reason for not taking part. Of these 22, 11 had been involved in compiling the original formulary in 1984–1985. The remainder were new recruits to undergraduate teaching. Nineteen practices were represented.

In April 1988 the group decided that 16 preparations should be added, and six dropped from the formulary. After the feedback in January 1989 a further two preparations were included (Table 1) bringing the total to about 160 drugs.

During the 2-week period the group recorded details of 5935 consultations (Table 2). The proportion of patients issued with a prescription varied from 46 % to 83 %, with an average of 65 %, similar to the national average. The proportion of items prescribed generically was 61 % compared with the national average of 37 % and the Newcastle Family Practitioner Committee (FPC) area average of 49 %.

Table 2. Prescriptions issued by 22 doctors

	Total		Range		Average
	n	%	*n*	%	
Number of patients consulted	5935		102–371		270
Number of patients issued script	3835	65	79–259	48–83	174
Total items prescribed	5103		107–456		232
Items prescribed generically	3107	61	60–243	24–92	141
Items for newly diagnosed problems	2909		62–228		132
"New" items in existing formulary	2323	80	50–169	63–100	106
"New" items in amended formulary	2378	82	50–171	62–100	108
Items prescribed as repeat scripts	2194		21–273		100
"Repeat" items in existing formulary	1693	77	18–200	56–99	77
"Repeat" items in amended formulary	1731	79	18–198	62–93	79
Overall compliance existing formulary		79		63–99	
Overall compliance amended formulary		81		65–94	

The group succeeded in prescribing within the existing formulary for 80 % of items (2323 out of 2909) for new (previously undiagnosed) conditions, and within the amended formulary for 82 % of these items (2378 out of 2909). The group performed almost as well with repeat prescriptions (items for previously diagnosed conditions), achieving 77 % compliance (1693 out of 2194) with the existing formulary, and 79 % compliance (1791 out of 2194) with the amended formulary.

The overall compliance of the group for all prescriptions was 79 (4016 out of 5103) with the existing formulary and 81 % (4109 out of 5105) with the amended formulary. Compliance with the amended formulary would have been better if the group had adhered to its decision to exclude co-trimoxazole.

Discussion

On average the 22 doctors who recorded their prescribing achieved 79 % compliance with the existing formulary and 81 % compliance with the amended version. In particular they achieved 77 % compliance with the existing formulary when prescribing for established conditions (repeat prescriptions), a marked increase on the 61 % compliance achieved in 1985 during the original development of the formulary [10]. Although a number of the doctors involved in the current exercise had not been involved in the original formulary, it seems that involvement in compiling a formulary can generate changes that affect not only prescribing for acute conditions but also long-term medication, but it may take several years for such changes to become manifest.

Our experience in compiling the original formulary demonstrated that general practitioners working in groups are able to select drugs rationally. Only minor amendments had been suggested by our clinical pharmacologist adviser. However, where dilemmas cannot be resolved impartial expert adivce is invaluable.

There is general agreement on the criteria for rational prescribing – the prescribed drug should be necessary, effective, safe and economic – but no single method has yet been devised to promote or evaluate good prescribing behaviour [11]. As formularies include drugs selected on the basis of safety, efficacy and economy there is reason to believe that compliance with a formulary could be an index of prescribing competence.

The original Newcastle formulary was compiled over the period of a year, and involved a series of evening meetings, a residential weekend and two prescription recording exercises. Updating the formulary has not been so arduous, but we have relied heavily on the dedication and enthusiasm of the undergraduate clinical tutors. Health authorities and FPCs will need to take account of the commitment required of doctors if "agreed local formularies" are to become a reality.

The study provides a model for the development and updating of such formularies. This does not infringe clinical freedom and offers an alternative to imposed restricted lists or financial sanctions as a means of improving the quality of prescribing and reducing the cost. The model includes the construction of agreed criteria, experimentation in clinical practice, feedback of results and discussion by the participating doctors.

Finally, much attention has been focused on prescribing and the cost of drugs within the National Health Service. The problems in Britain are minor compared to those in other parts of Europe. Drug costs in West Germany, for example, for a similar population are treble those in Britain. In consequence we are collaborating with colleagues from a number of European countries to compile a model European general practice formulary. For this the criteria originally constructed by the Newcastle doctors has been adapted.

References

1. Anonymous (1989) Local drug formularies: are they worth the effort? Drug Ther Bull 27 : 13–16
2. Beardon PHG, Brown SV, Mowat DAE, et al. (1987) Introducing a drug formulary to general practice: effects on prescribing costs. J R Coll Gen Pract 37 : 305–307
3. Field J, Freeman GK (1987) Ten years' prescribing costs at Aldermoor Health Centre. Practitioner 231 : 701–704
4. Grant GB, Gregory DA, van Zwanenberg TD (1985) Development of a limited formulary for general practice. Lancet I : 1030–1032
5. Grant GB, Gregory DA, van Zwanenberg TD (1987) A basic formulary for general practice. Oxford University Press, Oxford
6. Green PE (1985) The general practice formulary: its role in rational therapeutics. J R Coll Gen Pract 35 : 570–572
7. Jolles M (1980) Why not compile your own formulary? J R Coll Gen Pract 31 : 372
8. Knox JDE (1988) Westgate Formulary Project. Final report to the Chief Scientist Organisation. Department of General Practice, University of Dundee
9. Lothian Liaison Committee. Co-ordinator Gilleghan JD (1987) Lothian Formulary No 1
10. Roy Coll Gen Pract, Northern Ireland Faculty. Practice Formulary 1988–90
11. van Zwanenberg TD, Grant GB, Gregory DA (1987) Can rational prescribing be assessed? J R Coll Gen Pract 37 : 308–310

Medical Audit of Prescribing in General Practice

Philip M. Reilly

Some definitions are helpful in minimising jargon and in clarifying what audit means. Audit is the *Enumeration* and *Evaluation* of aspects of medical care against criteria of good practice as developed by the practising general practitioners (GPs) involved. Peer review is the use of medical audit by a group of doctors, all practising in comparable situations in order to measure the quality of care given by each of them and to help each other remedy any defects revealed, in short to try to achieve optimal care.

Peer review in general practice is most acceptable if it is internal to the practice and clinical in content. The working conditions and the type of problems encountered lend themselves to an approach that is informal, voluntary and educational with no sanctions, rather than being formal, statutory, and regulatory with sanctions [9]. This does not imply any lack of rigor by the participants.

Pre-Requisites for Audit

For an audit to lead to improvements in effectiveness or efficiency of medical care it is necessary to complete the following tasks [4, 5]:

1. Define desirable standards, criteria, targets or protocols for good practice (e.g. prescribing) against which performances can be compared.
2. Gather objective evidence about performance systematically.
3. Compare results against standards and/or among peers; negotiating change.
4. Identify deficiencies and taking action to remedy them; mobilising resources.
5. Monitor the effects of action on quality reviewing and renewing the process.

The above sequence is often depicted as a continuous cyclical process, known as the "audit cycle", a cycle reiterating the following steps:

1. Find out what is happening.
2. Decide what should be happening.
3. Introduce change and monitor effects.

Frequently this sequence is left incomplete (e.g. step 3 is never properly carried out) with the production of so-called "orphan" data [7]. All the steps in the sequence are of equal importance. To reap the benefits of audit the full cycle must be completed and repeated [11].

Rationale Pharmakotherapie in der Allgemeinpraxis
Rational Pharmacotherapy in General Practice
M. M. Kochen (Hrsg.)

It is essential that the following propositions be addressed [1]: (a) information produced from an audit will not automatically lead to change, (b) setting a standard may not be easy and may pose practical difficulties, (c) data collection may be laborious especially when added to ordinary day-to-day activities, and (d) active involvement of all participants is not guaranteed.

There is still a major question about feedback [6]. Passive feedback seems to have little effect on clinical practice. Active feedback (implying judgement by recipient), particularly when used in conjunction with guidelines (protocol) does have an impact on clinical practice.

In the current context of prescribing in the UK, even the detailed but passive feedback of prescribing data about one's practice may not alter behaviour or may do so in an undesirable way. This feedback of prescribing data is called PACT (Prescribing Analysis and Cost) and is given to general practitioners at regular intervals, together with a statement of the cost of that prescribing. Prescribing above a certain level of cost will incur a financial penalty to the doctors while prescribing below a certain level, i.e. resulting in savings when compared to the average level of prescribing cost in the area, will result in those savings being spent, not in the practice of the doctors concerned, but in the primary care services of that area. The danger in this situation lies in the possibility of doctors making indiscriminate cuts in their prescribing costs. Such cuts will be much more likely to be attempts at saving, especially when confronted with "high-cost" (in prescribing terms) patients. There is also a possibility that patients with more common but "low-cost" illness would not get the medications they require. The evidence for this latter possibility is poor and comes from sources which might not be entirely objective [13]. But if doctors prepare themselves through making selections of drugs for the various illness they diagnose then it is very likely that prescribing would be appropriate, not just in cost terms, but also in terms of efficacy, safety and acceptability. Such selections of drugs should of course be voluntary and flexible. The essential point is that the very exercise of selection will educate the doctors and develop a constructive policy which will be adhered to especially if the doctors involved have participated actively [3].

What Impedes Change?

Clinical and administrative review in general practice is unsuccessful if the following features are not dealt with successfully [12]: (a) poor/impractical design, (b) excessive servicing of project required, (c) unsatisfactory response by recipients, and (d) unsatisfactory protocol construction.

But even it both design and maintenance of the audit – (a) and (b) above – are acceptable there is still no guarantee that participation leading to effective protocol construction will emerge. This is an important and, as yet, unanswered question in the context of UK prescribing, where detailed feedback systems are already operating.

Undoubtedly points (a) and (b) above do not apply in audits of prescribing as the feedback system is reasonably well-designed and does not require servicing by the general practitioner. Appropriate prescribing will therefore depend on how effectively general practitioners evolve sound prescribing policies and also how well they function as a group.

Levels of group activity occur as follows:

- Defensive and other comments: The group members frequently comment that they are not much good at the task in hand.
- Projective comments: Before long, however, one or more members make more assertive comments: "we are the sort of practice which ..."
- Deficiency acknowledgement: This is especially seen when the group has its own data in front of it.
- Dialogue: As above, especially when everybody knows each other's data.
- Agreement/disagreement: How productive this exchange really is depends on how this group handles the range of committed and other views.
- Construction of protocol: The group needs some form of working consensus as well as knowledge so that members may do specific tasks.
- Implement change: The change must be carried out efficiently and in a committed manner.
- Check that change has taken place: This needs practice organisation as well as commitment.

Groups will not progress beyond the stage of agreement/disagreement unless they work together regularly (at least monthly) and in a manner that caters for the needs of the members as well as the task in hand [8].

What will Increase Changes of Successful Audit in General Practice?

Medical audit will be much more likely to work when the following conditions pertain [10]:

- *Purpose:* relevant to patient care.
- *Control:* by peers, participation voluntary.
- *Method:* non-threatening, interesting, objective, repeatable (i.e. follow-up).
- *Resources:* cheap, simple, causing minimal disturbance to work.
- *Records:* adequate clinical content, retrieval systems essential.
- *Standards:* set locally by participants.

The widespread use of microcomputers in UK general practice may well help develop effective audit of prescribing if the feedback data on prescribing (PACT) come in the form of a hard/soft disc and also give the user an opportunity to manipulate such data and question it imaginatively. Such tasks are quite formidable even then, though groups of peers may be able to determine criteria for audit, they may not be able to adhere to them [2]. A false consensus is reached, apparently to avoid disagreements in the group. There is therefore a failure to work through to the adoption of stringent criteria which the group would then consider its "own" as well as a reluctance to return to cover the particular topic in the future.

In reality [7] only a small proportion of approximately 20 % may actually do the work of setting criteria and applying them to themselves and their colleagues. The majority could later challenge the validity of the chosen criteria when, for example, the data collected shows an unacceptable level of compliance. In attempting to generate a feeling of responsibility for the criteria chosen, the group enlarges and lengthens them. Such developments result in criteria that are less precise and usually less easily audited. Precise criteria are essential if variable quantities of data are to be used and not left unused and even unconsidered – the so-called "orphan" data.

Participants in audit respond best to specific items which, if not attained, are remedied by an education programme which is focused, personal and occurs soon after the audit exercise has stopped. Success is most likely when involvement has been active, addressing an issue documented by clinical research and selected for its importance to patient well-being and for correctability by doctor performance.

Medical audit of prescribing in general practice will require the development of desirable criteria using objective evidence. Where results fall short of selected standards then change will have to be negotiated. A process of education and monitoring are basic to effective audit. Such processes have resource implications but represent a sound investment in the development of competent professionals.

References

1. Crombie DL, Fleming DM (1988) Practice Activity Analysis: Occasional Paper 41. RCGP. London
2. Freeling P, Burton RH (1982) General practitioners and training by audit. J Roy Coll Gen Pract 32:231–237
3. Grant GB, Gregory DA, Van Zwanenberg TD (1985) Development of a limited formulary for general practice. Lancet 1:1030–1032
4. Hughes J, Humphrey C (1990) Medical audit in general practice. King's Fund Centre. London
6. Mitchell MW, Fowkes FGR (1985) Audit renewed: Does feedback on performance change clinical behaviour. J Roy Coll Physicians (London), 19:251–254
7. Nelson AR (1976) Orphan data and the unclosed loop. New Engl J Med 295:617–619
8. Reilly PM (1985) An audit of prescribing by peer review. MD Thesis. The Queen's University of Belfast
9. Shaw CD (1980a) (1) The background. Brit Med J 1:1256–1258
10. Shaw CD (1980) Looking forward to audit. Brit Med J 2:1509–1511
11. Smith T (1990) Medical audit. Brit Med J 300:65
12. Stott NEH, Davis RH (1975) Clinical and administrative review in general practice. J Roy Coll Gen Pract 25:888–896
13. Teeling-Smith G (1991) Patterns of prescribing. Office of Health Economics, London

Plenum 3/Plenary Session 3

A European Formulary for General Practice: State of the Art and Future Developments

George B. Grant

Before dealing with formularies it is good to be reminded of the irrationality in prescribing which often occurs in practice. A few examples will illustrate this. These may be familiar to the readers and if this is the case they do bear repetition. They are taken from three widely different countries. This is no reflection on the countries concerned as many other countries could have been quoted. In each case there is a small text saying why they are irrational, useless for the conditions in which they are used, sometimes addictive, and possibly dangerous.

Notes on Doubtful International Prescribing

Norway

Dimethicone is still used as an over-the-counter drug for colicky babies, although of doubtful efficacy. Combination drugs for migraine containing ergotamine tartrate, caffeine, and an antiemetic with a barbiturate or meprobamate, are widely used and as much as 0.4 defined daily dose (DDD) per 1000 persons are consumed – enough for 430 million persons. These drugs are therefore probably being used excessively in spite of the fact that barbiturates are very addictive and ergotamine very dangerous in excessive dosage. Some other drugs are still registered in Norway despite their dangers, e.g. labetalol.

Germany

Persumbran is a quite well-known proprietary combination drug used quite extensively for angina pectoris. It contains: dipyridamole (25 mg) and oxazepam (10 mg). Dipyridamole is an antiplatelet drug and the British National Formulary warns under cautions: "worsening angina". In fact it is not listed for treating angina. Oxazepam is a benzodiazepine which, although not the most addictive, has bad withdrawal effects that are not desirable, particularly in patients with angina. This preparation is not a good one to use against angina.

Myocardon is another proprietary combination drug used for angina. It consists of: theophylline, phenobarbitone, papaverine, atropine, and glyceryl trinitrate. There is no indication for the use of theophylline against angina and indeed among its cautions and side effects are tachycardia and arrhythmias. There is also a narrow margin between the therapeutic and toxic levels. Phenobarbitone is addictive

Rationale Pharmakotherapie in der Allgemeinpraxis
Rational Pharmacotherapy in General Practice
M. M. Kochen (Hrsg.)

and should not be used. Papaverine is an opium derivative which can produce vascular muscle relaxation but is mostly used after surgery and is most effective by injection. Opiates are liable to misuse. Atropine, an antimuscarinic, has no indication in angina. Hip hip hurrah! Our old and trusted friend glyceryl trinitrate gains a rightful place! In fact, it should be used alone for more effectiveness at much less expense and danger.

Italy

Mucolytics account for about 40 % of drugs prescribed for respiratory conditions. Although they may liquefy the sputum to some extent there is no good evidence that they are better than placebo in improving symptoms. Of all drug packages prescribed in Italy 38 % are for so-called neurotropic drugs or cerebroactive drugs. They are from a rather heterogenous collection of substances and their indications are described as "for peripheral and cerebrovascular conditions". There is no good evidence that these conditions are improved by these widely prescribed drugs. The most commonly prescribed antibiotics by GPs are ceftriaxone and piperacillin. These are only justified in exceptional circumstances. The latter is indicated in infections due to pseudomonas aeruginosa.

These are random and specific examples to illustrate one reason for using a formulary. They may not be typical of whole countries. The following section lists some other reasons.

Drug Formulary

The reasons for employing a formulary include:

- To rationalise a clinician's prescribing.
- To review the use of drugs and their effectiveness.
- To concentrate study in depth to a limited number of drugs.
- To know and balance side effects with therapeutic benefit.
- To study the cost of drugs and their pharmacological equivalents.
- To have a treatment protocol for all doctors in a multidoctor practice.
- To use it for teaching trainee general practitioners (GPs) and students.
- To *promote safety* in prescribing.

The procedure two colleagues and I followed to produce a formulary was:

1. While teaching GP prescribing to students it was necessary to compile a list of drugs for treating particular conditions that could act as an example and a focus for discussion. We did this for a number of common conditions encountered in general practice, e. g. asthma, angina pectoris, throat infections, urinary tract infections, and contraception (in all, for a total of 40 conditions).
2. One of our team, Tim van Zwanenberg, had worked in an underdeveloped country, Papua New Guinea, for some years. Qualified medical doctors were few and far between there and to gain access to a doctor could mean flying

over mountainous rain forests. Therefore, there were trained paramedics who had the main responsibility for primary care. A document was produced which contained the signs and symptoms of conditions likely to be encountered along with their appropriate drug treatment. Dr. van Zwanenberg postulated that about 90 % of conditions in 90 % of the patients met in the average general practice in the UK could be similarly and adequately treated by reference to a limited list of drug preparations. Many of these conditions are self-limiting and only require simple, well-tried, and cheap drugs.

3. We then drew up a list of common conditions in general practice (about 40) which we hoped would cover the 90 %. We wrote short notes about them and made a list of the appropiate drug treatment with dosage, cautions and cost. At a weekend meeting in the English Lake District with about twenty willing and cooperative GP colleagues the list was modified to meet suggestions which had been made by them. We then asked the colleagues to record their prescribing for two weeks using our formulary in treating their patients. They also gave details of age, sex, diagnosis, etc. We had a control group of ten GPs who were not involved with the formulary but who kept a 2-week record also. The draft formulary was discussed again with the group and further modified. Another 2-week record was kept and the results showed that about 75 % of the conditions encountered were on our list and that the members of the special group were able to treat their patients from our formulary in 75 % of cases, whereas the control group used our drugs in only 34 % of cases. The draft was again discussed and modified. It was presented for comment to a professor of clinical pharmacology, Mike Rawlins, who gave it full approval.

The final list contained 137 drugs out of 3000–4000 possible prescribable ones under the National Health Service. It was subsequently published, reprinted, and a second edition published following a revision and review by the larger group (as in the first edition) as "A Basic Formulary for General Practice".

The importance of consultation with colleagues and consultants where appropi-ate cannot be over-emphasised if a formulary is to be accepted by other doctors. This was the lynchpin of our work, of great importance in its acceptance and success.

In 1987 there was a meeting in Bielefeld organised by the Bundeskongress Entwicklungspolitischer Aktionsgruppen (BUKO). In a meeting at a GP workshop the possibility of producing a European Formulary was mooted. Several months later I wrote to the participants inviting their interest. There was enough support and enthusiasm to set up the first meeting in Bremen in June 1988. Five countries were involved at that time and at that meeting it was decided to go ahead. We have since had meetings in Bremen, Newcastle, Stockholm, and Rouen; and editorial meetings in Holland and Belgium. There are now fourteen countries involved: Austria, Belgium, Czechoslovakia, Eire, France, Germany, Holland, Italy, Norway, Poland, Portugal, Spain, Sweden and United Kingdom (with England, Scotland, and Northern Ireland represented). We call ourselves the *European Formulary Group* (EFG).

Since we had a larger group than was manageable for detailed study we formed an editorial committee representative of the following areas: Scandanavia, the Low Countries, Germany, UK, and southern Europe. Although each country had only one or two representatives they had a team behind their representatives at home who all contributed to the work of producing the formulary. The method of working which we adopted was quite simple. Each country took a disease or symptom complex and produced a protocol for treating it, e. g. Germany took "pain and terminal care", and the UK the "gastrointestinal system". These protocols were studied in detail first by the editorial committee, which was representative of each of the five aforementioned general geographical areas, and subsequently by the whole EFG, which suggested changes etc. and which, of course, determined general policy. This system works well and agreement was usually reached quite easily.

Last year the WHO agreed to support the EFG. This was a major breakthrough. Their help was to consist of support for the publication of the European Formulary. They laid down, however, two important conditions on which their support depended. The EFG thought that they were very reasonable and agreed to them. They were, first, that a separate appendix to the formulary should be published relative to it, giving reasons for the prescribing of particular drugs and giving the appropriate references in the literature or reports of clinical trials, and second, that when completed these texts should be scrutinised by university departments of clinical pharmacology and general practice or their equivalents. The recommendations of these expert authorities would be taken into consideration by the EFG and alterations made where necessary. The completed formulary would then be acceptable to the WHO and published.

A detailed working plan for the formulary was drawn up and following the meeting in Rouen (June 1990) contributions were written in the new format and the appendix was supplemented. It means in fact that the formulary, in addition to being a handy and usable tool in general practice and teaching, will be backed up in the appendix by references which point to the scientific reasoning behind the recommendations. The language adopted in meetings, letters and all documents is English, being the one most favoured by the EFG members and also the most practicable. However, the formulary will require translating into other languages in countries where the medical and pharmaceutical professions are not very conversant with English.

It is hoped that the formulary will be distributed widely so that as many doctors in general practice in Europe as possible will have the opportunity to use it.

If accepted there could be far-reaching effects such as:

1. To enable patients requiring ongoing drug treatment who migrate across European frontiers to continue with their concurrent treatment.
2. To reduce the number of identical drugs used internationally.
3. To encourage drug manufacturers to review their policies.
4. Hopefully, to drastically reduce national drug costs which are very often too high for the benefits obtained, e. g. in the UK £2 500 000 000 per annum.

5. To direct the thoughts of prescribers to the doubtful benefit of using a new drug over a well-tried and satisfactory one.

What of the Future?

It will be necessary to update the EF regularly, perhaps producing a quarterly bulletin. Doctors should be encouraged to produce their own formulary, but they do need expert back-up in many cases, to make the right decisions. They also have not the time to start a formulary from the very basics. Using the EF as a basis and receiving advice from the EFG would make this simpler and safer. This would require the setting up of an advice centre. It in turn would need a secretariat to deal with these functions. The educational advantage of this course of action would be very great. Perhaps in each country, or centrally, lecturers could run short courses for GPs to update their pharmacological knowledge.

Our aim is to have the EF published and widely accepted. This in my view will only be possible if as many people as possible contribute advice and criticism. This was how we did it in 1987 in Newcastle and we should follow that pattern in Europe.

References

1. Grant GB, Gregory DA, van Zwanenberg TD (1985) Development of a limited formulary for general practice. Lancet 1: 1030–1033
2. Grant GB, Gregory DA, van Zwanenberg TD (1987) A basic formulary for general practice. Oxford University Press, Oxford

Rational Discussion as a Guide to More Cost-Effective and Scientific Prescribing in General Practice: 15 Years of Experience in Northern Ireland

Hugh McGavock

Introduction

Northern Ireland is a province of the United Kingdom of about 170 km^2. Its population of ca. 1.6 million is located in one medium-sized city, one small city, a series of small towns and a fertile and beautiful countryside. Medical care (of a high standard) and prescriptions are free for most people at the point of delivery, paid for by a levy on all salaries.

There are 955 general practitioners (GPs), working in 347 practices, of which about 15 % are single-handed. Most GPs are graduates of the universities of Belfast or Dublin and professional relationships are generally friendly and cooperative. Since 1976, all practices have received a prescribing analysis visit about once every 3 years. High-cost practices have been visited annually. The prescribing visitor has always been a government doctor with wide previous experience of general practice. Visits have always been voluntary. Not once in 15 years has a prescribing visitor been refused a 1-h appointment. All partners in a practice are usually present for the prescribing visit. The result has been GP self-regulation, so that Northern Ireland has among the most economical prescribing in Europe – only Denmark and Great Britain have lower drug costs.

Why Bother with GP Prescribing Analysis?

GP prescribing analysis and the self-regulation which it stimulates are important for two reasons. The first is the ethical dilemma of the 1990s, i.e. no nation can now afford to offer all its citizens the full range of medical care currently available. Governments, medical insurance companies and doctors therefore have a duty to maximize cost-effectiveness in medical care to make available resources stretch as far as possible – to offer as much medical care to as many people as possible. The second reason is the ethical and legal demand that prescribing must be as rational and scientific as possible. For the GP using almost the entire range of medicines, this is a very difficult task. One of the best ways of achieving it is to feed back to doctors an analysis of their own prescribing, which has been scrutinized and annotated by a knowledgeable doctor, pharmacist or clinical pharmacologist. Experience in Northern Ireland shows that this feedback is most powerful when the scrutineer accompanies his/her scrutiny!

Rationale Pharmakotherapie in der Allgemeinpraxis
Rational Pharmacotherapy in General Practice
M. M. Kochen (Hrsg.)

What are the Essential Prerequisites for Success in GP Prescribing Feedback?

There are three essential prerequisites for success in feedback: First, there must be an accurate, comprehensive, and up-to-date computerized prescribing data base from which to extract doctors' prescribing profiles. Second, the GPs must be willing to cooperate. This should be a voluntary self-regulation exercise, not a coercive one. Third, the prescribing visitor must have a good knowledge of clinical pharmacology, adequate experience of general practice or community pharmacy and must also have the ability to stimulate doctors' interest in and commitment to self-regulation. He must be a true evangelist! All these desiderata exist in Northern Ireland, and the remainder of this paper describes what has been done there over the past 10 years.

Achieving More Cost-Effective Prescribing

This is the easiest part of the prescribing visit, because it is self-evident. It does not matter whether a doctor's prescribing is above or below the national average in frequency or cost, it can always be made more cost-effective, as Table 1 shows. We call it our 'best buys' list, and the savings shown were those of a four doctor practice approved for training young GPs in their final year before accreditation. This practice was already quite cost-effective – 5 % below the national average. Yet Table 1 shows that those doctors could have saved £33 852 per annum (ca. DM 100 000), and improved the quality of prescribing in the process. The first part of Table 1 shows the benefits of using generic drugs whenever a medicine's patent has elapsed. The second part is on a more scientific basis, but still with a view to cost-effectiveness.

Most doctors accept Table 1 quite quickly, but only a minority of practices implement it fully. When they do, the results are dramatic, as Table 2 shows. This shows that after two prescribing analysis visits, five inner-city GPs in a deprived area reduced their prescribing costs from 39 % above average to 5 % above average, with a similar trend in frequency of prescribing. Table 3 is more typical. It shows a 3 % reduction in GP prescribing costs following prescribing analysis visits carried out in May 1990. No visits have been omitted from Table 3, and in 21 matched but unvisited practices, there was a 2 % (seasonal) reduction. Hence, the prescribing visits achieved a 1 % improvement in cost-effectiveness, £1 000 000 p.a. for Northern Ireland.

Achieving More Rational Prescribing

A study I did in 1984 [1] showed a wide variation in the ways GPs used different drug groups, as Tables 4 and 5 show. The disturbing feature is that this variation occurs not only in drugs used to treat symptoms (Table 4), but also in important powerful therapeutic agents used only after careful diagnosis (Table 5).

Table 1. 'Best buys' list applied to a four doctor inner-city practice, resulting in annual savings of £33 852

Cost-effective uses of generic drugs		Approximate saving/month (£)
Central Nervous System		
Amitriptyline BP	Tryptizol costs 3 times as much	10
Haloperidol BP	Serenace cost 3 times as much	
Imipramine BP	Tofranil costs 3 times as much	
Temazepam BP	Other short-acting hypnotics cost 2–3 times more	46
Cardiovascular system		
Dispersible aspirin BP	Other antiplatelet drugs cost 7–12 times more	
Frusemide BP	Lasix costs 3–10 times as much	35
Methyldopa BP	Aldomet costs twice as much	57
Oxprenolol BP	Trasicor costs twice as much	
Propranolol BP	Inderal costs 4–6 times as much	39
Spironolactone BP	Aldactone costs 3 times as much	82
Peripheral vasodilators 'Not worth giving'	See BNF note, please	503
Respiratory System		
Salbutamol tabs BP	Ventolin tabs costs 25% more	
Pseudoephedrine BP	Sudafed costs twice as much	28
Gastrointestinal tract		
Metoclopramide BP	Maxolon costs 4 times as much	39
Nonsteroidal anti-inflammatory drugs		
Ibuprofen BP	Brufen costs twice as much	129
Indomethacin BP	Indocid cost upt to 5 times as much	22
Naproxen BP	Naprosyn costs 50% more	85
Antibiotics		
Ampicillin BP	Penbritin cost twice as much	24
Amoxycillin BP	Amoxil cost 20% more	66
Co-trimoxazole BP	Septrin costs 4 times as much } Bactrim costs 3 times as much }	64
Erythromycin tabs	Erymax costs 4 times as much	
Metronidazole BP	Flagyl costs 3 times as much	20
Exytetracycline BP	Imperacin costs twice as much	
Tetracycline BP	Achromycin costs twice as much	5
Trimethoprim BP	Ipral + Monotrim costs up to 80% more	
Others		
Allopurinol BP	Zyloric cost up to 7 times as much	161
Subtotal saved		1 415 per month

Table 1 (continued)

Medical reasons for cost-effective drug choices	Approximate saving/month (£)
1. Most elderly patients on Moduretic for mild hypertension could be prescribed bendrofluazide 2.5 mg as a safer and cheaper alternative (see BNF).	30
NB Hyponatraemia is a greater risk in elderly patients given Moduretic than those treated with a thiazide alone. Most patients on treatment with a low dose thiazide do not need a potassium-sparing diuretic, or a potassium supplement.	
2. Elderly patients on Frumil are at risk of hyperkalaemia. Frusemide with a potassium supplement may be better in the majority of cases.	13
3. Most patients on Natrilix could be prescribed bendrofluazide 2.5 mg as a cheaper alternative, effective in treating mild hypertension.	168
4. Safety note: Do not use a potassium supplement or K^+ sparing diuretic with an ACE inhibitor, or cyclosporin or in renal impairment.	
5. For most general practice infections, cephalosporins are not recommended as first choice (see BNF). Apply saving to a better therapy	595
6. The new, potent, broad-spectrum oral cephalosporin, cefuroxime (Zinnat) should not be used in general practice without very good reason, and never presumptively.	
7. Ampicillin caps BP should be prescribed in place of amoxycillin caps BP which are 4 times more expensive. (They now have similar antibacterial spectra).	
8. The new 4-quinolone, ciprofloxacin (Ciproxin), should not be used in general practice without very good reason, and never presumptively (see BNF).	
9. Cimetidine (Tagamet or Dyspamet) remains by far the most cost-effective H^2-blocker. Ranitidine (Zantac) need only be considered where cimetidine is contraindicated. (See BNF, Appendix 1, Histamine section).	600
Monthly total	2821/month ×12
Total yearly savings of about ⟶	33 852 pa

All the above generics are available to all community pharmacists. All the above generics are subject to the same statutory quality surveillance and legal constraints as the more costly proprietaries.
BNF, British National Formulary; BP, British Pharmacopoeia.

Table 2. The effect of good prescribing feedback. This table shows how effective a yearly visit was to a busy inner-city practice in a relatively deprived area of Belfast

Year	Prescribing cost (% above national average)	Prescribing frequency (% above national average)	
1984	39	40	Visit 1
1985	11	29	Visit 2
1986	5	14	

Table 3. Gross prescribing costs for practices visited during June 1990. (Cost comparison for month before and month after visit)

Practice no.	Above or below Northern Ireland average (%)	Gross costs May 1990 (£)	Gross costs July 1990 (£)	Gross costs Results (£)	Change as % of May
1	+32	26 994.13	25 973.21	–1 021	– 4.8
2	+ 7	10 362.41	9 476.52	– 886	– 8.6
3	+13	9 228.67	9 202.48	– 26	– 0.3
4	+ 7	44 089.69	51 952.61	+7 863	+17.8[a]
5	+10	28 998.22	27 990.17	–1 008	– 3.5
6	+15	60 724.58	57 794.00	–2 930	– 4.8
7	+16	10 247.96	9 329.78	– 916	– 9.0
8	– 8	26 080.65	33 084.52	+7 004	+26.9[a]
9	+ 3	45 149.00	41 603.56	–3 546	– 7.9
10	+17	44 937.69	43 838.74	–1 099	– 2.4
11	– 9	32 814.67	29 402.19	–3 412	–10.4
12	+ 3	14 785.54	13 950.73	– 835	– 5.6
13	+47	11 801.18	11 541.52	– 260	– 2.2
14	+ 3	63 021.43	60 606.21	–2 415	– 3.8
15	+22	42 169.87	39 209.93	–2 960	– 7.0
16	–	39 644.44	38 393.69	–1 251	– 3.2
17	– 8	16 528.38	15 577.80	– 951	– 5.8
18	+17	23 111.20	21 436.55	–1 675	– 7.2
19	–47	22 639.92	22 646.88	+ 7	0
20	+ 9	70 541.17	65 029.42	–5 512	– 7.8
21	+33	37 101.15	31 295.78	–5 805	–15.6

Net = 18(–) £ 36 510
3(+) £ 14 874

Total = –£ 21 636

% Change, May-July 1990, visited practices = –3.2 %

[a] Practices 4 and 8 told the visiting doctor that they intended to *increase* costs in protest against government policy.

Table 4. Differences in 'symptomatic' prescribing between low-cost and high-cost doctors

Type of Medicine	Additional prescriptions of high-cost doctors (%)[a]	Additions according to drug form (%)[b]
Hypnotics	80	94 more tablets
Minor analgesics	45	55 more tablets 75 more liquid
Antacids	39	67 more tablets 46 more liquid
Laxatives	47	40 more tablets 70 more liquid
Cough medicines	32	48 more liquid
Anti-rheumatics (NSAID)	44	42 more tablets
Vitamins	69	49 more tablets 37 more liquid

[a] Prescriptions per 1000 patients per month.
[b] Quantity per 1000 patients per month.

Table 5. Differences in 'specific' prescribing (drugs given to remedy identified pathology, low-cost vs. high-cost doctors)

Type of Medicine	Additional prescriptions of high-cost doctors (%)[a]	Addition according to drug form (%)[b]
All heart drugs (except antihypertensives)	48	37 more tablets
Diuretics	57	51 more tablets
Anti-Asthmatics	39	66 more tablets 87 more liquid 20 more inhalters
Hypoglycaemics	40	37 more tablets 61 more insulin
Thyroid and anti-thyroid drugs	64	50 more tablets

[a] Prescriptions per 1000 patients per month.
[b] Quantity per 1000 patients per month.

Table 6. The main therapeutic groups in a teleological classification reflecting perceived use in general practice

Drug type	Therapeutic group
Specific	Anticonvulsants Antiparkinson drugs Antidepressants Heart preparations Diuretics Antihypertensives Asthma preparations Hypoglycaemic agents Corticosteroids Thyroid/Anti-thyroid agents Anticoagulants Vaginal preparations Eye preparations Dressings Appliances
Symptomatic	Hypnotics Analgesics minor Antacids Laxatives Expectorant/cough suppressants Anti-inflammatory (rheumatism) Vitamins Antihistamines Hosiery
Often Presumptive	Sedatives/tranquillisers Tagamet/Zantac etc. Vasodilators/vasoconstrictors Penicillins Other anti-microbials Topical skin preparations

As a result, I constructed a new drug classification (Table 6) for the purpose of analysing the teleological use of drugs. We now have this computerized and can produce such analyses once a month for every practice in Northern Ireland. Table 6 classifies drugs according to the degree of specificity of their use in general practice. The potential of such teleological classification for revealing patterns of prescribing was demonstated in 1988 [1]. In that study, prescribing was divided into:

1. *Specific prescribing*. The criteria for inclusion of a drug or drug group in this catgory were that (a) before a drug is used there is always an accurate diagnosis, often confirmed by laboratory or other investigations and often by a specialist; (b) the drug must be known to intervene in a specific and well-understood manner to alter the pathophysiology in the patient's favour.

2. *Symptomatic prescribing*. Here, the criterion is that such drugs relieve symptoms with no effect or slight effect on the disease process.

Numerous discussions with GPs in different parts of the UK revealed the need for the addition of at least one further group to this classification. Many colleagues agreed that there are several important, potent therapeutic groups which ought correctly to be used only as specifics, with firm diagnoses, but which they were in the habit of using on the basis of a presumptive diagnosis on "therapeutic trial". They included several expensive preparations with well-recognised side effects, like antibiotics, the histamine H_2-antagonists and the peripheral vasodilators. Often, but not always, there was no intention of conducting laboratory, x-ray or other studies to verify the presumptive diagnosis. That is, the indication for these drugs is "*often presumptive*". The premise is that the quantity of 'specific' drugs should be a function of the amount of serious pathology diagnosed and treated in a practice. The 'symptomatic' drugs should reflect the practices' response to patients' symptoms. The problem with the interpretation of the 'presumptive' drugs is that we do not know what proportion was used for an exact diagnosis, and what proportion was used without adequate verification. We are currently using this specific/symptomatic/presumptive (SSP) classification on a trial basis during our prescribing visits. We use it in two ways: (a) aggregated and (b) by individual therapeutic group.

Figures 1–4 show the aggregated histograms for SSP analysis in four very different practices. Figure 1 shows the prescribing frequencies of a single-handed GP with high prescription frequency for specific drugs and low frequency for both symptomatic and often presumptive drugs. Figure 2 shows a practice of five doctors with high prescription frequency for specific drugs but also high in symptomatic and often presumptive medication. Figure 3 shows a practice with four doctors whose specific prescribing frequency is low but whose use of symptomatic and often presumptive drug groups is high. Figure 4 shows a practice of three doctors whose frequency of prescribing is low in all drug groups. Our initial interpretation of these very different patterns would be that, prima facie, Fig. 1 is optimal, Fig. 2 good but could be improved considerably, particularly by reviewing the use of the often presumptive drug group. Figures 3 and 4 should probably give the doctors cause for concern. Before using such graphs routinely in a feedback mode to GPs however, two further steps are required:

1. Quantity per prescription must be specified. These data are not at present available to us. The best we can do is to assume that if the cost per prescription is similar to average, then the quantity per prescription is probably likewise average. Figures 1–4 have been selected on this basis.
2. The "specific" category must be calibrated against recorded morbidity and workload in an adequate sample of practices, before we may assume that prescribing in this category is a function of screening, diagnosis and treatment of serious illness.

While aggregated feedback may be useful, it is the feedback by therapeutic group which is the more powerful and specific stimulus for the prescribers. Table 7

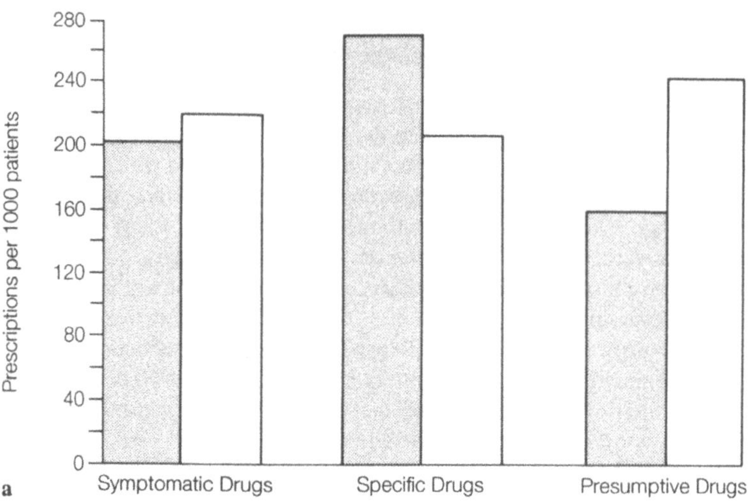

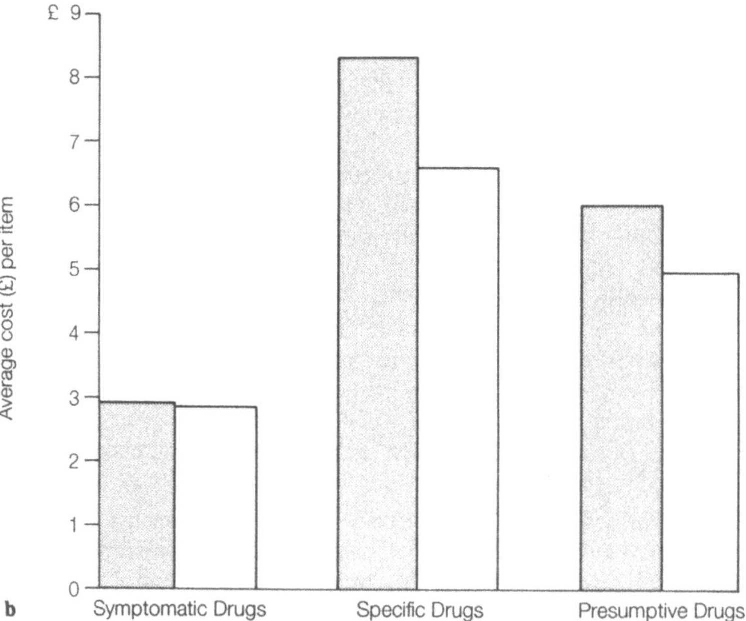

Fig. 1. Monthly prescribing frequency (**a**) and prescribing cost (**b**) in a single-handed practice as compared with Northern Ireland as a whole. The single-handed practice has an average frequency of symptomatic drugs, but 28 % above average for specific drugs and 35 % below average for presumptive drugs. Cost per prescription is £2 greater than average, for specific drugs, £1 greater, for presumptive drugs. *Dark bars*, practice; *light bars*, Northern Ireland

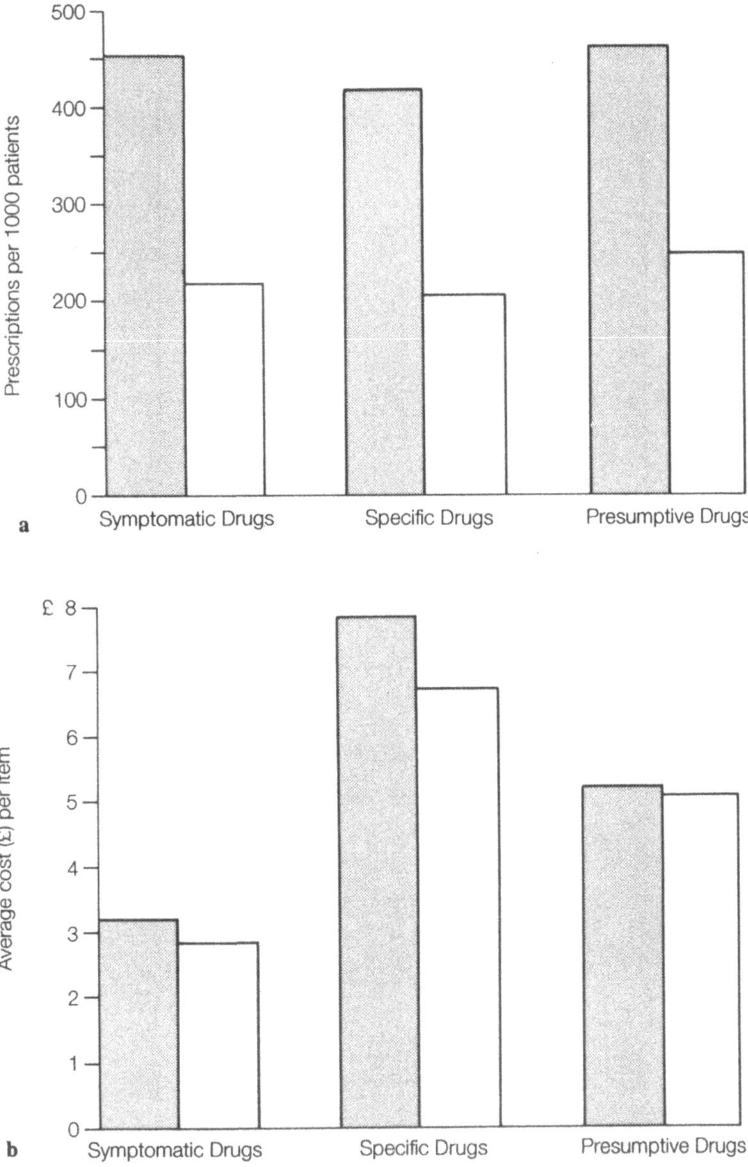

Fig. 2. Monthly prescribing frequency (**a**) and prescribing cost (**b**) of a five-doctor practice as compared with Northern Ireland as a whole. The practice has a prescribing frequency over 100% higher than average in all groups, and cost for specific drugs over £1 per scrip greater than average. ***Dark bars***, practice; ***light bars***, Northern Ireland

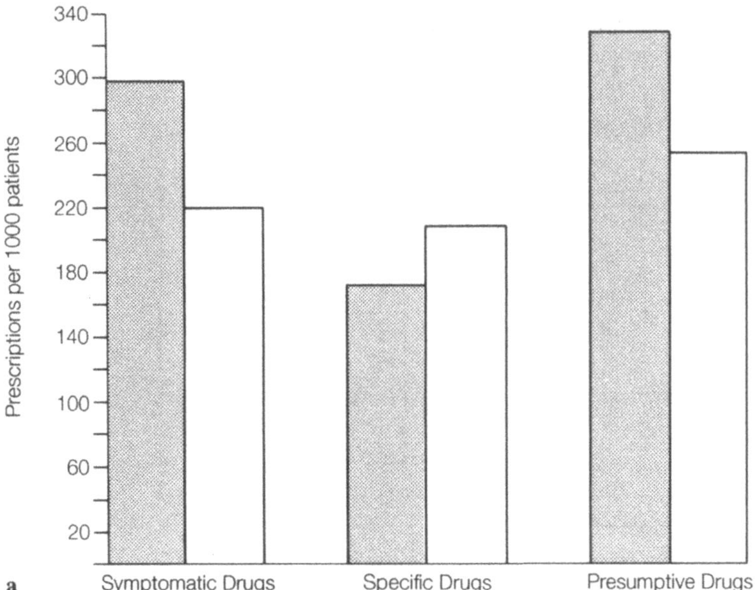

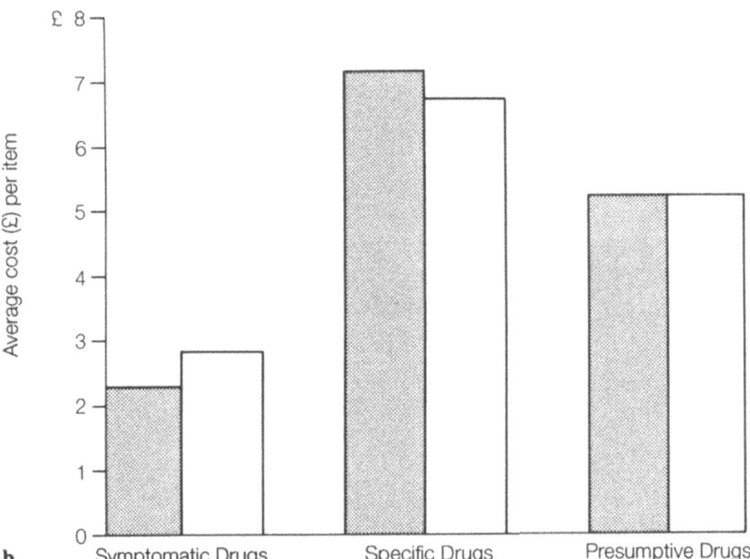

Fig. 3. Monthly prescribing frequency (**a**) and prescribing cost (**b**) of a four-doctor practice as compared with Northern Ireland as a whole. The practice has a prescribing frequency 36 % above average for symptomatics, 32 % above for presumptives but 17 % below average for specific drugs

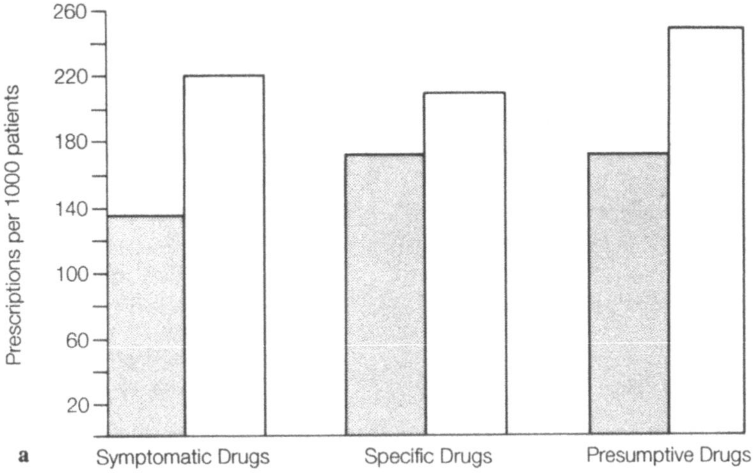

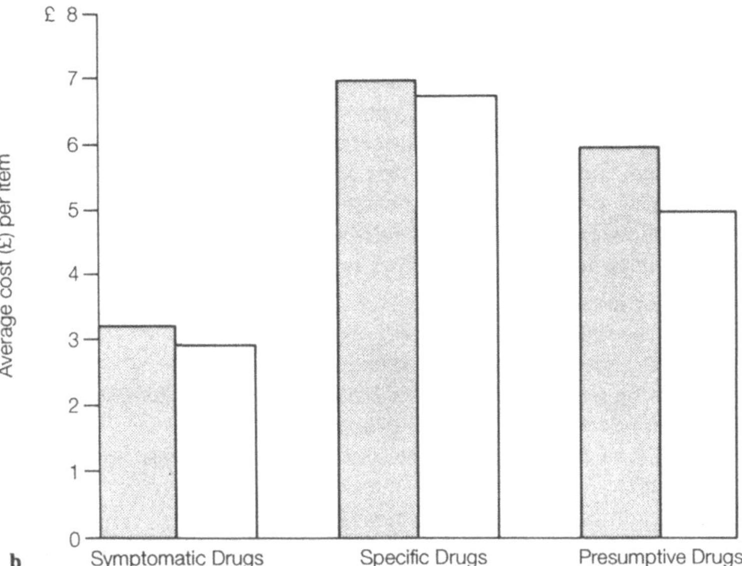

Fig. 4. Monthly prescribing frequency (**a**) and prescribing cost (**b**) of a three-doctor practice as compared with Northern Ireland as a whole. The practice has a prescribing frequency below average by 39% for symptomatics, 17% for specifics and 30% for presumptive drugs. Cost for presumptives was 95p per scrip greater than average. *Dark bars*, practice; *light bars*, Northern Ireland

Table 7. How you might use comparative prescribing data

Your data show that you are:	Discussion topic – should you, the GP:
↓	↓
High on particular symptomatic treatments	Review your policies re patients' symptoms?
Low on insulin prescribing	Screen for glycosuria?
High on oral hypoglycaemic prescribing	Check whether patients are complying with their non-drug regimen?
High on NSAID prescribing	1. Start practice policy on prescribing for joint pain? 2. Check hemoglobin of all on NSAID?
High on antibiotic prescribing	Audit your criteria for antibiotic prescribing?
Low on antiasthmatic inhaler prescribing	Measure peak expiratory flow rate every time you auscultate a chest?

shows a few of the suggestions we make to our colleagues from analysis of their own prescribing patterns. If this could be done at least once a year, there should be a great national increase in rational prescribing over the next decade – and all by self-regulation.

At every prescribing analysis visit, we also give the GPs an up-to-date booklet containing 50 pages of important therapeutic notes directly relevant to everyday family medicine. We tell them if they are using outdated drugs, giving the reasons for changing to more effective or safer drugs.

The following gives a few examples of some questions often raised by feedback of prescribing patterns. Are the doctors aware of:

- Changes in antibiotic spectra?
- Drugs that induce liver enzymes?
- Problems with low-dose oral contraceptives?
- Misuse by patients of oral hypoglycaemic agents or lipid-lowering agents?
- Their levels of benzodiazepine prescribing?
- The risk of inadvertent self-poisoning with slow-release theophylline/aminophylline?
- Cardiac drugs that can cause heart failure?
- The relationship between the half-life of nonsteroidal antiinflammatory agents and gastrointestinal symptoms/ulceration/haemorrhage?
- Their ratio of symptomatic to 'specific therapeutic' prescribing?

We advise our colleagues on using a practice formulary. Our visits to doctors are supported by an occasional television and radio campaign to the public, advising people not to expect a medicine for every little malaise, to use their doctors' time considerately and to seek information about medicines from their community pharmacist. Doctors express their appreciation of this publicity, which helps them to refuse a prescription when necessary.

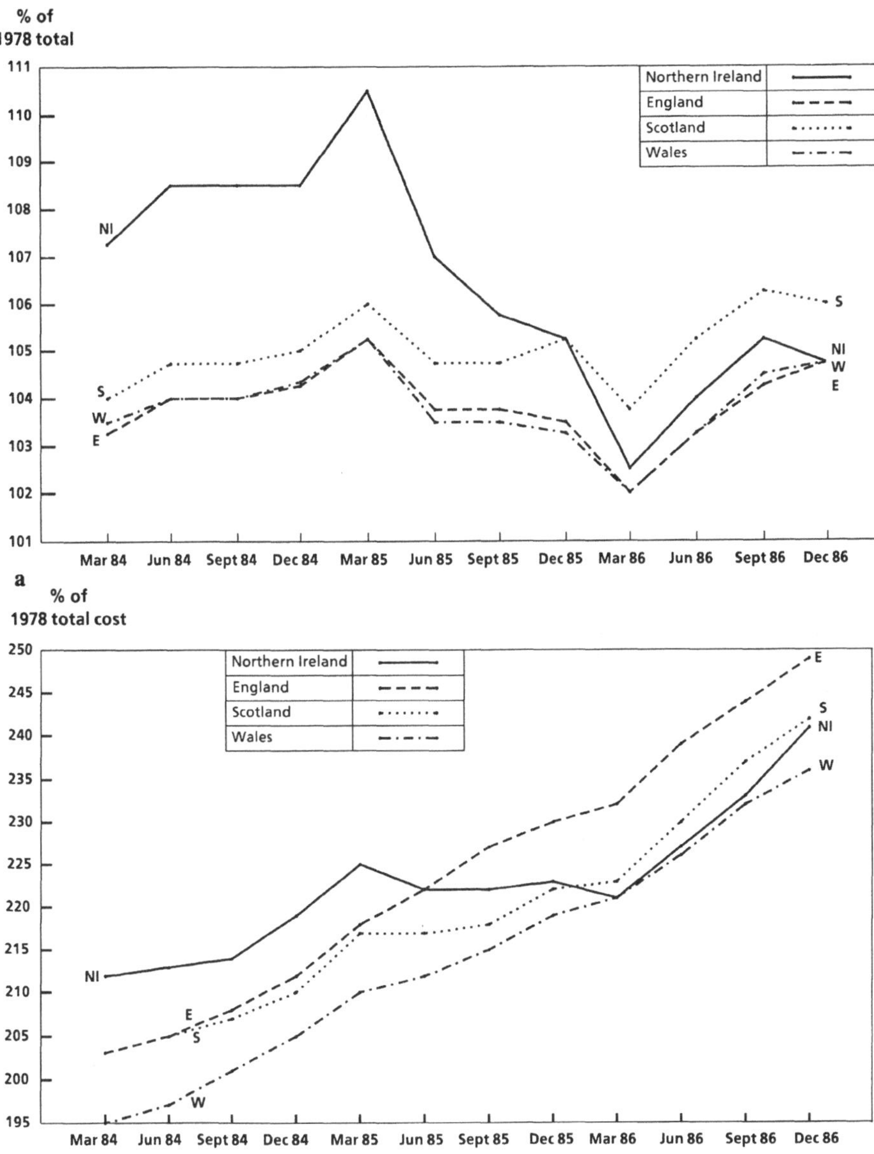

Fig. 5. Quarterly percentage increase in **a** total numbers of GP prescriptions and **b** gross GP prescribing cost in Northern Ireland as compared with England, Wales and Scotland, 1978–1986 (numbers and cost in 1978 = 100 %)

Do the Prescribing-Analysis Visits Work?

Tables 2 und 3 show that the prescribing analysis visits do work. Figure 5 shows the power of this technique by comparing prescribing frequency (Fig. 5a) and cost (Fig. 5b) in Northern Ireland with those in England, Wales and Scotland (where only very high-cost practices are visited, on the basis of economy alone). The techniques described here were used from 1984 to 1986 and only one visit was possible to each practice. The result, in the three years shown, was a notional saving, vis-à-vis England and Wales, of £6.4 million, and all of this money was used for other medical services in GP and hospital. Our Minister of Health wrote to all GPs in Northern Ireland congratulating and thanking them for their remarkable achievement.

Conclusion

Over a 10-year period, we in Northern Ireland have shown that cost-effectiveness and rationality of prescribing by GP's can be improved by regular accompanied feedback of their own prescribing records, suitably analysed and interpreted. We believe that a similar response could be achieved wherever there is a suitable computerized data base. Great Britain has adopted the Northern Ireland model as part of its current major National Health Service reorganisation.

Reference

1. McGavock H (1988) Some patterns of prescribing by urban general practitioners. Br Med J 296 : 900–902

Möglichkeiten und Grenzen des Wirksamkeitsnachweises beim niedergelassenen Allgemeinarzt aus der Sicht der medizinischen Biometrie

Joerg Hasford

Die Phasen der klinischen Prüfung

Bevor ein Arzneimittel in der Bundesrepublik Deutschland vom Bundesgesundheitsamt zugelassen werden kann, muß es in einer Reihe von Studien auf seine Wirksamkeit und Verträglichkeit untersucht worden sein. Diese Untersuchungen am Menschen *vor* der Zulassung werden international in die Phasen I–III der klinischen Prüfung gegliedert [4].

In der *Phase I* der klinischen Prüfung wird das Arzneimittel zum ersten Mal am Menschen angewendet. An kleinen Gruppen meist gesunder Probanden wird die Pharmakokinetik, Bioverfügbarkeit, Toleranz und Verträglichkeit bei ein- und mehrfacher Gabe verschiedener Dosierungen des Arzneimittels untersucht. Auch erste orientierende Untersuchungen zur Eignung für die geplante Indikation können stattfinden. Phase-I-Studien werden – wegen des erforderlichen Diagnose- und Beobachtungsaufwandes sowie der Notwendigkeit, mögliche unerwünschte Wirkungen unverzüglich optimal behandeln zu können, – unter stationären Bedingungen durchgeführt.

In der *Phase II* wird das Arzneimittel an etwas größeren Kollektiven (Fallzahl ~ 50–300) sorgfältig ausgewählter Kranker im angestrebten Indikationsgebiet bezüglich Wirksamkeit, Verträglichkeit und Dosierung untersucht. Auch die Studien dieser Phase finden überwiegend im stationären Bereich statt, wobei es jedoch bereits – indikationsabhängig – Ausnahmen geben kann.

In der *Phase III* werden Wirksamkeit und Verträglichkeit in der breiteren Anwendung geprüft (Fallzahl ~ 300–3000) wobei die Studienbedingungen der angestrebten Anwendungssituation *nach* der Zulassung deutlich stärker entsprechen. Die untersuchten Kollektive sind größer, die Behandlungs- und Beobachtungsdauer jeweils länger. Die Patienten können Begleiterkrankungen haben und entsprechende Begleittherapien erhalten. Werden die Patienten später überwiegend ambulant behandelt, so werden Studien der Phase III auch mit niedergelassenen Ärzten und deren ambulanten Patienten durchgeführt.

Die folgenden Ausführungen konzentrieren sich dementsprechend auf die Möglichkeiten, Phase-III-Studien beim niedergelassenen Allgemeinarzt gemäß dem Stand der Wissenschaft durchzuführen.

Rationale Pharmakotherapie in der Allgemeinpraxis
Rational Pharmacotherapy in General Practice
M. M. Kochen (Hrsg.)

Juristische Vorbedingungen

Die klinische Prüfung ist eine im zweiten Arzneimittelgesetz verankerte Voraussetzung für die Zulassung von Arzneimitteln in der Bundesrepublik Deutschland [2]. Insbesondere §§40–42 befassen sich mit den Anforderungen, denen klinische Prüfungen genügen müssen. Der Arzt, der sich an einer klinischen Prüfung beteiligt, leistet also einen Beitrag, der zur Erfüllung gesetzlicher Vorschriften erforderlich ist. Die Teilnahme von Ärzten an klinischen Prüfungen ist zudem ein wichtiger, weil unverzichtbarer Beitrag zur Erkenntisgewinnung. Ohne klinische Prüfung kein arzneimitteltherapeutischer Fortschritt.

Die im Bundesanzeiger veröffentlichte Bekanntmachung von Grundsätzen für die ordnungsgemäße Durchführung der klinischen Prüfung von Arzneimitteln vom 9. Dezember 1987 regelt rechtlich verbindlich die Planung, Durchführung, Auswertung und Dokumentation klinischer Prüfungen [1].

Die Berufsordnungen für Ärzte aller Bundesländer schreiben vor, daß der Prüfplan einer unabhängigen und sachkundigen Ethikkommission zur Beratung vorgelegt werden muß.

Die Phase-III-Studie

Konzeption

Typischerweise werden die Studien der Phase III randomisiert durchgeführt: der Patient erhält, nachdem vom Arzt geprüft wurde, ob er den Aufnahmekriterien der Studie genügt (s. Anhang) und nachdem der Patient seine informierte Zustimmung zur Teilnahme an der Prüfung erteilt hat, per Zufallsverteilung eine der Studientherapien. Dieser Vorgang wird mit dem Ausdruck Randomisierung bezeichnet. Die Patienten werden dann prüfplangemäß behandelt und beobachtet. Die Kenngrößen, die über den Therapieerfolg Aufschluß geben sollen (= Zielkriterien- oder -größen), werden erhoben und zwischen den Gruppen der unterschiedlich behandelten Patienten statistisch verglichen. Die Quelle der Erkenntnis der Therapieforschung ist immer der Vergleich zwischen unterschiedlich behandelten Patienten.

Die Aussagekraft dieses Vergleichs und somit der klinischen Prüfung hängt ganz wesentlich von 2 Faktoren ab, auf deren Bedeutung und Realisierbarkeit beim niedergelassenen Allgemeinarzt näher eingegangen wird: von der Randomisierung und der Beobachtungsgleichheit.

Randomisierung und Strukturgleichheit

Der Vergleich zwischen unterschiedlich behandelten Patienten ist nur dann aussagekräftig, wenn die Patienten zu Anfang der Studie vergleichbar waren. Unter dieser Eigenschaft, die auch als Strukturgleichheit bezeichnet wird, versteht man, daß sich die Patienten der verschiedenen Behandlungsgruppen in Bezug auf all die Faktoren, die den weiteren Krankheitsverlauf bestimmen, gleichen. Solche den weiteren Krankheitsverlauf determinierenden Faktoren können z. B. sein: Alter, Allgemeinzustand, Grad der Herzinsuffizienz oder Höhe des Cholesterinspiegels. Nur wenn die Gruppen zu Anfang vergleichbar sind, können die im Verlauf bzw. nach der Behandlung beobachteten Unterschiede bei den Zielgrößen auch sicher auf die unterschiedliche Behandlung zurückgeführt werden. Die statistisch zufällige Zuteilung gewährleistet als einziges uns bekanntes Verfahren, daß – ein ausreichend großer Stichprobenumfang vorausgesetzt – die Verteilung der bekannten und unbekannten Faktoren, die den weiteren Krankheitsverlauf determinieren, zwischen den Gruppen nur zufällig variiert.

Diese Randomisierung stellt jedoch kein großes Hindernis dar, denn sie ist auch beim niedergelassenen Allgemeinarzt technisch leicht durchzuführen. Nachdem der Patient auf seine Eignung für die Studie untersucht worden ist und – über die Studie aufgeklärt – seine Zustimmung zur Teilnahme gegeben hat, wird eine zentrale Stelle angerufen und der Patient für die Studie angemeldet. Daraufhin erhält der Arzt sofort am Telefon die Information, welche der Studientherapien dem Patienten zu verordnen ist. Diese zentrale Randomisierung per Telefon bereitet nach unseren mehrjährigen Erfahrungen auch für niedergelassene Ärzte keine Schwierigkeiten. Wird die Studie doppelblind durchgeführt, d. h. weiß weder Arzt noch Patient, welche Therapie im Einzelfall verordnet wird, so erhält der Arzt fortlaufend numerierte, patientengerecht abgepackte Arzneimittel, die vom Hersteller der Randomisierungssequenz entsprechend vorbereitet worden sind. Die aus methodischer Sicht für die Aussagekraft einer Therapiestudie absolut essentielle Randomisierung ist also ohne größere Schwierigkeiten auch beim niedergelassenen Allgemeinarzt durchzuführen.

Beobachtungsgleichheit

Strukturgleichheit allein reicht jedoch für einen aussagekräftigen Vergleich der Zielgrößen zwischen den Behandlungsgruppen nicht aus. Alle randomisierten Patienten müssen in gleicher Weise im Verlauf der Behandlung und ggf. auch danach beobachtet werden. Um diese Beobachtungsgleichheit erreichen zu können, ist eine wesentliche Voraussetzung, daß im Prüfplan die erforderlichen Untersuchungen genau festgelegt sind. Diese Festlegungen betreffen v. a. die zu erhebenden Befunde, die Art der einzusetzenden Diagnostik, die Untersuchungszeitpunkte, die Art und Weise, wie und von wem die Untersuchungen durchzuführen sind. Die Meßverfahren sollten in aller Regel standardisiert sein. Gegebenenfalls müssen die Untersucher eigens geschult werden.

Auch wenn die Verlaufsuntersuchungen eine große Erfahrung oder einen erheblichen apparativen Aufwand erfordern, so spricht das nicht prinzipiell gegen die Durchführung einer solchen klinischen Studie beim niedergelassenen Allgemeinarzt. Die Patienten können von einem speziellen Projektarzt in der Praxis des niedergelassenen Kollegen untersucht werden [3], oder sie werden zu den festgelegten Untersuchungszeitpunkten gebeten, den in erreichbarer Nähe befindlichen Spezialisten, z. B. einer Universitätsklinik, zu konsultieren. Der Allgemeinarzt sollte eine solche Vorgehensweise nicht als Mißtrauen gegenüber seinen Fähigkeiten interpretieren. So führen wir auch mit Universitätskliniken eine Reihe von Studien mit zentralisierter Diagnostik durch.

Auch das bereits erwähnte doppelblinde Prüfdesign ist ein wichtiger Beitrag für die Unabhängigkeit der Beobachtung und der Diagnostik vom Wissen um die Therapie und somit *für* die Beobachtungsgleichheit. Stehen Laborparameter im Mittelpunkt des Erkenntnisinteresses, so bietet sich das Einsenden der entsprechenden Proben an ein zentrales Referenzlabor an. Die für die Aussagekraft der Studie erforderliche Beobachtungsgleicheit läßt sich also prinzipiell auch beim niedergelassenen Allgemeinarzt realisieren. Allerdings erfordert dies oft eine aktive Mitarbeit, eine gewisse Flexibilität und die Bereitschaft von seiten des Arztes Neues zu lernen.

Compliance

Selbstverständlich müssen die Studientherapien in den verschiedenen Behandlungsgruppen prüfplangemäß angewendet werden. Dies ist im stationären Bereich sicher einfacher als im niedergelassenen.

Die Compliance der Patienten kann auch in Therapiestudien so mangelhaft sein, daß das Erreichen der Ziele der klinischen Prüfung allein dadurch gefährdet wird. Leider stehen, entgegen der oft verbreiteten Meinung, zuverlässige Verfahren zur Sicherstellung einer guten Compliance nicht bereit. Der Compliance des Patienten dürfte eine sorgfältige Aufklärung und Information förderlich sein, weiterhin entsprechende Erinnerungsstützen sowie eine gewisse Privilegierung des Studienpatienten, z. B. erkennbar verringerte oder keine Wartezeiten. Darüber hinaus stehen heute spezielle „zählende" Tablettendosen zur Verfügung, die eine in vielen Fällen treffende Messung der Compliance ambulanter Patienten zulassen. Studiendesigns, die nur Patienten zur Randomisierung zulassen, die in einer Vorlaufsphase eine zufriedenstellende Compliance gezeigt haben, werden z. B. in den USA oft eingesetzt. Probleme mit der Compliance sind im ambulanten Bereich bei von Patienten selbst anzuwendenden Therapien kaum zu vermeiden. Daher sollte der Compliance und ihrer Förderung schon bei der Planung der Studie besondere Aufmerksamkeit gewidmet werden.

Schlußfolgerungen

Therapiestudien, die den wesentlichen Qualitätskriterien eines Wirksamkeitsnachweises entsprechen, lassen sich auch bei Allgemeinärzten realisieren. Sie sollten in der Phase III der klinischen Prüfung gerade bei den Indikationen stattfinden, die bevorzugt von Allgemeinärzten behandelt werden. Dazu zählen Herz-Kreislauf-Erkrankungen, Hochdruck, Erkrankung des rheumatischen Formenkreises und Stoffwechselerkrankungen, um nur einige wichtige zu nennen.

Klinische Prüfungen beim niedergelassenen Allgemeinarzt versprechen wichtige Erkenntnisse, die im stationären Bereich nicht gewonnen werden können. Der Patient des niedergelassenen Arztes lebt meist in seinem angestammten Umfeld und ist dort in entsprechendem Umfang aktiv. Therapeutisch erwünschte und unerwünschte Wirkungen können unter den Bedingungen des üblichen Anwendungsmodus nach der Zulassung untersucht und erkannt werden. Wichtige unerwünschte Wirkungen, z. B. Müdigkeit, Konzentrationsstörungen, hypotone Episoden oder Schwindel, werden oft erst bei ambulanten Patienten bemerkt. Auch der Einfluß auf die Lebensqualität, die insbesondere bei chronischen Erkrankungen eine wesentliche Behandlungsindikation und zugleich ein wichtiges Therapieziel darstellt, kann bevorzugt beim ambulanten Patienten in seinem häuslichen, beruflichen und sozialen Umfeld untersucht werden. In diesem Zusammenhang sei auch darauf hingewiesen, daß die amerikanische Arzneimittelbehörde, die Food and Drug Administration, Maße der Lebensqualität als Hauptzielgrößen akzeptiert.

Gute Studien zum Wirksamkeitsnachweis können und sollten daher auch beim Allgemeinarzt durchgeführt werden. Wenn es bislang nur vereinzelt solche Studien gibt, so liegen die Gründe vermutlich auch in der mangelnden Bereitschaft niedergelassener Ärzte begründet, randomisierte Studien durchzuführen. Hier dürfte noch ein erheblicher Aufklärungsbedarf vorliegen, was die Methodik, Ethik und Durchführbarkeit solcher Studien im Praxisalltag betrifft. Nur ein Arzt, der das Modell des Wirksamkeitsnachweises ebenso verstanden hat wie die Fragestellung der aktuell anstehenden Arzneimittelprüfung, wird auch seine Patienten entsprechend zur Studienteilnahme motivieren und die Studie erfolgreich durchführen können.

Anhang

Gesichtspunkte zur Entscheidung über die Teilnahme an einer klinischen Prüfung

Liegt ein Prüfplan vor, der über folgende Punkte genauen Aufschluß gibt?
- Aktueller Stand des Wissens,
- Fragestellung und Zielgrößen,
- Studiendesign (kontrolliert, randomisiert, multizentrisch etc.),
- Prüf- und Vergleichstherapien,
- Ein- und Ausschlußkriterien für die Studienpatienten,
- erforderlicher Stichprobenumfang (Fallzahlenschätzung),
- Basis-, Verlaufs- und Abschlußdiagnostik einschließlich Zeit- und Ablaufplan,
- Dokumentation,
- statistischer Auswertungsplan,
- Organisation des Studienablaufs,
- ethische und rechtliche Bewertung der Studie einschließlich Patientenversicherung,
- Inhalt der erforderlichen Aufklärung der Patienten.

Ist die Fragestellung für mich interessant und ist sie medizinisch relevant?
Kann ich Patienten überzeugend über die Studie aufklären und zur Teilnahme raten?

Kann ich die erforderliche Diagnostik in meiner Praxis durchführen?
Läßt sich der studienbedingte Arbeitsaufwand (Einweisung in die Studie, Aufklärung der Patienten, Basis-, Verlaufs- und Abschlußdiagnostik, Dokumentation, Prüfertreffen etc.) mit meiner sonstigen Belastung vereinbaren?
Ist der Leiter der klinischen Prüfung erkennbar kompetent?
Sind die Verhandlungspartner fachlich kompetent?
Ist ein Dossier über die präklinischen und bisherigen klinischen Erfahrungen mit dem zu prüfenden Arzneimittel erhältlich?
Wie sieht das Votum der Ethikkommission aus?

Literatur

1. Bundesminister für Jugend, Familie, Frauen und Gesundheit (1987) Bekanntmachung von Grundsätzen für die ordnungsgemäße Durchführung der klinischen Prüfung von Arzneimitteln. Bundesanzeiger 39, 30. 12. 1987
2. Bundesminister für Jugend, Familie, Frauen und Gesundheit (1990) Gesetz zur Neuordnung des Arzneimittelrechts (2. AMG). Bonn
3. Linden M (1987) Phase-IV Forschung. Springer, Berlin Heidelberg New York Tokyo
4. Victor N, Schäfer H, Nowak H et al. (1991) Arzneimittelforschung nach der Zulassung. Springer, Berlin Heidelberg New York Tokyo

Plenum 4 / Plenary Session 4

Lebensalter, Geschlecht und Psychopharmaka

Ursula Sehrt

Arzneiverbrauchsprofile

Die Arzneiverbrauchsprofile, unterteilt nach Alter und Geschlecht (in Abb. 1 dargestellt für 1989 in rechnerischen Tagesdosen je Versicherten: DDD, für „daily defined doses"), weisen seit Jahren einen konstanten Anstieg mit zunehmendem Lebensalter auf. Dabei überwiegt deutlich das weibliche Geschlecht [4].

Dies gilt für den größten Teil der Indikationsgebiete der Roten Liste, an denen sich die Arzneiverbrauchsprofile orientieren. So gibt es keine Indikationsgruppe, in der die DDD nicht analog zum Versichertenalter ansteigen würden und ganz wenige ohne geschlechtsspezifische Unterschiede (z. B. Antibiotika/Chemotherapeutika). Nur sehr selten überwiegen die männlichen Versicherten, z. B. bei Broncholytika/Antiasthmatika, Gichtmitteln und Urologika [10].

Eine besonders ausgeprägte, dazu altersabhängige Dominanz der weiblichen Versicherten findet sich z. B. in den Indikationsgruppen Analgetika/Antirheumatika, Antihypnotika, Dermatika, durchblutungsfördernde Mittel – dies bereits im 4.

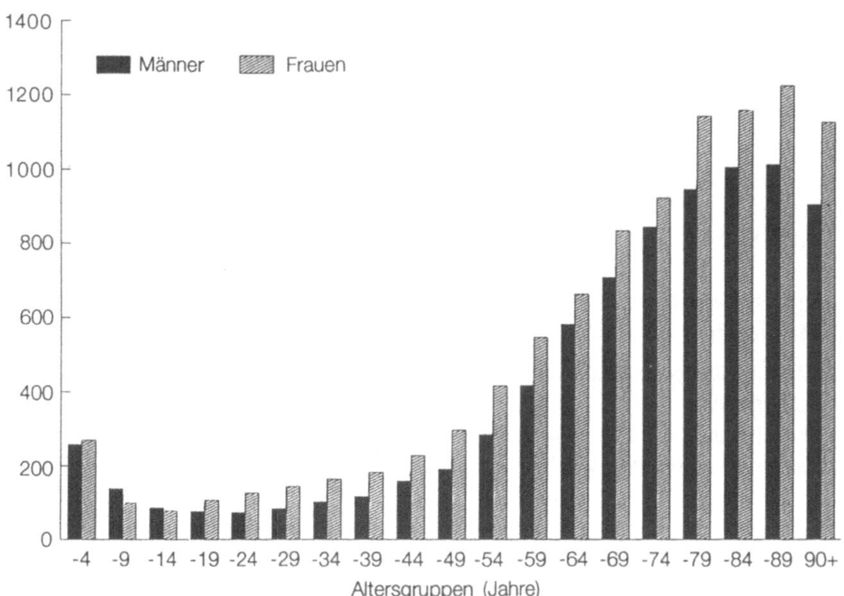

Abb. 1. Arzneiverbrauchsprofile nach Alter und Geschlecht: alle Arzneimittel. (Aus [5])

Rationale Pharmakotherapie in der Allgemeinpraxis
Rational Pharmacotherapy in General Practice
M. M. Kochen (Hrsg.)

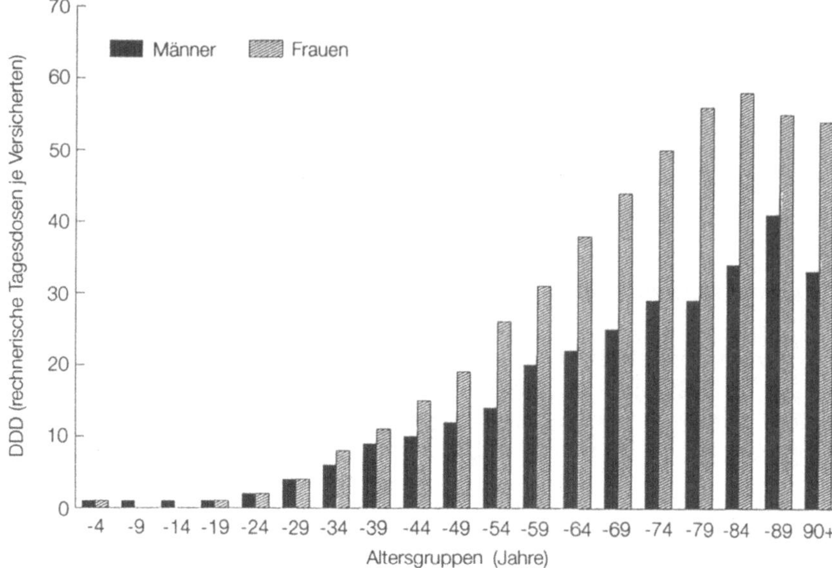

Abb. 2. Arzneiverbrauchsprofile nach Alter und Geschlecht 1989: Psychopharmaka. (Aus [5])

Lebensjahrzehnt! – , Migränemittel, Venenmittel sowie Hypnotika/Sedativa und Psychopharmaka.

Abbildung 2 zeigt den Anstieg der DDD für Psychopharmaka in Abhängigkeit von Lebensalter und Geschlecht. Dabei fällt auf, daß dieser Anstieg für männliche Versicherte im Vergleich zur Zunahme des Gesamtverbrauchs an Arzneimitteln in den höheren Dezennien flacher verläuft, während der ohnehin größere Psychopharmakaverbrauch der weiblichen Versicherten in den höheren Altersgruppen ganz rapide weiter zunimmt.

Fragestellung

Ausgehend von diesen Daten aus dem GKV-Arzneimittelindex interessieren folgende Fragen:

1. Welche Rolle spielen Psychopharmaka für die Arzneitherapie in der Allgemeinpraxis?
2. Welche auch in einer Allgemeinpraxis gängigen Psychopharmaka werden bevorzugt verordnet bzw. eingenommen?
3. Gibt der GKV-Arzneimittelindex Hinweise auf verordnungslenkende Einflüsse bezüglich des Umgangs mit Psychopharmaka in der Allgemeinpraxis?
4. Ist der mit dem Lebensalter ansteigende und bei weiblichen Versicherten auffällig hohe Verbrauch an Psychopharmaka rational, d. h. morbiditätsbedingt unter Einbeziehung psychosozialer Faktoren begründbar?

5. Gibt es irrationale, aber unabänderliche Gründe für den hohen Konsum von Psychopharmaka – in höheren Altersklassen – bei weiblichen Versicherten?

Die Rolle von Psychopharmaka in der Allgemeinpraxis

Vorab sei betont, daß Hypnotika/Sedativa bei den nachfolgenden Ausführungen nicht näher berücksichtigt werden, weil sie in der offiziellen Klassifizierung einem anderen Indikationsgebiet zuzuordnen sind. (Näheres dazu s. Beitrag „Über den Umgang mit Benzodiazepinen in der Allgemeinpraxis", S. 251 ff.).

Allgemeinärzte und Praktiker rezeptieren 53 % aller zu Lasten der GKV verordneten Psychopharmaka. Über 27 % werden von anderen Arztgruppen verordnet und nur knapp 18 % durch die sog. indikationsspezifische Fachgruppe der Ärzte für Neurologie und Psychiatrie [4].

Diese Zahlen veranschaulichen mehr als alle Worte, welch wichtige Rolle Psychopharmaka in einer Allgemeinpraxis spielen.

Spektrum verordneter Psychopharmaka

Abbildung 3 zeigt, daß Tranquillanzien, und zwar so gut wie ausschließlich in Form von Benzodiazepinen, vor Antidepressiva und Neuroleptika die mit weitem Abstand am häufigsten verwandte Gruppe von Psychopharmaka sind. Gleichzeitig

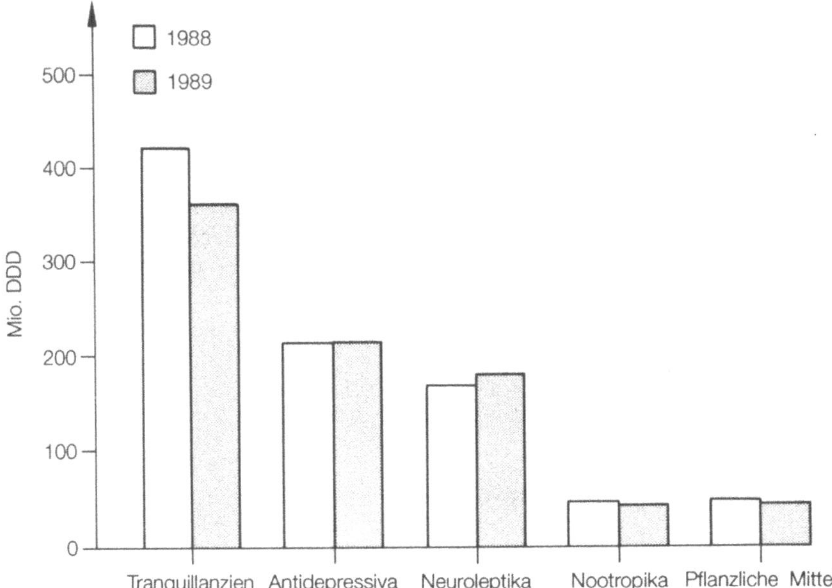

Abb. 3. Verordnung von Psychopharmaka nach definierten Tagesdosen (*DDD*). Vergleich 1988 und 1989. (Aus [5])

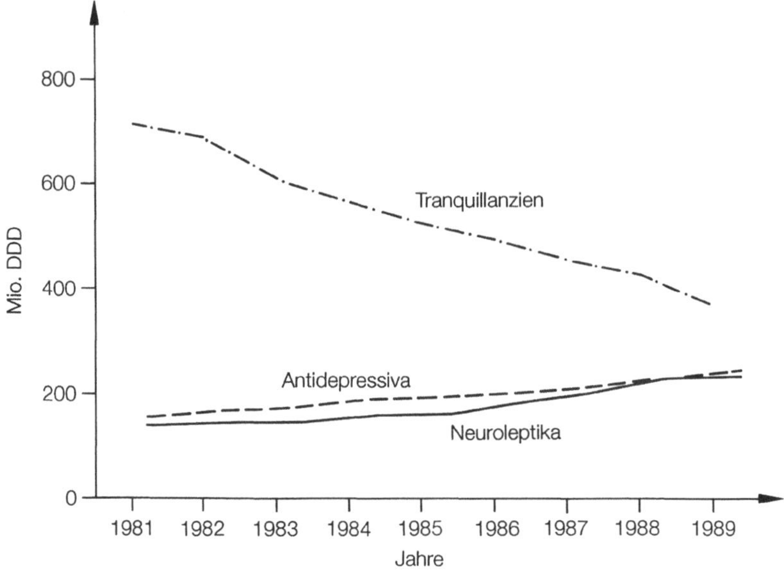

Abb. 4. Verordnungen von Psychopharmaka nach *DDD* (definierte Tagesdosen) 1981 bis 1989. (Aus [5])

ist jedoch ein deutlicher Rückgang der DDD bei den Tranquillanzien und ein leichter Ansteig der DDD für Antidepressiva und Neuroleptika im Jahre 1989 gegenüber 1988 zu verzeichnen.

Es wird immer wieder als begrüßenswert im Sinn von Rationalität hervorgehoben, daß die Verordnungshäufigkeit von Benzodiazepinen seit 1981 kontinuierlich rückläufig ist (Abb. 4), während sich im gleichen Zeitraum Antidepressiva und Neuroleptika auf dem Vormarsch befinden [4].

Wie sich dieser Trend im Vergleich der Jahre 1985 und 1989 in DDD ausdrückt, ist aus Tabelle 1 ersichtlich. Während in diesem Zeitraum die DDD für Tranquillanzien um 28 % sanken, stiegen sie für Antidepressiva um 72,9 % und für Neuroleptika um 52,4 % an. Unter dem Strich erhöhten sich die DDD dieser 3 Psychopharmakagruppen um 1,6 %.

Tabelle 1. Verordnungstrends Psychopharmaka (*DDD* = „daily defined doses“)

Gruppe	DDD 1985 [Mio.]	DDD 1989 [Mio.]	Differenz [%]
Tranquillanzien	505,0	362,9	–28
Antidepressiva	125,3	216,6	+72,8
Neuroleptika	120,1	183,0	+52,4
Gesamt	750,4	762,5	+ 1,6

Solche gewaltigen Sprünge der Verordnungsfrequenzen innerhalb weniger Jahre können sui generis nicht über eine plötzliche Wandlung von Morbiditätsspektren plausibel gemacht werden.

Außerdem hätte es eines enormen, angesichts der verfügbaren flankierenden Maßnahmen kaum nachvollziehbaren Kraftakts insbesondere der Hausärzte als Hauptverordner bedurft, den DDD-Einbruch von 28 % bei den Benzodiazepinen ersatzlos zu kompensieren. Dies hätte rein rechnerisch bedeutet, rund 388 000 von 1 384 000 GKV-Versicherten, die unter einer Dauertherapie mit Benzodiazepinen stehen, erfolgreich zu entwöhnen, (und zwar ohne Berücksichtigung ihres Einsatzes unter dem Indikationsgebiet Hypnotika/Sedativa).

Potentiell verordnungslenkende Einflüsse und ihre Konsequenzen

Insbesondere seit Vorliegen der Empfehlungen und Warnungen des Sachverständigenrates der Bundesregierung [1] werden Verordnungsfrequenz und Dauer der Anwendung von Benzodiazepinen wegen der bekannten Abhängigkeitsrisiken zunehmend kritisiert. Daraus resultieren logischerweise verordnungslenkende Einflüsse, die sich nicht nur auf das Pro und Kontra einer evtl. erstmals anzusetzenden Benzodiazepintherapie bezogen.

In Tabelle 2 sind exemplarisch die DDD-Entwicklungen von 1985 und 1989 für 4 marktführende Vertreter der Benzodiazepine angegeben. Wiederholt tauchen Warnhinweise auf, z. B. bei Bromazepam in Bezug auf sein hohes Mißbrauchspotential, bei Diazepam bezüglich seiner Phase-I-Reaktion, seiner substanzeigenen langen Halbwertszeit (und v. a. wegen der seiner Metaboliten), wodurch unter pharmakokinetischen Aspekten insbesondere ältere und alte Patienten erhöhten Risiken ausgesetzt werden. Drastisch rückläufige DDD erscheinen in diesen beiden Fällen somit durchaus rational.

Tabelle 2. Verordnungstrends Benzodiazepine (*DDD* = „daily defined doses")

Substanz	DDD 1985 [Mio.]	DDD 1989 [Mio.]	Differenz [%]
Bromazepam	185,0	126,2	–31,8
Oxazepam	76,8	96,1	+25,1
Diazepam	135,7	51,8	–61,8
Lorazepam	29,5	29,9	+ 1,4

Lorazepam scheint, bezogen auf den Beobachtungszeitraum, eine unerschütterliche Anhängerschaft zu haben, wobei abzuwarten bleibt, inwieweit sich hier ein deutsches Politikerschicksal in Zukunft auswirkt[1]. Was den DDD-Anstieg der Anti-

[1] Gemeint ist der ehemalige Ministerpräsident von Schleswig-Holstein, Uwe Barschel, der dieses Medikament eingenommen hatte.

depressiva zwischen 1985 und 1989 um 72,8 % veranlaßt haben könnte, läßt sich nur vermuten, und zwar dann, wenn man den Weg einzelner Substanzen verfolgt:

Psychomotorisch aktivierende Substanzen spielen im ambulanten Versorgungsbereich praktisch keine Rolle, weder 1985 noch 1989 [3].

Bei den psychomotorisch stabilisierenden Substanzen ist zu berücksichtigen, daß sich unter ihnen Arzneistoffe mit fließendem Übergang zu psychomotorisch sedierenden Eigenschaften gemäß Kielholz-Schema befinden. Genau diese Antidepressiva haben deutliche Zuwächse zu verzeichnen (Tabelle 3).

Tabelle 3. Verordnungstrends Antidepressiva (*DDD* „daily defined dosis")

Substanz	DDD 1985 [Mio.]	DDD 1989 [Mio.]	Differenz [%]
Clomipramin	4,0	5,4	+ 35,0
Maprotilin	14,4	21,1	+ 46,5
Opipramol	2,8	14,2	+407,1
Amytriptylin	17,5	32,8	+ 87,4
Amytriptylin-N-Oxid	6,8	15,0	+120,6
Doxepin	12,2	39,4	+223,0

Hierher gehören Clomipramin (Anafranil) mit +35 %, Maprotilin (Ludiomil) mit +46,5 % und Opipramol (Insidon) mit +40,7 %.

Ferner sind beachtliche Zuwachsraten für die marktführenden psychomotorisch sedierenden Antidepressiva festzustellen: +87,4 % für Amitriptylin (Saroten, Generika), +120,6 % für Amytriptylin-N-Oxid (Equilibrin) und +223 % für Doxepin (Aponal).

Eine im Prinzip analoge Entwicklung läßt sich für die Neuroleptika aufzeigen (Tabelle 4). Hier findet man bei den Phenothiazinen mit stark sedierender Wirkungskomponente zwischen 1985 und 1989 DDD-Zuwachsraten von rund 63 % für Promethazin (Atosil, Generika) sowie von über 33 % für Thioridazin (Melleril, Melleretten). Gleiches gilt für die Butyrophenone Haloperidol (Haldol, Generika) mit +35,6 %, Melperon (Eunerpan) mit +151,1 % und Pipamperon (Dipiperon) mit +207,7 %. Ferner ist die DDD-Zunahme von 38,6 % bei den Fluspirilen-Zubereitungen (Imap 1,5 und Imap) auffällig.

Tabelle 4. Verordnungstrends Neuroleptika (*DDD* „daily defined dosis")

Substanz	DDD 1985 [Mio.]	DDD 1989 [Mio.]	Differenz [%]
Promethazin	14,0	22,8	+ 62,9
Thioridazin	13,8	18,4	+ 33,3
Haloperidol	26,4	35,8	+ 35,6
Melperon	4,5	11,3	+151,1
Pipamperon	1,3	4,0	+207,7

Die beschriebenen Verordnungstrends von Psychopharmaka sprechen dafür, daß heute vielfach Antidepressiva (v. a. psychomotorisch sedierende), sowie einschlägig wirksame Neuroleptika (vermutlich oft unter der sog. neuroleptischen Schwelle dosiert) an Stelle der Benzodiazepine eingesetzt werden, und zwar bevorzugt bei älteren Frauen.

Fragen der Rationalität

Eine wissenschaftlich anerkannte Indikation zur Langzeit- oder gar Dauertherapie mit Benzodiazepinen besteht für kein Lebensalter. Offiziell heißt es dazu:

> Über das Nutzen-Risiko-Verhältnis einer langfristigen Benzodiazepin-Medikation (über 2 Monate) bei Patienten mit behandlungsbedürftigen chronischen Angstzuständen liegen bislang keine wissenschaftlich allgemein anerkannten Erkenntnisse vor [1].

Die Mehrzahl der als Psychopharmaka angewandten Benzodiazepine ist mit Anwendungsempfehlungen etwa folgenden, vom BGA zugelassenen, Inhalts ausgestattet:
- akute und chronische Angst-, Erregungs-, Spannungs- und Unruhezustände;
- Schlafstörungen;
- (bei sehr variationsreicher Terminologie) für Beschwerdebilder, die heute üblicherweise unter dem Krankheitsbegrifff der funktionellen Syndrome subsumiert werden.

Die Angstneurose wird heute gemäß der ICD-9 in das Paniksyndrom und in das generalisierte Angstsyndrom unterteilt, dem in der Allgemeinpraxis eine ungleich größere Bedeutung zukommt. Aus der unbewußten krankhaften Angstverarbeitung entstehen die für die Allgemeinpraxis bedeutsamen psychosomatischen Störungen in Form der funktionellen Syndrome bzw. „echte" Psychosomatosen und larvierte Erschöpfungsdepressionen (Abb. 5; [2]).

Eine Studie an 7825 Patienten der Gießener Medizinischen Poliklinik, d. h. an einem selektierten Krankengut, ergab, daß bei 22,4 % der männlichen und bei 29,2 % der weiblichen Patienten ausschließlich funktionelle Syndrome vorlagen. Man kann hier also von einer gewissen Dominanz des weiblichen Geschlechts ausgehen [8].

Ferner ist bekannt, daß funktionelle Syndrome als somatisierte Folgezustände einer chronischen Angstreaktion meist bei jüngeren Patienten mit einem Gipfel im 3. und 4. Lebensjahrzehnt anzutreffen sind. Vom 50. Lebensjahr an sinkt die Häufigkeit funktioneller Syndrome beträchtlich, jenseits des 65. Lebensjahres sind sie eine Rarität.

In einer eigenen Untersuchung wiesen 45 % aller 515 Patienten mit psychischen und psychosomatischen Störungen funktionelle Syndrome auf, 31 % litten an unterschiedlichen Formen von Depressionen, 6,5 % hatten Paniksyndrome. Drei Viertel aller funktionellen Syndrome fanden sich bei Patienten zwischen 20–49 Jahren. Erwähnenswert ist, daß annähernd die Hälfte aller Patienten mit funktionellen Syndromen beim Erstkontakt mit der Allgemeinpraxis bereits iatrogen fixiert war. Wenn man von den Altersdepressionen mit einem Anteil von 13 % am Gesamtkol-

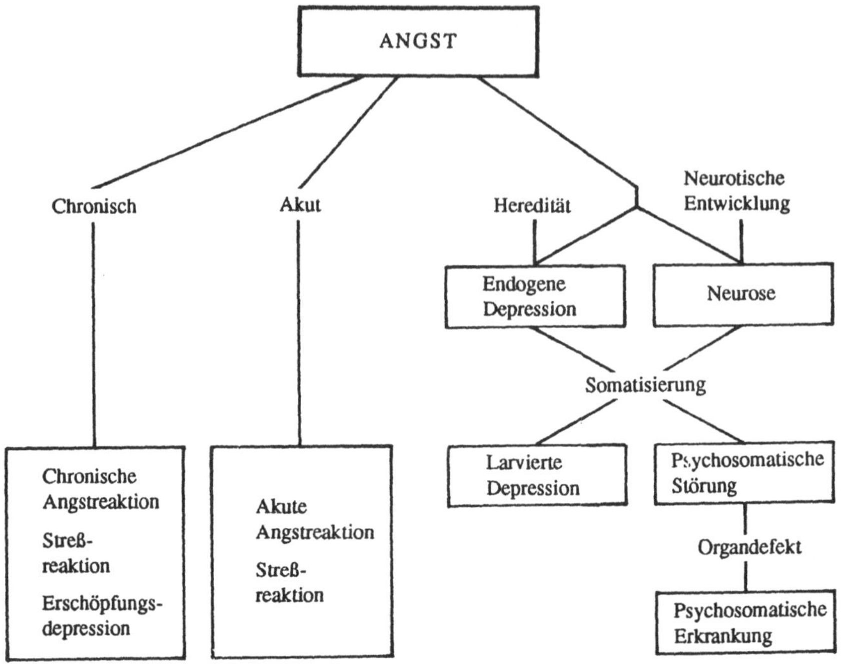

Abb. 5. Angst und Symptomentwicklung. (Aus [2])

lektiv absieht, fanden sich drei Viertel aller Depressionen bei Patienten zwischen 30–59 Jahren.

Fast bei der Hälfte der 515 Patienten mit psychischen und psychosomatischen Störungen lagen gravierend konfliktbesetzte Beziehungen vor, v. a. zwischen Partnern und zwischen Eltern und Kindern [5]. In einer anderen Untersuchung wurde nachgewiesen, daß bei 46 % von 226 geriatrischen Patienten psychische Probleme von Krankheitswert vorlagen, bei denen gleichzeitig konfliktgeladene, oft destruktive Beziehungsstörungen bestanden, was sich regelhaft auch auf die Patient-Arzt-Beziehung negativ auswirkte [6].

Vor diesem psychosozialen Hintergrund ist es wichtig zu wissen, daß sich derzeit 17 % der Bevölkerung – bezogen auf Deutschland-West – im Sinn regelmäßiger Hilfe und Pflege um ältere Angehörige kümmern. 80 % aller Pflegeleistenden sind Frauen. In der bereits zitierten eigenen Untersuchung gehörten 61 % der pflegenden Frauen der sog. Sandwichgeneration an. Die psychischen und psychosomatischen Störungen in diesem Kollektiv korrelierten eindeutig mit dem Schweregrad der Pflegebedürftigkeit der zu versorgenden Angehörigen. Großen Einfluß hatten dabei auch chronifizierte Beziehungskonflikte, klimakterische Ausfallerscheinungen sowie Individualkonflikte.

In der erwähnten Studie, die im übrigen keinerlei Anhaltspunkte für einen Zusammenhang zwischen somatischer Morbidität bzw. Multimorbidität und psychischen Störungen der älteren und alten Patienten ergab, waren 21 % des männlichen gegenüber 67 % des weiblichen Kollektivs verwitwet.

Diese Beobachtung korreliert mit den epidemiologischen Daten, daß der Anteil weiblicher GKV-Versicherten altersabhängig ansteigt. Er beträgt in der Altersgruppe zwischen 50–59 Jahren 50,9 %, in der Altergruppe zwischen 80–89 Jahren 70,7 % [4].

Somit wäre der Ansatz einer rationalen Begründung für den mit dem Lebensalter und bei weiblichen GKV-Versicherten besonders auffälligen Anstieg des Psychopharmakaverbrauchs allenfalls an psychosozialen Faktoren festzumachen. Reicht das – v. a. im Hinblick auf die biopsychosoziale Kompetenz des Allgemeinarztes?

Unabänderliche Irrationalität?

Anhand der Daten der Verbrauchsprofile von Psychopharmaka sowie der erwähnten Untersuchungen bleibt festzustellen:

- Unzählige einschlägige Patientenkarrieren, insbesondere bei Frauen, starten bereits im 4. Lebensjahrzehnt.
- Bereits in jüngeren Altersklassen häufen sich organisierte psychische und psychosomatische Störungen bis zur iatrogenen Fixierung.
- Führend und bedeutsam für die künftige Entwicklung ist in der Mehrzahl der Fälle die Beziehungsproblematik.
- Die Wirksamkeit des Patient-Arzt-Gesprächs, die Potenz der „Droge“ Arzt wird zu wenig genutzt.
- Keine andere Arztgruppe als die der Allgemeinärzte verfügt über vergleichbar große Chancen, der Entwicklung von Psychopharmakakarrieren frühzeitig Einhalt zu gebieten, da
  a) 80 % seiner Patienten mitbetreuten Familien angehören,
  b) gut zwei Drittel seiner Patienten länger als 5 Jahre in seiner Behandlung stehen,
  c) er jederzeit die unermeßlich großen Informationsquellen des Hausbesuchs und der erlebten Anamnese nutzen kann.
- Die Abnahme der Benzodiazepinverordnungen zugunsten des Einsatzes von psychomotorisch sedierenden Antidepressiva und Neuroleptika erweckt den Eindruck eines Konsumaustausches.
- Einer bereits organisierten Psychopharmakakarriere jedwerder Art ist unter den Arbeitsbedingungen einer Allgemeinpraxis schwerlich Einhalt zu gebieten.

In diesem Zusammenhang sei auf die potentiellen *Nebenwirkungsprofile* von Benzodiazepinen, Neuroleptika und Antidepressiva speziell in höheren Altersklassen, verwiesen [7, 9], die nachfolgend aufgeführt sind.

Benzodiazepine:

- Ataxie,
- Mundtrockenheit,
- Alpträume,
- verwaschene Sprache,

- Pruritus, flüchtige Exantheme,
- Arthralgien,
- Schwindel,
- verschwommenes Sehen,
- Depression,
- Verwirrtheit,
- Gedächtnisstörungen,
- paradoxe Reaktionen:
  Halluzinationen,
  akute Verwirrtheitszustände,
  delirante Zustände.

Neuroleptika:

- Blutdruckabfall bis zum schweren orthostatischen Kollaps,
- Herzrhythmusstörungen wie Tachykardien, komplexe Arrhythmien und Blockierungen,
- extrapyramidale Symptome, u. U. hyperkinetisches Dauersyndrom,
- depressive und delirante Zustände,
- anticholinerge Effekte.

Antidepressiva mit Praxisrelevanz:

- Mundtrockenheit,
- Akkomodationsstörungen,
- Schwitzen,
- Schwindel,
- Pruritus,
- orthostatischer Kollaps,
- kardiotoxisches Risiko (Rhythmusstörungen),
- extrapyramidale Symptome (meist direkt),
- Sedierung,
- Verwirrtheits- und delirante Zustände,
- anticholinerge Effekte.

Da die Inzidenz von unerwünschten Arzneimittelwirkungen mit zunehmendem Lebensalter drastisch ansteigt, wäre – unabhängig von der Psychopharmakagruppe – insbesondere bei älteren und alten Patienten eine streng individuell dosierte und überwachte Therapie erforderlich. Komplizierend kommt hinzu, daß im Senium gemäß Arzneiverbrauchsprofilen oft Kombinationstherapien mit psychisch wirksamen Substanzen durchgeführt werden. Es sei nur an den hier nicht näher beschriebenen hohen Konsum von Hypnotika/Sedativa erinnert, deren Nebenwirkungsspektren sich, wie oben dargestellt, in mannigfacher und vielfach fataler Weise überlappen. Dies wirkt sich um so gravierender aus angesichts der alters- und morbiditätsbedingt eingeschränkten Regulationsbreite veschiedenster Organsysteme im Senium.

Diskussion

Es wurde ausführlich dargestellt, daß der Psychopharmakaverbrauch mit wachsendem Lebensalter deutlich, bei weiblichen Versicherten sogar drastisch ansteigt. Mit einem Verordnungsanteil von 53 % spielen Allgemeinärzte und Praktiker eine Schlüsselrolle für den Psychopharmakaeinsatz. Die daraus resultierende Verantwortung dieser Anwendergruppe spiegelt sich in der Tatsache wider, daß trotz des rückläufigen Einsatzes von Tranquillanzien die Gesamt-DDD von Benzodiazepinen, Antidepressiva und Neuroleptika in den vergangenen Jahren leicht angestiegen sind. Hier ist von verordnungslenkenden Einflüssen auf die Verschreibungsgewohnheiten gerade der Allgemeinärzte und Praktiker als Hauptverordner auszugehen. Die Rationalität muß hinterfragt werden.

Auffällig erscheint die Konsumverlagerung von den Benzodiazepinen (Oxazepam ausgenommen) zu überwiegend psychomotorisch sedierenden Antidepressiva und Neuroleptika. Daraus kann abgeleitet werden, daß die gleiche therapeutische Zielrichtung, nämlich die pharmakologisch induzierte Ruhigstellung der Patienten, heute z. T. mit anderen Mitteln angesteuert wird.

Vor dem Hintergrund der entscheidenden Frage nach der Indikation einer medikamentösen Behandlung sowie nach dem Vorliegen nichtmedikamentöser Therapiemöglichkeiten kann dieser Trend aus rein pharmakologischer Sicht – und ungeachtet aller gegen die Benzodiazepine vorgebrachten Bedenken – nicht als rational bezeichnet werden. Hinzukommt, daß Benzodiazepine, Antidepressiva und Neuroleptika im Senium, d. h. in dem Lebensabschnitt, in dem sie am häufigsten appliziert werden, auch die häufigsten alterstypischen, oft schweren unerwünschten Wirkungen aufweisen. Deren Spektren überlappen sich vielfach, was angesichts häufiger Kombinationstherapien mit psychisch wirksamen Substanzen in den höheren Altersklassen von großer praktischer Bedeutung ist [7]. Jede Therapie mit Psychopharmaka, erst recht bei älteren und alten Patienten, müßte wegen ihrer Risikopotentiale maßgeschneidert sein, zumal im Senium Ausmaß und Muster vorhandener Funktionseinbußen einer an keinem anderen Kollektiv zu beobachtenden Variationsbreite unterliegen.

Abseits dieser pharmakologischen Überlegungen gibt die Häufigkeit psychischer und psychosomatischer Störungen auch jüngerer Patienten einer Allgemeinpraxis ebenso zu denken wie die hohe Frequenz und die Auswirkung gravierend gestörter Beziehungsnetze.

Es wurden psychosoziale Faktoren beschrieben, die geeignet sind, mit zunehmendem Alter und insbesondere beim weiblichen Geschlecht Psychopharmakakarrieren zu starten und zu unterhalten. Dem steht das spezifische Instrumentarium der Allgemeinpraxis entgegen, mit dessen Hilfe frühzeitig verbale Interventionsstrategien eingesetzt werden können. Dabei hat der Allgemeinarzt auch Ersatzfunktionen für die heute im natürlichen Patientenumfeld weitverbreitete Kommunikationsschwäche wahrzunehmen. Zu seinem sozialen Verantwortungsbereich gehören Bemühungen um die gesellschaftliche Reintegration älterer Patienten sowie um die maximale Nutzung aller Möglichkeiten zur sog. aktivierenden Pflege. Der Allgemeinarzt stellt mit seiner Art der Intervention die Weichen für den weiteren Verlauf zahlloser Patientenkarrieren. Aber er kann nicht an allen Fronten kämpfen und nicht ohne angemessene Unterstützung psychisch bzw. psychosozial determinierte Konfliktsituationen bewältigen.

Angesichts der bestehenden Pflege- und der oft chronifizierten Beziehungsproblematik gilt dies in besonderem Maß für die Betreuung geriatrischer Patienten.

Trotz allen Respekts vor pharmakologischer Rationalität bleibt dem Allgemeinarzt unter dem Druck der Realität oft nur die Wahl zwischen einem Neuroleptikum für die „querulatorische Schwiegermutter" und einem Benzodiazepin für die ihr Angstsyndrom bereits somatisch umsetzende, „ungeliebte Schwiegertochter" in Sandwichsituationen.

Literatur

1. Bundesverband der Pharmazeutischen Industrie e.V. (Hrsg) (1991) Rote Liste 1991. Editio Cantor, Aulendorf/Württ.
2. Luban-Plozza B, Pöldinger W, Kröger F (1989) Der psychosomatisch Kranke in der Praxis. 5. Aufl. Springer, Berlin Heidelberg New York Tokyo
3. Schwabe U, Paffrath D (Hrsg) (1986) Arzneiverordnungsreport '86. Fischer, Stuttgart, New York
4. Schwabe U, Paffrath D (Hrsg) (1990) Arzneiverordnungsreport '90. Fischer, Stuttgart
5. Sehrt U (1989) Psychosomatische Grundversorgung in der Allgemeinpraxis. In: Bergmann G (Hrsg) Psychosomatische Grundversorgung. Springer, Berlin Heidelberg New York Tokyo
6. Sehrt U (1990) Der alternde Patient, sein Umfeld, sein Hausarzt. In: Luban-Plozza B (Hrsg) Der alternde Mensch und sein Arzt. Springer, Berlin Heidelberg New York Tokyo
7. Sehrt U, Weber E (1986) Besonderheiten der Pharmakotherapie im Senium. Münch Med Wochenschr 35:595–598
8. Uexküll T von (Hrsg) (1986) Psychosomatische Medizin, 3. Aufl. Urban & Schwarzenberg, München Wien Baltimore
9. Weber E (Hrsg) (1989) Taschenbuch der unerwünschten Arzneiwirkungen, 2. Aufl. Fischer, Stuttgart New York
10. Wissenschaftliches Institut der Ortskrankenkassen (WIdO) (Hrsg) (1990) GKV-Arzneimittelindex: Arzneiverbrauch nach Altersgruppen

Allgemeinärztliche Therapiefreiheit – ein Mythos?

Ivan Nemitz

Grundlagen

Die 3 Grundelemente meines Themas, Freiheit – medikamentöse Therapie – Mythos, sollen zunächst definiert werden.

Freiheit: Sie ist ein grundlegender Begriff des abendländischen Denkens und unserer Zivilisation, den jedes menschliche Wesen für sich beansprucht. In Wahrheit ist der Begriff der Freiheit aber gar nicht so alt. Er stammt aus dem alten Griechenland, aus dem Athen vor 2500 Jahren.

Das französische Gegenstück zum *Duden*, der *Petit Robert* definiert Freiheit „als Situation einer Person, die in keiner Weise von jemandem abhängig ist" ([3], S. 1090).

Medikamentöse Therapie:
J.L. Schelling, Profesor für klinische Pharmakologie in Lausanne, gibt folgende Definition: „Das Verschreiben eines Medikamentes ist eine einfache Handlung, oft automatisch, dessen Ausführung der Arzt im allgemeinen nicht kontrollieren kann" ([4], S. 119).

Mythos:
Er wird im *Petit Robert* [3] als „vereinfachtes, oft illusorisches Bild eines Individuums" beschrieben, „wobei eine menschliche Gruppe dieses Bild entwickelt oder akzeptiert und dieses eine bestimmende Rolle im Verhalten der Gruppe spielt" (S. 1251).

Im folgenden möchte ich auf die Frage nach den Unterschieden der ärztlichen Tätigkeit von Hippokrates einerseits und unserer Medizin am Ende des 20. Jahrhunderts andererseits eingehen.

Sehr schematisch könnte man sagen: Hippokrates war der erste Arzt, der den begrifflichen Rahmen schuf, um seinen Beruf, die Medizin, so frei wie möglich auszuüben.

Er konnte dies tun, weil er die Krankheit als ein natürliches Phänomen ansah (nicht als etwas Übernatürliches) und indem er die Medizin völlig von der Magie und der Religion abgrenzte. Obwohl der Freiraum, den er sich innerhalb der Arzt-Patienten-Beziehung so schuf, immens war, mußte er wohl trotzdem eingestehen, daß seine therapeutischen Möglichkeiten sehr begrenzt waren.

Heute stellen wir eine völlige Umkehr des Verhältnisses Freiheit – Wirkungsgrad fest. Wenn auch unsere therapeutischen Möglichkeiten in nur einem halben

Rationale Pharmakotherapie in der Allgemeinpraxis
Rational Pharmacotherapy in General Practice
M. M. Kochen (Hrsg.)

Jahrhundert sehr bedeutend geworden sind, hat sich doch der Freiraum, in dem Hippokrates die Medizin begründete, ständig verringert.

Dafür ist die medikamentöse Therapie, die Verordnung von Arzneimitteln, ein sehr gutes Beispiel, weil das Verschreiben von Medikamenten starken äußeren Einflüssen, vorwiegend ökonomischen, ausgesetzt ist, die sich der Kontrolle des Arztes entziehen.

Diese Einflüsse gehen einerseits von der Pharmaindustrie aus, die versucht, Gewinne zu realisieren, die nicht unerheblich sind, und andererseits von den Kostenträgern, die versuchen, ihre Ausgaben zu begrenzen.

Die therapeutische Freiheit des Arztes wird also zwischen diesen beiden gegensätzlichen Polen eingeengt.

Eine grundlegende Frage wäre es, nach den eigentlichen Interessen des Patienten zu suchen, aber dies wäre Thema eines eigenen Beitrags.

Ist das Verschreiben eines Medikaments wirklich eine freie und rationale Handlung oder handelt es sich dabei nicht eher um einen Mythos?

Meine Überlegungen basieren einerseits auf den Regelmechanismen des schweizerischen Gesundheitswesens im Bereich der Pharmakotherapie und andererseits auf unseren täglichen Erfahrungen als Allgemeinärzte, die Medikamente verschreiben.

Arzneimittelbestimmungen in der Schweiz

1988 gab es in der Schweiz ca. 8000 verschiedene Medikamente in 10 000 veschiedenen Formen, 13 000 verschiedenen Dosierungen und 25 verschiedenen Packungsgrößen.

Der Verkauf dieser Medikamente wird durch die Interkantonale Kontrollstelle für Heilmittel (IKS) reglementiert; interkantonal, weil in der Schweiz jeder der 26 Kantone seine eigene Gesundheitsgesetzgebung hat.

Die Verkaufsart ergibt sich aus einer Liste, die die Medikamente in 6 Kategorien aufteilt. Die Liste A umfaßt ca. 10 % der Medikamente, die Liste B ca. 38 %. Medikamente sowohl der Liste A als auch der Liste B werden in der Apotheke gegen Rezept verkauft, wobei bei Medikamenten der Liste A vor einem erneuten Medikamentenbezug auch ein neues Rezept ausgestellt werden muß, d. h. diese Substanzen unterliegen einer sog. verschärften „Rezeptpflicht".

Dies bedeutet, daß nur 48 % der auf dem schweizerischen Markt verfügbaren Medikamente aufgrund ärztlicher Verschreibung abgegeben werden; der Rest (52 %) wird frei in Apotheken, Drogerien oder sonst im Handel verkauft.

Wer übernimmt die Kosten für die so verordneten Medikamente?

Grundlage bildet die sog. Spezialitätenliste, die vom Bundesamt für Sozialversicherung aufgrund einer Bundesverordnung von 1968 herausgegeben wird. Diesem Bundesamt obliegt es, die Medikamente zu bestimmen, die von den Kostenträgern, d. h. von den 385 Krankenkassen unseres Landes, ebenso von den obligatorischen Unfallversicherern übernommen werden müssen. 1988 fanden sich 2666 Medikamente auf dieser Liste.

Dies ist ein sehr kurzer Hinweis auf die Bestimmungen, die den Pharmamarkt in der Schweiz definieren und an die sich auch der Arzt bei der Medikamentenverschreibung halten muß.

Betrachten wir die einzelnen Faktoren, die den Arzt sehr direkt beeinflussen, wenn er das Rezept schreibt und er sich für den Markennamen eines Medikaments entscheiden muß.

Es gibt mehrere Faktoren, die diesen Entscheid beeinflussen. Die wichtigsten sind:

- Pharmaindustrie,
- Krankenkassen,
- Patienten.

Der verschreibende Arzt befindet sich damit im Zentrum eines Spannungsfeldes, wobei jeder dieser 3 Faktoren eine bestimmende Rolle bei der Wahl eines Handelspräparats spielen kann.

Pharmaindustrie

Es scheint klar, daß pharmazeutische Unternehmen über ihr bedeutendes Kommunikationsnetz den stärksten Druck auf den Verschreibenden ausüben. Ihre Mittel dazu sind: Ärztebesucher, Abgabe von Musterpräparaten, Postaussendungen, Anzeigen und Artikel in der medizinisch-pharmazeutischen Fachpresse, wissenschaftliche Kongresse, Ausstellungen bei wissenschaftlichen Kongressen sowie audiovisuelle Mittel.

Bei den Postaussendungen an die praktizierenden Ärzte handelt es sich z. B. oft nur noch in zweiter Linie um eine eigentliche medizinische Information, sondern viel eher um eine wohlorganisierte Werbekampagne.

Nach Informationen der „Gruppe pharmazeutische Fachinformation der schweizerischen Gesellschaft für chemische Industrie", welche den Auftrag hat, das Gentlemen's Agreement für pharmazeutische Fachinformation von 1969 zu überwachen, erhielt der praktizierende Arzt allein im Jahre 1989 1604 Aussendungen mit einem Totalgewicht von 92,4 kg. Dieses Gentlemen's Agreement dient auch dazu, einen besonders traurigen Aspekt der Beziehung zwischen Pharmaindustrie und Arzt zu überwachen: Die Geschenke, die der Arzt entweder per Post oder auch durch den Ärztebesucher von der Pharmaindustrie erhält und die den Namen eines Medikaments auf Ewigkeit im Gedächtnis des Arztes verankern sollen.

Auch bei der Abgabe von Mustern gab es häufig Mißbräuche, so daß 1986 eine Marktordnung erlassen werden mußte, um den Sumpf trockenzulegen. Ziel dieser Marktordnung war es, „die Verteilung von Medikamenten mit einheitlichen und transparenten Bedingungen zu regeln, um eine ökonomische Versorgung der Bevölkerung mit den verordneten Medikamenten zu gewährleisten und den Bedürfnissen der Bevölkerung und der Krankenkassen Rechnung zu tragen".

In einer ökonomischen Magisterarbeit, die der Marketingstrategie für die Lancierung eines neuen pharmazeutischen Produkts gewidmet war [1], fand ich eine Klassifizierung der Ärzte in 3 Kategorien:

- der nicht Entwicklungsfähige,
- der langsam Entwicklungsfähige,
- der schnell Entwicklungsfähige.

Krankenkassen

Was sind nun die Einflüsse des Kostenträgers, d.h. wie beeinflussen die Krankenkassen die Wahlfreiheit des verschreibenden Arztes?

Seitdem es Generika oder – wie sie auch genannt werden – Synonym-Präparate auf dem Markt gibt, wird von dieser Seite immer mehr Druck auf den Arzt ausgeübt.

Es handelt sich um Medikamente, die durch Zweitfirmen nach Ablauf des Patents, welches das Originalpräparat schützt, hergestellt werden und die gleichen Wirkstoffe enthalten.

Die Krankenkassen interessieren sich deshalb so sehr für die Generika, weil der Preis einer „Kopie“ bei gleicher Dosierung mindestens 25% unter dem Preis des entsprechenden Originalpräparates sein muß, da für die Generika keinerlei Kosten für Forschung, klinische Prüfung und Markteinführung anfallen.

Es gibt 3 verschiedene Arten von „Kopien“:

- *Markengenerika:* Kopien mit einem Markennamen.
- *Wirkstoffgenerika:* der Arzt rezeptiert einzig den Wirkstoffnamen und die Dosierung.
- *Ersatzgenerika:* das Originalpräparat wird durch irgendeine Kopie ohne Markennamen ersetzt.

In der Schweiz wird ein Großteil der Kopien als Markengenerika verkauft, wobei diese auch bei der Interkantonalen Kontrollstelle für Heilmittel (IKS) registriert werden müssen.

1983 schrieb der Präsident des schweizerischen Krankenkassen-Konkordates an alle Ärzte des Landes und bat sie, Generika zu verschreiben.

In seinem Brief heißt es wörtlich:

> In der Beilage erhalten Sie eine Vergleichsliste von Original- und Synonym-Präparaten mit identischen Wirkstoffen oder Wirkstoffgruppen für die gleiche oder ähnliche Indikation. Nur Sie als Arzt können betimmen, welches Präparat zur Anwendung gelangen soll und welches die wirtschaftlichste Medikation ist. Wir bitten Sie, die von unserer Vertrauensapothekerin und von weiteren Fachleuten zusammengestellte Liste zu prüfen und zu überlegen, wo Sie allenfalls Einsparungen erzielen können. Die vorhandenen Mittel in der Krankenversicherung sind knapp, jeder heute nicht eingesparte Franken wird in naher Zukunft fehlen ...

Dieser Brief schlug hohe Wellen, und die Pharmaindustrie reagierte heftig, indem sie argumentierte, man wolle ihr die nötigen Mittel zur Forschung entziehen.

Somit steht also der verschreibende Arzt vor einem Gewissenskonflikt: Soll er die Forschung unterstützen, von der er sich weitere therapeutische Mittel erhofft? Oder: Soll er versuchen, die Kosten für die Krankenkasse zu dämpfen, da sonst die Krankenkassenprämien weiterhin steigen?

Es bleibt noch die Frage, welches der auf der Liste befindlichen Generika gewählt werden soll und nach welchem Kriterium?

Patienten

Zuletzt ist noch der Einfluß des Patienten auf die Freiheit der ärztlichen Verschreibung zu erwähnen. Ich möchte hier eine Studie zitieren, die ich in meiner Praxis durchführte. Ich untersuchte aufgrund von 1000 Erstkonsultationen das Verschreibungsprofil und die Nachfrage des Patienten nach Medikamenten.

25,6 % der Patienten erhielten kein Rezept während der Konsultation.

Die 744 ausgestellten Rezepte umfaßten 1759 Medikamente, d. h. im Mittel, 2,4 Medikamente pro Rezept. Im Durchschnitt erhielten Frauen nicht mehr Medikamente als Männer.

Diese 1759 Medikamente verteilten sich auf 52 verschiedene therapeutische Klassen, was 277 verschiedenen Medikamentenmarken entsprach.

Als ausdrücklich verlangte Medikamente bezeichne ich Medikamente, welche von den Patienten außerhalb des Hauptmotivs der Konsultation verlangt wurden, ohne daß ein entsprechendes Symptom erwähnt wurde und ohne daß ich die Verschreibung dieses Medikaments oder die Erneuerung der Verschreibung dieses Medikaments plante.

Setzen wir diese Nachfrage nach Medikamenten in Beziehung zum Geschlecht und zum Alter, dann stellen wir fest, daß 17 % der Medikamente bei den Frauen und 11 % der Medikamente bei den Männern ausdrücklich verlangt wurden und daß der Anteil der verlangten Medikamente mit zunehmendem Alter bei beiden Geschlechtern steigt. Bis zum Alter von 50 Jahren besteht nur ein geringer Unterschied, danach erhöht sich der Anteil der ausdrücklich verlangten Medikamente bei den Frauen relativ abrupt auf 30 %.

Es stellt sich nun die Frage nach den verschiedenen therapeutischen Klassen dieser 237 verlangten Medikamente, die 5 % aller verordneten Medikamente entsprechen.

Frauen verlangen v. a. Schlafmittel, Anxiolytika, Venenpräparate und Diuretika.

Männer dagegen verlangen vorwiegend Antazida, Spasmolytika und Antitussiva.

Wie sind diese Resultate zu interpretieren? Die große Nachfrage nach psychotropen Medikamenten durch Frauen erscheint als Resultat des Beziehungsfeldes, in der diese Frauen leben: Von der Gesellschaft in die Rolle der „Stütze der Familie" gedrängt, muß die Frau häufig wenig befriedigende Aufgaben übernehmen. Außerdem muß sie durch das Älterwerden mehrere Konflikte bewältigen, z. B. die Ablösung der Kinder, die Menopause, die Pensionierung oder auch den Verlust des Partners; also lauter Trennungssituationen. Dazu entwickeln sich oft parallel chronische Krankheiten, die das seelische Gleichgewicht stören können. Die Schlaflosigkeit, die Angst oder auch die depressive Reaktion sind Folgen davon. Bei Beziehungsproblemen hilft sich der Mann viel eher mit Alkohol, um die inneren Spannungen zu dämpfen. Die Frau wendet sich wohl wegen der soziokulurellen Barrieren viel lieber an den Arzt um Hilfe. Dieser, häufig ungenügend ausgebildet, um irgendeine andere Therapie als die medikamentöse zu wählen, begnügt sich mit der Verschreibung eines psychotropen Medikaments. Die Patientin kann, einmal erleichtert, kaum mehr ohne Medikamente leben, da ja die existentiellen Probleme ungelöst bleiben. Eine zumindest psychologische Abhängigkeit vom Medikament bildet sich aus. Aufgrund der Reglementierung über den Verkauf dieses Medikaments wird der Arzt das Ziel einer starken Nachfrage, der er sich kaum entziehen kann, ohne tiefschürfende Spannungen in der Arzt-Patienten-Beziehung zu provozieren [2].

Die Schlußfolgerung aus diesen Überlegungen lautet, daß die Feiheit der ärztlichen Verschreibung wohl eher eine *Illusion* ist. Zwar erfolgt die Wahl des wirkstoffes noch häufig nach rationalen Kriterien, die tatsächliche Verordnung aber eher nach emotionalen bzw. irrationalen Gesichtspunkten.

Litertur

1. Balleys C (1982) La communication marketing pour le lancement d'un produit pharmaceutique. Licence HEC. Universitè, Genève
2. Nemitz I, Melle G van (1983) Les médicaments en médecine générale. Etude des profiles de prescription et de la demande. Schweiz Med Wochenschr 113: 1719–1726
3. Petit Robert (1977) Dictionnaire de la langue française. Société du nouveau Littré, Paris
4. Schelling JL (1983) Thérapeutique médicale. Flammarion, Paris

Drugs and Placebos in General Practice: The View of a Sceptic

James S. McCormick

'General practice' requires some sort of definition if what follows is to make sense. For the purposes of this contribution it refers to those doctor-provided services which are directly accessible to the public and which are prepared to deal in the first instance with any problem which is presented. It has to deal not only with cancer and heart disease but also with 'my budgerigar has died'.

The decision to seek professional help is, by most people in most circumstances, not easily made. The reasons that people decide to come to general practitioners may be listed as reassurance, diagnosis, treatment, 'problems of living with the human condition', legitimisation of 'sick role', surveillance of chronic disease and prevention. The commonest reason for seeking help is to discover the meaning of symptoms rather than to seek treatment. Pains and discomforts between the top of the head and the genitals require an explanation. Unexplained they may herald heart disease, cancer, a hospital admission or imminent death. The first need is reassurance which may need to be coupled with a diagnosis, a label of some kind, which has some explanatory and prognostic power. 'This is a simple strain, not a symptom of arthritis'.

Treatment in general practice, usually by drugs of one kind or another, is instituted for a variety of reasons. Reasons for prescribing include:

Symptom relief
Patient's expectations
Maintenance of 'sick role'
Closing strategy
Being on the safe side
Cure or amelioration of disease

Symptom Relief

All treatments work! This is fortunate because it enabled me, for many years, to earn a livelihood in general practice. It is also fortunate because it underpins the growing success of absurdities which range from homoeopathy to acupuncture and aromatherapy. All treatments alleviate symptoms, only a relatively few alter the course of disease. It is a fallacy to assume that alleviating pain and discomfort is the same as curing disease, it is folly not taking the trouble to identify the difference.

Rationale Pharmakotherapie in der Allgemeinpraxis
Rational Pharmacotherapy in General Practice
M. M. Kochen (Hrsg.)

Identifying the difference is a recent phenomenon and rests on the placebo controlled double-blind randomised trial. Nothing else suffices because our experience is a fallacious guide. Learning by experience results in learning to make the same mistakes with increasing confidence. Because we are enthusiastic prescribers we forget that most human ills are self-limiting. What happended to the millions of women who suffered acute dysuria before the advent of antibiotics and mid-stream urine samples? Is the literature of the last century and the beginning of this full of the miseries of unrelieved frequency?

Those of a properly sceptical frame of mind find themselves caught by Asher's paradox. I cannot do better than quote the master himself. 'If you can believe fervently in your treatment, even though controlled studies show that it is quite useless, then your results are much better, your patients are much better, and your income is much better too. I believe that this accounts for the remarkable success of some of the less gifted, but more credulous members of our profession, and also for the violent dislike of statistics and controlled tests which fashionable and successful doctors are accustomed to display' [1].

The more dramatic the placebo the greater the benefit, red pills are better than white ones, needles better than physick, surgery better than medicine. Coronary artery by-pass surgery has major placebo effects. Imagine going through all that and not feeling restored! There are some effective drugs which alleviate pain in a non-specific way. That is they do not alter the course of the disease but act as analgesics or anaesthetics. While non-steroidal anti-inflammatory drugs are advertised and promulgated as more than analgesics, a very successful advertising ploy, in most instances their good effects are evident because of their analgesic potential. Alcohol has it uses and opiates suffer relative neglect because of unreal fears of the possibility of addiction.

Patient's Expectations

The commonest rationalisation in our society for foolish prescribing is that the patient expects a prescription. This is sometimes followed by the parenthetic remark that 'if I don't give them what they want they will go elsewhere'. While this is obviously set in the culture of particular societies at particular times and the previous experience of patients themselves, it is often exaggerated and often does not represent reality. Explanation and appropriate and effective reassurance will often obviate the need for medicine. It is also worth remembering that some prescriptions are never 'cashed' and that medicine cabinets throughout the Western world are full of uneaten and decaying tablets and capsules. Part of this waste is the result of prescribing courses of antibiotics for self-limiting conditions: when symptoms abate taking medicine is both hard to remember and difficult to justify.

Legitimisation of 'Sick Role'

In our society the only acceptable way of escaping social obligations, going to school, going to work, washing dishes, having sexual intercourse, is to declare oneself 'sick'. In return society demands that after a short time, in addition to expressing the desire to be well, a doctor must be consulted to 'legitimise' the sickness. In the case of those for whom pieces of paper certifying unfitness are not possible, legitimisation can only be sustained by 'being under treatment' or 'attending the doctor'. As a result the prescription is for many, the necessary proof of their illness and their right to be sick. Doctors are as a rule unaware of the many patients who come to them to be kept sick rather than to be made well and many repeat prescriptions are unwittingly written to meet this need.

'Closing Strategy'

Many practitioners are overworked in the sense that they attempt to see too many patients in a relatively brief time span. As a result consultations are carried out under severe time constraints. It therefore behooves doctors to develop good 'closing strategies' which offer the possibility of ending the consultation with honour. The writing and accepting of a prescription is one of the most effective and widely employed of these. It is much less time intensive than explanation and reassurance.

'Being on the Safe Side'

One of the major differences among doctors is their attitude to risk. Some are fearful of risk, and using the rationalisation of possible medico-legal consequences, try to cover themselves against every eventuality. This leads to over-investigation, with its burden of 'false-positive' results, over-referral to colleagues and indubitably to over-prescribing. The physician who shares his anxieties and uncertainties with his patients does them a disservice. 'This is almost certainly not heart pain *but* ...' negates reassurance and condemns the patient to further, often dangerous investigation, just 'to be on the safe side'. A recent letter to the *British Journal of General Practice* suggests a correlation between willingness to visit 'out of hours' and the rate of antibiotic prescribing for sore throats [3]. That is, those who were unhappy to take the risk of giving telephone advice were unlikely to take the risk of eschewing antibiotics for sore throats.

Cure or Amelioration

The scientific basis for rational prescribing is the identification of diseases for which proven effective therapies of low risk are now available. While in medical school the emphasis is properly on achieving an accurate diagnosis and much less on therapy, even the briefest exposure to general practice makes one aware that in about half the new problems which are presented no meaningful diagnosis is possible.

One of the feature that distinguish good medical practice from complementary or alternative medicine is the specificity of proven therapies. Cyanacobalamin is essential and effective therapy for vitamin B^{12} deficiency, insulin for some diabetics and for nothing else, thyroxine for endogenous deficiency of hormone production. Such responses are generalisable throughout the European Community and the Western world and rest on accurate diagnosis. However, such conditions, even when one includes surgical emergencies, are relatively rare in family practice. On the other hand there are large differences in prescribing between the various member states of the community which relate, for the most part, to the diagnoses or labels which are attached to those 50 % of consultations in which no clear reason for the patient's symptoms is immediately obvious. Prescribing for non-diseases is widespread and harmful. It is harmful because it suggests to people that they have a disease when they do not. In Ireland the commonest non-disease is hypertension, in Germany it is heart disorder and hypotension, in France it is disorders, unspecified, of the liver, in the United States it is probably hypercholesterolaemia. Having 'blood pressure' has markedly deleterious effects on self-image and well-being. Of those men given placebo in the Medical Research Council Trial 10 % became impotent [2]! It is also harmful in that none, or almost none, of the drugs used to treat these non-diseases is free from undesirable side effects, and all of them cost money and in most the cost is a continuing one. Lacking a respectable physical label for discomfort many are gratuitously given a mental disease, the worried are treated for 'anxiety neurosis' with benzodiazapines, the sad for 'depression' with tricyclics.

The other main reason for foolish prescribing is treating viral infections with antibiotics. Truly rational prescribing of antibiotics in general practice is an unrealistic goal in a 'speedy culture' where sensitivity is not readily available. Sensible prescribing must be based upon probabilities. For example the use of sulphonamides as first-line treatment for cystitis is justified by what is known of the sensitivities of common organisms. On the other hand to treat all sore throats with antibiotics because viral and bacterial causes are clinically indistinguishable, usually justified by recourse to the distant possibility that nasty streptococci may be involved, is not sensible. When did any of you last see a case of 'acute rheumatism' or 'rheumatic fever'?

Conclusion

Medicine abhors the vacuum of inactivity. Prescribing is the commonest and most widespread manifestation of mindles acitvism. If we as physicians were prepared to treat our patients as equal consenting adults, to confess our ignorance while reassuring them that their worst fears were groundless, and were we to be cautious of attaching dubious labels as a justification for using drugs, our patients would be healthier, the economy of our countries would benefit and we would be better abel to claim a scientific basis for our activities.

References

1. Asher (1972) Talking sense, Jones FA (ed). Pitman Medical, London, p 47
2. Medical Research Council Working Party (1981) Adverse reactions to bendrofluazide and propranolol. Lancet ii: 632
3. Pitts J, Whitby M (1990) Action tresholds. Br J Gen Pract 40: 350–3511

Problemorientierte Workshops
Problem-Oriented Workshops

Arzneimittelverordnung in Europa – Traditionen

Drug Prescribing in Europe: Can Traditions Be Overcome?

Drug Prescribing – Can Traditions Be Overcome?

Daniele Coen

Pinpointing the Problem

A survey published in 1986 showed a very strong negative correlation between the time since a physician graduated and the currency of his or her knowledge concerning the care of patients with hypertension [6]. In other words, physicians seem to treat disorders much in the way in which they were taught in formal training. If this is the sense that we want to give to the word "tradition", some corollaries follow:

First, the need to overcome tradition is directly proportional to the rate of real innovation in a field. The rate of real innovation in pharmacotherapeutics is not exceedingly fast, since most new drugs are actually "me-toos" that do not add much to what pre-existing drugs already offered. As an example, Table 1 shows the rate of relevant innovation in the drug market as assessed by three independent sources in recent years [1,2,5]. This observation is even truer if we restrict the field to general practice, where many time-honored remedies are still unexcelled (penicillin, thiazide, aspirin etc.). In this respect the need to overcome tradition does not seem to be that strong and the decision of many British general practitioners (GPs) not to include in their formularies drugs that have been on the market for less than five years seems wise and not backward.

Table 1. The quality of new drugs according to three independent bulletins

Bulletin	Evaluation		
	Effective and innovative	Effective but non-innovative	Ineffective and irrational
Scrip[a]	140		368
La Revue Prescrire[b]	18	314	28
Ricerca & Pratica[c]	9	63	28

[a] Reports evaluation by Rhone Poulenc Santé of 508 drugs marketed 1975–1985.
[b] Evaluated 360 drugs marketed in France 1981–1986.
[c] Evaluated 100 drugs marketed in Italy 1984–1986.

Second, in fact the wish to overcome tradition seems to be much more a characteristic of the pharmaceutical industry than of concerned pharmacologists, health

Rationale Pharmakotherapie in der Allgemeinpraxis
Rational Pharmacotherapy in General Practice
M. M. Kochen (Hrsg.)

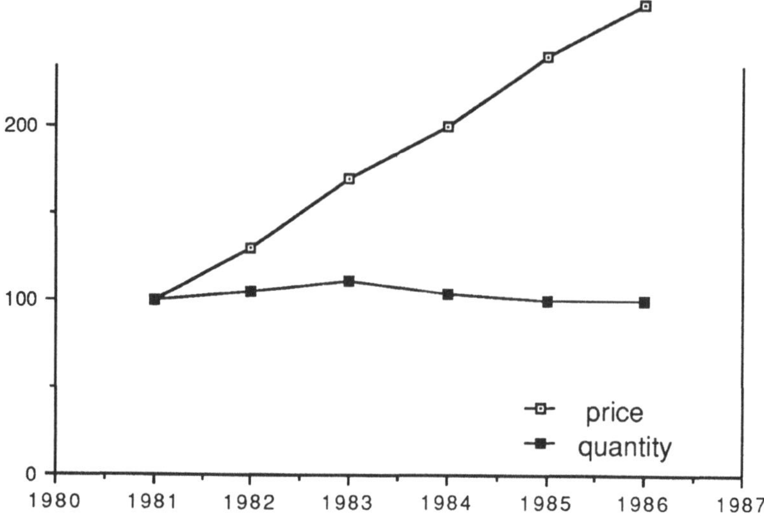

Fig. 1. Average price of drugs and drug consumption in Italy

bodies or the general public. As shown in Fig. 1, between 1981 and 1986 the total drug expenditure in Italy more than doubled, with consumption remaining steady. The rise in price was mainly due to the so called *price mix*, that is to the increasing use of new drugs of high price supported by strong marketing initiatives in place of older and cheaper drugs of equivalent efficacy.

Third, when new and effective therapeutic strategies come of age, doctors do not hesitate and, with few exceptions, adopt them quickly. The fast success of drugs like H^2-antagonists, beta blockers, and ACE inhibitors well exemplifies this statement. We could say that in some cases the enthusiasm for novelty is even excessive, and that the unjustified use of new, effective drugs becomes itself a problem.

If this is true, the question should be restated. *We should not ask ourselves how to overcome tradition but rather how to overcome bad therapeutic habits, regardless of their ancient or recent birth date.*

How to Overcome Bad Therapeutic Habits

A therapeutic option can be considered inappropriate for many different reasons. Here are the most common:

1. The symptom/illness does not need drug treatment.
2. The efficacy of the drug has not been proven beyond doubt.
3. Alternative drugs with a better benefit/risk ratio are available.
4. Alternative drugs with a better benefit/cost ratio are available.

5. No drugs are available to treat a symptom/illness, but preventive, psychological, nursing, social, economical steps should be taken to help the patient tackle his health problems.

These situations interact with one another within the wider context of uncertainty in medicine (i. e. the many clinical problems for which a widely agreed approach does not yet exist) to produce puzzling scenarios in drug use like those proposed in the following:

1. Comparative data from different culturally and epidemiologically heterogeneous countries demonstrate that the same, well-defined problem (diabetes, hypertension) is treated with a number of drugs that can vary two- to threefold (WHO-DURG).
2. Patients admitted to coronary care units with a diagnosis of myocardial infarction posed according to standard criteria, have been treated with completely different pharmacological approaches, apparently without any difference in mortality or outcome (ISIS-1) [15].
3. Elderly patients with memory and behavioural impairment do not receive any "specific" drug in many northern European countries, while they use up to 5 %–7 % of the whole drug market in some Mediterranean countries.
4. It is well known, from all reviews of hospital formularies, that it is enough to change department (or the head of a department) to see patients with a similar diagnosis being treated with radically different therapies. Again with no apparent difference in outcome.

It is not easy to figure effective solutions to the problem, but what seems to be clear by now is that simply providing doctors with good information is not enough. There seem to be two major limits to sheer information, even when independent and of good quality:

1. For as much of an effort as one can put into reaching doctors with drug bulletins, consensus statements and other written material, this will be but a drop in the ocean of industry-supported information (journals, high-quality press leaflets, meetings, personal contacts etc.). A competition in this field is neither foreseeable nor ultimately desirable. As G. Tognoni says: "The market that wins a market is a market" [12].
2. Information on single drugs is doomed to quick obsolescence, and it is doubtful that the strong efforts needed to reach some behavioural changes [4, 11] will pay in the long run. In fact, it will not be possible to keep pace with the fast turnover of drugs on the market and any improvement in the use of a single well-known drug (or class of drugs) will soon be replaced by the inappropriate use of the newest one.

The only hope for good quality information to be effective is being spread among doctors who have become reactive to it, that is, who can recognize it from the bulk of less-trustworthy data and who are able to usefully integrate it in their everyday practice. Some skills must be learned by doctors before this happens:

1. Therapeutics should be approached with a problem-oriented and not with a drug-oriented attitude. This means that all possible options of care/cure of an illness should be examined in terms of expected benefits, risks and costs before a choice is made. A drug-oriented approach, on the contrary, bypasses all this invaluable clinical work with the apparently simplifying question: "Will this drug do?" The following points are corollaries of a problem-oriented approach.
2. Any therapeutic problem should be faced considering first of all the natural history of the disease and the possible role of non-drug treatment. Epidemiological knowledge on expected risks and benefits of drug and non-drug treatment should be sought especially before engaging in long-term treatment of diseases like hypertension, hypercholesterolaemia, senile dementia, psychiatric syndromes, etc.
3. The efficacy of drugs should be evaluated on the basis of well-conducted clinical trials, which doctors should be able to seek, to read, to criticize, at least in the fundamentals of design and methodology. Side-effects of drugs should be evaluated on the basis of equally appropriate studies (case-control, cohort, in their absence spontaneous referral data).
4. Doctors should learn to live with uncertainty. Not every medical problem has an answer and fake drugs or impure placebos should not offer an easy way out from the daily recognition that this is true. Good sense, a compassionate attitude, open discussion with patients are important skills that should be mastered.

All what we have said this far could be summarised by saying that *the trend towards better prescribing must pass through a cultural (r)evolution that brings doctors to play an active, rather than a passive role in the game of drug information.*

Research and Formularies: The Tools

Formularies have been produced for decades both in industrialized and in less-developed countries at the local, regional and national levels. Some of the best known have been produced by central institutions such as WHO [13] or governments with the aim to offer doctors more or less strict guidelines to rational and economic prescribing. The cultural relevance of the first WHO list is doubtless, but most centrally produced formularies that followed this example met the hostility of doctors who felt constrained in their clinical freedom.

Locally produced formularies have flourished more recently in Europe, especially in Great Britain. One of their characteristics is that of featuring a sort of co-authorship between doctors or groups of doctors who work in a given area. In fact, although only few persons formally sign the formulary, often they are just those who put on paper what was discussed or actually experimented by a much larger group of colleagues [7,8]. The most valuable consequence of a formulary of this kind is that while it is being written, its contents progressively become "routine" for a good majority of its intended readers. Thus, in this case the (in)formation is found not so much in the reading, but in the writing of the formulary, a process that compels participating doctors to go through all the steps of a problem-oriented approach to therapy. Recent papers have argued that both hospital and general-practice formularies developed at a local level deserve the time and money spent for their production, since they improve the quality and reduce the cost of prescriptions [3, 14].

A European Formulary for General Practice is at this time being written under the auspices of the EEC by a group of practitioners and clinical pharmacologists from most European countries. When available (1992), it shall offer doctors who do not want to engage in the writing of a formulary the chance to work "backwards" from an already written formulary to the scientific and clinical reasoning that determined its contents. Doctors should indeed try to adopt the formulary, discuss its indications in a group of colleagues, propose possible modifications and confront finally their opinions and experience with the literature presented in the appendix of the European Formulary, a literature which is the basis for the determination and supporting of its indications. Again, this is a potentially fruitful way to promote the direct engagement of doctors in the development of their therapeutic skills.

There is no room here to engage in an in-depth discussion on the role, both scientific and educational, of research in general practice, about which interesting papers have been written [9, 10]. An example from outside the world of GP, coming again from Italy (Table 2), can nevertheless serve as a conclusion, suggesting that research done within the premises of clinical practice can produce immediate

Table 2. The impact of research trials on in-hospital mortality from myocardial infarction in Italy

Period or date	Mortality (%)	Setting or study
1955–1979	30	Before CCUs were widely available
1970–1983	12–15	Patients treated in CCU
1986	13	GISSI[a] mortality in control group
	10.7	GISSI mortality in patients treated with streptokinase
1990	8.8	GISSI-2[b]: overall mortality in patients treated with a fibrinolytic agent plus a package of recommended treatment (beta-blockers + ASA + nitrates)

CCU, coronary care unit.

[a] GISSI was a large-scaled clinical trial investigating the effectiveness of intravenous thrombolytic treatment in acute myocardial infarction. It involved 11 812 patients at 178 Italian CCUs, representing about 70% of all Italian CCUs.

[b] GISSI-2 compared alteplase with streptokinase and heparin with no heparin in 12 490 patients with acute myocardial infarction. 223 Italian CCUs participated in the study.

beneficial therapeutic effects. Conversely, introducing a research attitude within everyday practice recovers to scientific investigation a mass of observations and data that would otherwise have been wasted.

References

1. Anonymous (1985) Ten years of NCE discovery analysed. Scrip Dec 23 : 1062
2. Anonymous (1987) Les medicaments de l'année 1986. La Revue Prescrire 7(61) : 39–43
3. Anonymous (1989) Local drug formularies: are they worth the effort? Drug Ther Bull 27 : 13–16
4. Avorn J. Soumerai SB (1983) Improving drug therapy decisions through educational outreach. A randomized controlled trial of academically based drug "detailing". N Engl J Med 308 : 1457–1463
5. Devoto MA, Franzosi MG (1988) Vere e false novitá: tre anni di mercato italiano. Ricera e pratica 19 : 17–23
6. Evans CE, Haynes RB, Birkett NJ et al. (1986) Does a mailed continuing education program improve physician performance? Results of a randomized trial in hypertensive care. JAMA 255 : 501–504
7. Grant GB, Gregory DA, van Zwanenberg TD (1985) Development of a formulary for general practice. Lancet i : 1030–1032
8. Grant GB, Gregory DA, van Zwanenberg TD (1990) A basic formulary for general practice. Oxford University Press, Oxford
9. Howie JGR (1984) Research in general practice: pursuit of knowledge or defence of wisdom? Br Med J 289 : 1770–1773
10. Mushlin AI (1984) New knowledge for primary care: a glimpse at general practice research in Great Britain. Ann Intern Med 100 : 744–750
11. Schaffner W, Ray WA, Federspiel CF, Miller WO (1983) Improving antibiotic prescribing in office practice – A controlled trial of three educational methods. JAMA 250 : 1728–1732
12. Tognoni G (1988) Migliorare la qualità delle prescrizioni in medicina di base: un punto di vista antitetico. Ricerca e pratica 19 : 24–28
13. WHO Expert Committee (1977) The selection of essential drugs. WHO TRS 641, Geneva
14. Working for patients (1989) Working paper 4, The Health Service Review. HMSO, London
15. ISIS-1 Collaborative Group. Randomized trial of intravenous atenolol among 16 027 cases of suspected acute myocardial infarction: ISIS-1. Lancet 1986; ii : 57-66

Nootropika und „durchblutungsfördernde“ Pharmaka: Eine Pille für alle Alten?

Nootropics and Drugs for “Better Circulation”: A Pill for All Aged?

Hausärztliche Verordnungsweise von Nootropika und durchblutungsfördernden Pharmaka

Ulrich Rendenbach

Einleitung

Ein Fünftel der Bevölkerung der Bundesrepublik Deutschland ist heute 60 Jahre und älter. Die Tendenz ist steigend. Die Zahl der in Westdeutschland an einer Demenz leidenden alten Menschen wird auf 700000 geschätzt, wobei dem Hausarzt eine Schlüsselrolle bei der Versorgung dieser Patienten zukommt [3.]. Da von allen Schwächen des Alters die beeinträchtigte Leistung des Gehirns vom Kranken und seinen Angehörigen als die schlimmste empfunden wird und „ganze Heerscharen von medizinischen Assistenz - und Fachberufen" [3] zur Behandlung nötig sind, ist verständlich, wenn Arzt und alter Mensch mit allen Mitteln versuchen, die Hirnfunktion möglichst lange zu erhalten. Unter Ärzten jedoch gibt es gegenteilige Auffassungen über den rechten Weg. Die einen, meist Pharmakologen, lehnen jegliche stoffliche Beeinflußbarkeit eines „verkalkten Gehirns" ab, andere, meist Hausärzte, verordnen Nootropika und durchblutungsfördernde Pharmaka. Eine Besserung sei aber höchstens durch Gehtraining für die arterielle Verschlußkrankheit (AVK) und durch „zerebrales Jogging" [9] für die vaskuläre Zerebralsklerose zu erreichen – so die einen [8, 10]. Die anderen sind vorsichtiger, weniger ablehnend, versuchen wissenschaftlich zu begründen, was sie an Wirkung vermuten [6, 11]. Hier soll der Versuch einer Standortbestimmung gemacht werden. Dabei muß es zu Kontroversen kommen – diese sind beabsichtigt.

Im Arzneiverordnungsreport 1990 liegen die „durchblutungsfördernden Mittel" mit 19,2 Mio. Verordnungen auf Rang 12 und bei den Kosten an 4. Stelle mit 1,2 Mrd. DM [9]. In der Rangliste der führenden Arzneimittel hält *Tebonin* den 8. Platz mit 3,3 Mio. Verordnungen für 1989 (101,3 Mio. Tagesdosen). Rein rechnerisch kann man ermitteln, daß im Jahre 1989 280000 Menschen Tebonin eingenommen haben. Hat ein Arzt 28 Patienten Tebonin verordnet, so müssen in den westlichen Bundesländern wenigstens 10000 Ärzte dieses Mittel verschrieben haben. Eine ähnliche Rechnung könnte man mit den weiteren häufig verschriebenen Präparaten aufstellen.

Die nach Verordnungen führenden Arzneimittel dieser Indikationsgruppe [9] waren auf Rang

8 – Tebonin,
10 – Dusodril,
56 – Trental,
72 – Sibelium.

Rationale Pharmakotherapie in der Allgemeinpraxis
Rational Pharmacotherapy in General Practice
M. M. Kochen (Hrsg.)

Trotz massiver öffentlicher Kritik (z. B. der Bremer Pharmakologe, Prof. Schönhöfer, in „Panorama" am 12. 12. 89) sind die Verordnungen der „durchblutungsfördernden Mittel" nur um 15 % zurückgegangen. Man könnte vermuten, daß der Zuwachs von 24 % bei den Salicylaten genau diese Lücke füllt, seit die prophylaktische Gabe von Acetylsalicylsäure bei drohenden Gefäßverschlüssen empfohlen wird.

Warum also werden Nootropika und durchblutungsfördernde Pharmaka verordnet? Es gilt, das Verordnungsverhalten der Hausärzte zu analysieren. Dazu eignet sich jedoch der Arzneiverordnungsreport 90 weniger, weil er lediglich Auskunft über Verschreibungshäufigkeiten vermittelt, aber nicht über Gründe dazu.

Auch der unverhohlene Vorwurf an den Arzt, er verordne durchblutungsfördernde Pharmaka „wie vielfach üblich, zur symptomatischen Monotherapie, die zudem unter unzutreffenden oder unbewiesenen pathogenetischen Vorstellungen erfolgt" [9], ist zur Beantwortung der gestellten Frage nicht geeignet. Der Hinweis schließlich, Tebonin habe sich „als Spitzenreiter in der Indikationsgruppe halten können" und „das Marketing sei offenbar gezielt auf die phytopharmakologische Marktlücke für dieses Indikationsgebiet gerichtet (z. B. Verteilung von Ginkgobäumen)" [9], ist eine Spekulation. Einmal liegt ein Rückgang um 15 % gegenüber 1988 vor, und schließlich sind Werbefeldzüge anderer Firmen von ungleich höherer Aggressivität.

Nosologie

Sich krank fühlen, ist ein subjektives Phänomen, das von einer Vielzahl von äußeren und inneren Faktoren abhängt. Ein naturwissenschaftlich exakter Befund korreliert mit dem subjektiven Krankheitsgefühl nur locker. Als geheilt gilt ein Mensch, wenn die Krankheit oder deren Ursache beseitigt wird, die Symptome wesentlich gemildert werden oder die Einstellung zur Krankheit verändert wird. Dieser Heilungsprozeß ist nachprüfbar oder durch Meinungsäußerung des Kranken zu messen. Demnach kann als primäres Ziel ärztlicher Handlung entweder subjektives Wohlbefinden im Vordergrund stehen oder der objektive Befund.

Leistungsminderungen des Gehirns im Alter werden in einer Allgemeinpraxis oft beklagt. In vielen Fällen ist trotz hohen technischen Aufwands lediglich eine Ursachenvermutung möglich. Durchblutungsstörungen des Gehirns, oft eine Verlegenheitsdiagnose des Hausarztes, ist gesellschaftsfähig, wenn sie auch nur knapp 30 % aller Demenzen verursacht [11]. Andere Diagnosen sind angstbesetzt (Alzheimer-Krankheit, Schlaganfall).

Plazeboeffect

Ein Placebo hat eine Wirkung, die nicht chemisch oder physikalisch zu erklären ist, die aber dennoch ins therapeutische Denken einfließt. Bei Art und Stärke der Wirkung ist die Erwartungshaltung des Kranken, vermittelt durch die Suggestion des

Heilers, von entscheidender Wichtigkeit. Placebo- und Wirkstoffeffekt sind also nicht zu trennen. In der Praxis wird häufig mit unreinen (oder Pseudo)placebos gearbeitet, das sind Medikamente, deren Inhaltsstoffe für unwirksam gehalten werden. Die Übergänge sind fließend. Gibt der Arzt unreine Placebos, läßt er den Patienten im Glauben an die Wirkung, er selbst weiß um die Täuschung und akzeptiert sie (oder er selbst glaubt an die Substanz).

Ginkgo biloba folium

Die Droge besteht aus getrockneten Blättern des Ginkgobaumes sowie aus deren Zubereitungen. Inhaltsstoffe sind Flavonoide, Procyanidine, Diterpenoide, Ginkgolide, Bilobalid. Für standardisierte Extrakte aus Ginkgoblättern (Tebonin, Generika) wurde sowohl eine Förderung der Durchblutung festgestellt als auch eine Senkung der Blutviskosität [4]. Eine erhöhte Hypoxietoleranz wurde nur tierexperimentell nachgewiesen. Als Anwendungsgebiete des Arzneimittels wurden zerebrovaskuläre Insuffizienz mit den Symptomen Schwindel, Ohrensausen, Konzentrationsschwäche im Rahmen eines organischen Psychosyndroms sowie arterielle periphere Durchblutungsstörungen infolge degenerativer Gefäßerkrankungen angegeben [4].

Eigene Untersuchungen

Die wachsende Kritik an der Pharmakotherapie der Hausärzte veranlaßte mich, in meiner Praxis das eigene Verordnungsverhalten und die Reaktionen meiner Patienten am „Spitzenreiter" Tebonin zu überprüfen. Es handelt sich um eine Kleinstadtpraxis mit ländlichem Einzugsgebiet und 1280 Krankenscheinen pro Quartal. Zu beantworten waren folgende Fragen:

1) Warum haben Sie Tebonin verordnet bekommen?
2) Seit wann nehmen Sie Tebonin?
3) Wer hat es Ihnen empfohlen?
4) Es gibt gute Ärzte, Spezialisten, die Tebonin genau untersucht haben. Sie behaupten, Tebonin habe keine Wirkung. – Sehen Sie das genauso?
5) Wenn es stimmt, was diese Ärzte sagen, daß Tebonin keine Wirkung hat, möchten Sie es trotzdem weiter einnehmen oder wollen wir einen Auslaßversuch machen?
6) Wieviel Tebonin haben Sie eingenommen?

Aufgenommen wurden alle Patienten, die im 2. und 3. Quartal 1990 Tebonin als Wiederholungsrezeptur erhielten. Insgesamt waren das 35 Patienten von 1280 (= 2,7 %; Prozentzahlen gerundet): 22 Patienten waren älter als 70 Jahre, 13 jünger, der jüngste 48 Jahre; 23 waren Frauen, 12 Männer.

Zur Frage 1:
Die *Symptome*, die zur Verordnung führten, lassen sich nicht in einer Statistik nor-

mieren, sie sind sehr individuell. Einige charakteristische Patientenaussagen seien wörtlich angegeben:

„Ich kann mich besser konzentrieren."
„Mein Hörsturz ist besser."
„Ich habe keinen Herzdruck mehr."
„Meine Kopfschmerzen sind besser."
„Wegen meiner Durchblutungsstörungen, ich merke aber nichts."
„Die Leere im Kopf ist weg."
„Ich habe Durchblutungsstörungen der Beine und kann besser laufen."
„Mein Schwindel ist weg."
„Meine Ohrgeräusche sind weg."
„Mein nächtlicher Beinschmerz ist weg."

Diese Liste ließe sich fortsetzen.
Als *Diagnosen* wurden angegeben:

Durchblutungsstörungen,
Zerebralinsuffizienz,
Tinnitus,
Zephalgie, Migräne.

Zu Frage 2:
Die Dauer der Einnahme schwankte zwischen einigen Monaten und 12 Jahren.

Zu Frage 3:
- Empfehlung aus dem Umfeld des Patienten (Freunde, Verwandte): 11 Patienten (31,5 %),
- von einem anderen Arzt bereits verordnet: 6 Patienten (17 %),
- Empfehlung vom Heilpraktiker: 7 Patienten (20 %),
- Erstverordnung auch von mir: 11 Patienten (31,5 %).

Zu Frage 4:
5 Patienten (14 %) gaben an, sie hätten keinerlei Wirkung bemerkt. Nur einer davon hatte auch seine Erstverordnung von mir.

Zu Frage 5:
Meinung zu einem Auslaßversuch:
- Ablehnung: 25 Patienten (71 %);
- Zustimmung: 9 Patienten (26 %);
  2 Patienten (6 %) verlangten nach mehrtägigem Auslaßversuch eine erneute Verordnung, weil es ihnen schlechter gehe.
- Keine Meinung: 1 Patient (3 %).

Zu Frage 6:
Die Dosis war fast immer Tebonin forte 3 Tbl. tgl. oder 3mal 20 Trpf. Die Regelmäßigkeit der Einnahme wurde von den Patienten als sehr hoch angegeben. In keinem Fall wurden gröbere Verstöße gegen die Einnahmevorschrift registriert.

Diskussion

In der Praxis des Hausarztes beginnt jede Konsultation damit, daß ein Mensch sein Befinden schildert. Von diesem subjektiven Erleben – so lehrt uns die naturwissenschaftliche Medizin – muß ein Arzt schnell zum objektiven Befund kommen, denn nur der ist „das Eigentliche", was Wert hat. Wir sind der Ansicht, Befinden könne trügen, Befunde aber seien „wissenschaftlich". Geht man von dieser Prämisse aus, so bleiben in einer Allgemeinpraxis viele Patienten übrig, bei denen eben kein „objektiver Befund" erhoben werden kann oder dieser zu geringfügig ist, um therapiewürdig zu sein. Im Arztbrief des Spezialisten steht dann, es könne kein pathologischer Befund erhoben werden; bei anhaltenden Beschwerden könne eine symptomatische Therapie versucht werden. Was darunter konkret zu verstehen sei, wird jedoch meist verschwiegen. Längst aber hat sich fern von Universitäten draußen in den Praxen ein Umgang mit dieser Problematik etabliert, der erst nach Erstellung von Statistiken und Kosten-Nutzen-Analysen langsam ins Bewußtsein der Öffentlichkeit dringt. Es wird oft vergessen, daß auch in der Praxis des Hausarztes wissenschaftliche Methoden (Beobachten, Hypothesen erstellen, Experimentieren) zur Anwendung kommen. Dies ist auch dann der Fall, wenn der Arzt seinem Patienten nach einer lebhaften, jedoch befundlosen Schilderung seines Befindens eine Therapie empfiehlt und nach Tagen fragt, ob es geholfen habe. Die Medizinwissenschaft denkt inkonsequent, wenn sie solchermaßen gewonnene (Er)kenntnisse als Erfahrungsmedizin belächelt. Stellt also ein Arzt fest, daß ein hoher Prozentsatz seiner Patienten in der „Sprech"stunde ein wesentlich gebessertes Befinden angibt, warum soll er dann den eingeschlagenen Therapieweg verlassen? Auch bei fehlendem Wirksamkeitsnachweis [8] – oder vielleicht doch nachgewiesener Wirkung [5] – ist eine generelle Ablehnung von Nootropika und durchblutungsfördernden Mitteln nicht zu rechtfertigen. Keinesfalls ist es richtig, daß geschickte Werbefeldzüge [9] oder gar mangelnde Sachkenntnis der Hausärzte (Schönhöfer in der Fernsehsendung „Panorama" am 12.12.89) die Ursache der Verordnungshäufigkeit sind. Immer verlangt der Erkrankte eine Behandlung, oft genug bringt er Therapievorschläge gleich mit. Hat er nicht auch ein Anrecht auf seine durchblutungsfördernde Medikation, wenn er sagt, es gehe ihm besser nach der Einnahme? Ist eine Wirkung erst dann hinreichend belegt, wenn es sich nicht nur um die eines unreinen Placebos handelt? Das jedoch scheint mir bei einigen Medikamenten noch lange nicht sicher zu sein.

Bei meinen eigenen Untersuchungen konnten nach intensiven Gesprächen lediglich 8 von 35 Patienten dazu überredet (überzeugt?) werden, auf Tebonin ersatzlos zu verzichten, davon hatte die Hälfte es auch als Erstverordnung von mir. Es scheint so, daß der Hausarzt auf die Fremdempfehlungen einen geringeren Einfluß hat als auf seine eigenen Verordnungen. Aus einer Einzelpraxis lassen sich zwar keine globalen Rückschlüsse ziehen, sicher aber vermitteln sie einen Eindruck der Problematik.

Der Hausarzt begleitet seine Patienten, die unter Schwindel, Wadenkrämpfen oder unterschiedlich ausgeprägten Hirnleistungsstörungen ein Leben lang leiden. Auch am Ende einer angiologischen „Patientenkarriere" steht der Hausarzt und muß irgendwie helfen. Oft genug bleibt ihm nur ein Medikament, mit dem er die Suggestion einer Besserung verbindet. Und geht es dem Kranken dann besser, wer vermag zu sagen, daß nicht sein darf, was nicht sein kann? Hier ist noch Forschungsarbeit zu leisten. Auch kann die Empfehlung, lediglich schwerwiegende Zielsymptome wie Schwindel, Störung der zirkadianen Rhythmik, Depressionen und psychomotorische Erregungszustände medikamentös zu behandeln (1979 in [7] und unkorrigiert 1986 wiederholt), nicht akzeptiert werden [11]. Sie läßt – konsequent angewendet – den Kranken *und* seinen Hausarzt im Stich. Zumal die Gefahr besteht, daß solche Empfehlungen schnell in den Negativlisten [1] als „nicht verordnungsfähig" eingestuft werden. Juristisch ist eine Verordnung solcher Substanzen aber derzeit möglich: Im § 27 des SGB V heißt es „... oder Krankheitsbeschwerden zu lindern." Die Linderung bestimmt nur der Patient. Und im § 35 heißt es: „Bei der Beurteilung von Arzneimitteln der besonderen Therapierichtungen ist der besonderen Wirkungsweise Rechnung zu tragen." – Hier muß noch diskutiert werden.

Fühlt sich ein Mensch krank, ist Hilfe vonnöten, und wenn es keine andere gibt, warum nicht ein Medikament mit einem schönen Beipackzettel, auf dem eine „Indikationslyrik" [8] die Symptome aufzählt, die der Kranke schon immer hat?

Literatur

1. Bundesausschuß der Ärzte und Krankenkassen (1985/86) Preisvergleichsliste 1. 10. 85, erweiterte Preisvergleichsliste 13. 3. 86. Köln
2. Capra F (1990) Wendezeit. Bern, Scherz
3. Clade H (1991) Wachsende Herausforderung an die Geriatrie und Gerontologie. Dtsch Ärztebl 88 : 23–24
4. Fintelmann V, Menßen HG, Siegers CP (1989) Phytotherapie Manual. Hippokrates, Stuttgart
5. Haas H, Witte S (1990) Leserzuschrift zu Schönhöfer et al. 1989. Kassenarzt 13 : 56–61
6. Mörl H (1989) Gefäßkrankheiten in der Praxis. Edition Medizin, Weinheim
7. Schönhöfer PS, Füllgraff G (1986, 1979) Arteriosklerose und Durchblutungsstörungen. In: Füllgraff G, Palm. Pharmakotherapie. Klinische Pharmakologie. Fischer, Stuttgart, 103–113, und 1986 : 111–119
8. Schönhöfer PS, Schulte-Sasse H, Manhold C, Werner B (1989) Sind Extrakte aus den Blättern des Ginkgobaumes bei peripheren Durchblutungs- und Hirnleistungsstörungen im Alter wirksam? Tägl Prax 30 : 585–601
9. Schwabe U, Paffrath D (1990) Arzneiverordnungsreport 90. Fischer, Stuttgart, S 199–208
10. Transparenztelegramm 1990/91 (1990) Arzneimittelverlag, Berlin
11. Trübestein G (1988) Periphere und zerebrale arterielle Durchblutungsstörungen. Perimed, Erlangen
12. Vester F (1980) Denken, Lernen, Vergessen. dtv, München

Schlaflosigkeit – Benzodiazepine – Abhängigkeit

Sleeplessness – Benzodiazepines – Addiction

Über den Umgang mit Benzodiazepinen in der Allgemeinpraxis

Ursula Sehrt

Statistische Grundlagen

Dem GKV-Arzneimittelindex, jährlich unter dem Titel „Arzneiverordnungsreport", vom WIdO (Wissenschaftliches Institut der Ortskrankenkassen) herausgegeben, ist zu entnehmen, daß rechnerisch von sämtlichen 54 732 100 GKV-Versicherten aus dem Bereich der alten Bundesländer täglich 1 Mio. Menschen Hypnotika/Sedativa im Sinn einer Dauertherapie einnehmen. Diese Zahl ist seit Jahren praktisch konstant.

Der GKV-Arzneimittelindex darf als zuverlässigste Aussagequelle gelten, da er nicht nur die Verordnungsgepflogenheiten sämtlicher Kassenärzte, sondern auch die Einnahmemodalitäten und in gewissem Umfang auch die Verordnungswünsche der Patienten widerspiegelt (rund 95 % der Bevölkerung gehören der GKV an und das WIdO erfaßt die Pharmadaten aller GKV-Versicherten [5].

Das statistische Faktum, daß in Deutschland-West täglich 1 Mio. GKV-Versicherte Schlafmittel – und dies bevorzugt in Form von Benzodiazepinen – einnehmen, ist alarmierend genug. Um jedoch die tatsächliche Tragweite des Problems einschätzen zu können, muß man berücksichtigen, daß zentral wirksame Pharmaka schlechthin in den Altersgruppen unter 30 Jahren (17 283 200 Personen, ca. 36 % aller GKV-Versicherten) eine völlig untergeordnete, quantitativ vernachlässigbare Rolle spielen [9].

93 % der Hypnotika/Sedativa werden also fast ausschließlich von den 37 448 900 Personen (= 64 % der GKV-Versicherten) ab 30 Jahren eingenommen, wobei die applizierten DDD analog zum Alter bis ins hohe Senium kontinuierlich ansteigen.

Der überproportional hohe Verbrauch von Schlafmitteln in höheren Altersklassen wird noch deutlicher bei Betrachtung der ab 50jährigen, die lediglich knapp 36 % der Versicherten stellen, auf die aber 83 % aller zu Lasten der GKV verordneten Hypnotika/Sedativa entfallen (Tabelle 1; [9]).

Dabei führt mit weitem Abstand das weibliche Geschlecht (was die verordneten DDD betrifft) mit einem Anteil von 70,5 % in diesem Indikationsgebiet. Einzelheiten sind Tabelle 2 zu entnehmen.

Bei diesen statistischen Angaben sind folgende Tatsachen zu berücksichtigen:

- Bereits ab der Altersgruppe von 50–59 Jahren sind Frauen in der GKV überrepräsentiert, was sich in den noch höheren Altersgruppen drastisch fortsetzt (Abb. 1).
- Speziell für Allgemeinpraxen ist durch die Untersuchungen von Hamm bekannt, daß rund zwei Drittel der dort betreuten Patienten Frauen sind [2].

Rationale Pharmakotherapie in der Allgemeinpraxis
Rational Pharmacotherapy in General Practice
M. M. Kochen (Hrsg.)

Tabelle 1. Verbrauch von Hypnotika/Sedativa in höheren Altersgruppen (m. + w.) in definierten Tagesdosen (*DDD*)

Alter (Jahre)	DDD [%]	Versicherte [%]
50–59	13,3	13,4
60–60	22,5	11,0
70–79	25,5	7,0
80–89	19,7	3,8

Tabelle 2. Anteil weiblicher Versicherter am Gesamtverbrauch von Hypnotika/Sedativa in definierten Tagesdosen (*DDD*)

Alter (Jahre)	DDD [%]	Weibliche Versicherte [%]
50–59	66,4	50,9
60–69	68,0	58,8
70–79	73,0	66,2
80–89	78,1	70,7

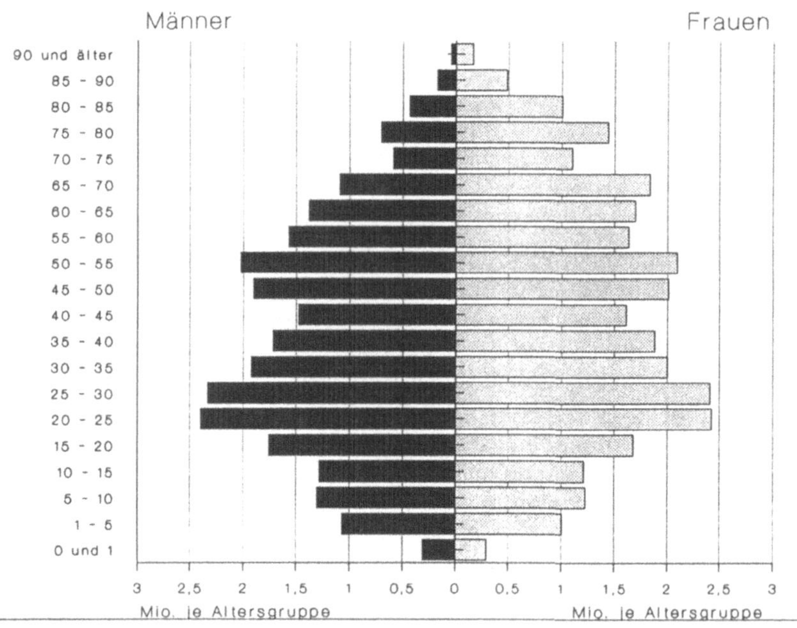

Abb. 1. Alters- und Geschlechtsstruktur der GKV-Versicherten 1989. (Aus [5])

Auch nach Bereinigung der Altersstatistik mittels geschlechtsgetrennter Versichertenzahlen bleibt aber die deutlich überhöhte Einnahme von Schlafmitteln durch weibliche Patienten nachweisbar, unabhängig von der Altersstufe (Tabelle 2).

Im Zusammenhang mit den vorgestellten Zahlen sind folgende Fragestellungen von besonderem Interesse:

1. Was wird überwiegend verordnet?
2. Welche Verordnungsanteile entfallen auf allgemeinärztliche Praxen?
3. Sind die bestehenden Verordnungspraktiken und Einnahmemodalitäten rational und rationell, d.h. medizinisch begründet und ökonomisch vertretbar?
4. Warum können so viele GKV-Versicherte nicht ein- und/oder durchschlafen?
5. Aus welchen Gründen konzentriert sich der Schlafmittelkonsum in diesen eklatanten Ausmaßen auf ältere bzw. weibliche Versicherte?

Marktführende Präparate

Wie aus Abb. 2 ersichtlich, führen bei der Verordnung von Hypnotika/Sedativa mit weitem Abstand die Benzodiazepine. Dies gilt seit etlichen Jahren, wenngleich seit 1987 ein leicht rückläufiger Trend zu beobachten ist. Dabei muß man berücksichtigen, daß – wie noch ausgeführt wird – als Schlafmittel auch Tranquillanzien eine wichtige Rolle spielen (trotz ihrer deutlich sinkenden Verordnungsfrequenz).

Während der vergangenen 5 Jahre wurden folgende Benzodiazepine unter der Indikation Hypnotika/Sedativa am häufigsten eingesetzt: Flunitrazepam (Rohypnol), gefolgt von Triazolam (Halcion) und Flurazepam (Dalmadorm, Generika), ferner Lormetazepam (Noctamid, Generika), Nitrazepam (Mogadan, Generika),

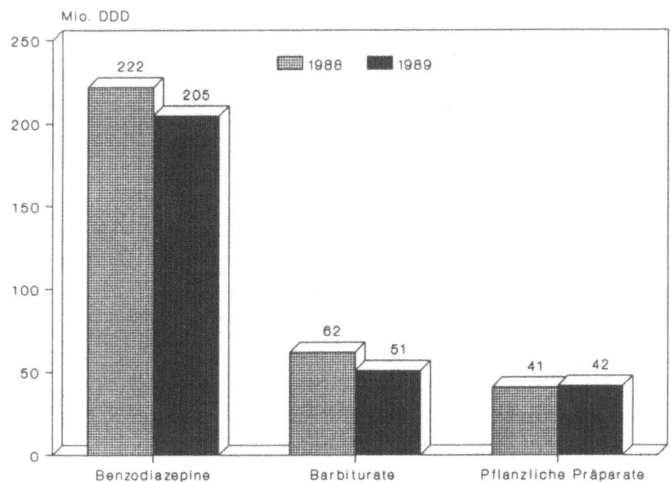

Abb. 2. Verordnung von Hypnotika und Sedativa 1989 in definierten Tagesdosen (*DDD*). (Aus [5])

Temazepam (Planum, Remestan), Brotizolam (Lendormin) und Lorazepam (Pro Dorm, unter der Indikation Psychopharmaka Tavor, Generika).

Es gibt zu denken, in welcher Hartnäckigkeit sich trotz leicht rückläufiger Tendenz Benzodiazepine mit langer Wirkdauer (Flunitrazepam, Flurazepam, Nitrazepam) unter den Marktführern halten, weil dies den heute gewünschten pharmakokinetischen Eigenschaften eines Schlafmittels widerspricht.

Flunitrazepam führt mit annähernd 47 Mio. DDD im Jahr 1989 noch immer die Rangliste im GKV-Index an – trotz seiner hohen Halbwertszeit von 10–20 h und der seines aktiven Metaboliten von 20–30 h.

Zahlen des WIdO von 1987 belegen, daß Flunitrazepam trotz seiner speziell im Senium ungeeigneten pharmakologischen Eigenschaften mit zunehmendem Patientenalter ständig häufiger verordnet wird (Tabelle 3).

Tabelle 3. Verbrauch von Flunitrazepam in höheren Altersgruppen [9]

Alter (Jahre)	DDD (Mio.)	GKV-Index (Rang)
51-60	5671	32
61–70	9331	16
71–80	14 215	14
≥ 81	6528	12

Erwähnenswert erscheint hier das Ergebnis einer Studie, in der sich herausstellte, daß von 390 über 65jährigen Patienten mit Femurfraktur durch nächtliche Stürze fast alle durch lange Halbwertszeiten (HWZ) gekennzeichnete Barbiturate als Hypnotikum benutzten [8]. Analoge Untersuchungen liegen für lang wirkende Benzodiazepine vor [4]. Dieser Umstand sollte die weitgehend ungetrübte Verordnungs- und Einnahmeeuphorie gegenüber Benzodiazepinen mit langer HWZ eigentlich spürbar bremsen.

Es ist zu betonen, daß die unter der Indikation Hypnotika/Sedativa angesiedelten Benzodiazepine nur einen Bruchteil der Substanzen darstellen, die faktisch auch zur Behandlung von Schlafstörungen verordnet bzw. eingenommen werden. Eine Differenzierung mit gebührender Trennschärfe zwischen Einsatz als Tranquillanzien oder/und Schlafmitteln ist für die unter der Indikation Psychopharmaka aufgelisteten Benzodiazepine praktisch unmöglich.

Um so mehr ist an dieser Stelle die Sorgfaltspflicht der Allgemeinärzte und Praktiker gefordert, die (s. Abb. 3) mehr als die Hälfte (53 %) aller Psychopharmaka, zuvorderst Benzodiazepine, verordnen.

Benzodiazepine, die offiziell unter dem Indikationsgebiet Psychopharmaka, Untergruppe Tranquillanzien, geführt, tatsächlich aber in unabsehbar großem Umfang als Schlafmittel eingesetzt werden, sind Präparate mit den Wirkstoffen Bromazepam, Oxazepam, Diazepam und Lorazepam. Die HWZ beträgt für Bromazepam 10–20 h, für Oxazepam 6–12 h (bei protrahierter schlafinduzierender Anflutung), für Diazepam 20–40 h (aktive Metaboliten unberücksichtigt), für Lorazepam 10–24 h.

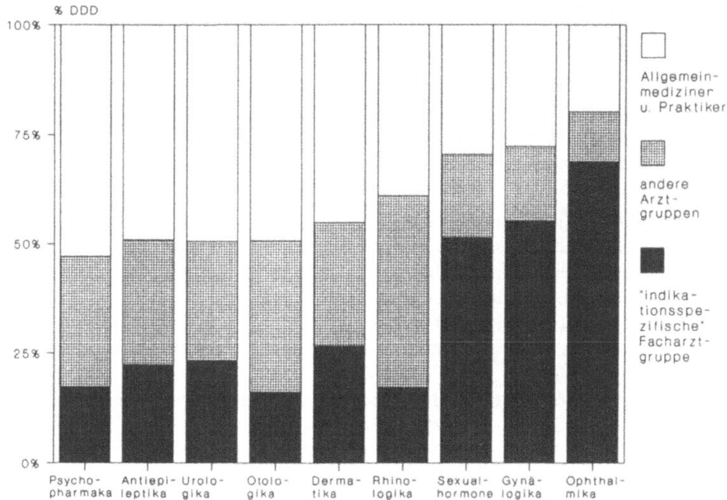

Abb. 3. Verordnungen nach Arztgruppen für ausgewählte Indikatiosngruppen nach definierten Tagesdosen (*DDD*, in Prozent) 1989. (Aus [5])

Insgesamt wurden 1989 in den alten Bundesländern rund 363 Mio. DDD an Tranquillanzien verordnet. Auch sie werden mit Abstand am häufigsten in den höheren Altersgruppen und schwerpunktmäßig bei Frauen eingesetzt, entsprechend den Ausführungen zu Hypnotika/Sedativa. Rein rechnerisch steht in Deutschland-West jeder fünfte GKV-Versicherte ab 80 Jahren unter einer Dauertherapie mit Tranquillanzien, die auch als Schlafmittel verwendbar wären [5].

Folglich findet man auch bei den unter Tranquillanzien angesiedelten Benzodiazepinen eine Entwicklung der DDD, die sich gegenläufig zur Ausdünnung der Altersgruppen verhält.

Benzodiazepinverordnungen in der Allgemeinpraxis

Wenn die Verordnungshäufigkeit von Benzodiazepinen, sei es unter der offiziellen Indikation Hypnotika/Sedativa oder als Tranquillanzien, so eindeutig ansteigt, obwohl die Besetzung der jeweiligen Altersgruppen kontinuierlich abnimmt, sind folgende Auslöser denkbar:

- eine medizinisch begründete Zunahme des Bedarfs,
- eine Dosissteigerung infolge Abhängigkeit,
- ein unreflektiertes Verordnungs- und Einnahmeverhalten.

In den Empfehlungen des Sachverständigenrats der Bundesregierung zur sachgerechten Anwendung von Benzodiazepinen ([1]; orange Teil, S. 23) heißt es:

> Benzodiazepine stellen einen Fortschritt in der Arzneitherapie von schweren Angstzuständen und den meisten medikamentös zu behandelnden Schlafstörungen dar. Sie

sind „kurzfristig" (4–6 Wochen) bei ausgeprägten Angstzuständen, die durch ärztliches Gespräch nicht zu beheben sind, indiziert. ...
Über das Nutzen-Risiko-Verhältnis einer langfristigen Benzodiazepin-Medikation (über 2 Monate) bei Patienten mit behandlungsbedürftigen chronischen Angstzuständen liegen bislang keine wissenschaftlich allgemein verbindlichen Erkenntnisse vor. ... Neuerdings geben Mißbrauch und Abhängigkeit auch bei niedriger Dosierung Anlaß zur Besorgnis. Benzodiazepine werden nach bisherigen Erkenntnissen nicht zu häufig, sondern zu lange Zeit verordnet. Deshalb sind die Ärzte aufgerufen, ... zu beachten:

1. Sorgfältige Indikationsstellung!
2. Bei Patienten mit einer Abhängigkeitsanamnese ist besondere Vorsicht geboten, in der Regel keine Verschreibung.
3. In der Regel kleinste Packungseinheit verordnen.
4. In möglichst niedriger, aber ausreichender Dosierung verordnen; Dosis möglichst schon in der ersten Behandlungwoche reduzieren bzw. Dosierungsintervall vergrößern.
5. Therapiedauer vor Behandlungsbeginn mit dem Patienten vereinbaren und Behandlungsnotwendigkeit in kurzen Abständen überprüfen ...
8. Aufklärung des Patienten, daß Benzodiazepine keinesfalls an Dritte weiterzugeben sind.
9. Alle Abhängigkeitsfälle über die jeweiligen Arzneimittelkommissionen ... dem Bundesgesundheitsamt zur Kenntnis bringen.
10. Benzodiazepin-Verschreibungen sollten vom Arzt stets eigenhändig ausgefertigt werden.

Wünsche und Erwartungen von Patienten

Gemäß den Empfehlungen des Sachverständigenrats sind die Patienten ausdrücklich vor den Abhängigkeitsrisiken der Benzodiazepine zu warnen. Folgende Faktoren sollen u. a. besonders vom Patienten beachtet werden:

- keine Einnahme länger als 4 Wochen ohne Rücksprache mit dem Arzt;
- keine eigenmächtige Dosiserhöhung wegen nachlassender Wirksamkeit;
- keine Einnahme von Benzodiazepinen bei anamnestischen Abhängigkeiten von Alkohol, Medikamenten oder Drogen;
- keine Einnahme aufgrund von Laienempfehlungen;
- keine Weitergabe von Benzodiazepinen;
- Hinweise auf Entzugssymptome wie Unruhe, Angstzustände, Schlaflosigkeit.

Angesichts der vorgelegten Zahlen muß man davon ausgehen, daß diese Empfehlungen zum sachgerechten Umgang mit Benzodiazepinen auch unter der Indikation der Behandlung von Schlafstörungen nur lückenhaft eingehalten werden, sowohl von den Versicherten als auch von den Verordnern.

Die bekannten Daten legen auch den Verdacht nahe, daß abhängigkeitsbedingte Dosissteigerungen häufig vorkommen müssen, weil sich der tatsächliche Verbrauch anders nicht hinreichend erklären läßt.

Die horrenden Mengen der hierzuzlande als Schlafmittel eingenommenen Benzodiazepine lassen auch warnen vor der verharmlosenden bis verniedlichenden Darstellung der sog. stabilen „ low-dose-dependence". Nach eigenen, über 10jährigen Erfahrungen in einer Allgemeinpraxis kommt es ohne konsequente ärztliche

Aufmerksamkeit und ohne permanente ärztliche Interventionsstrategien häufig zu Dosissteigerungen.

Es soll hier nicht bestritten werden, daß es Fälle von stabiler „low-dose-dependence" gibt. Aber weitaus häufiger begegnet der Hausarzt der bereits eigenmächtig vollzogenen Dosissteigerung, die dem Patientenwunsch entspringen, das Ausmaß der anfänglich als wohltuend empfundenen Wirkung zu erhalten. Besonders auffällig wird dieser Umstand bei neu in die Behandlung übernommenen Patienten, die z. B. 2 Einzeldosen Flunitrazepam, 4–6 Einzeldosen Oxazepam oder Nitrazepam, 6–8 Einzeldosen Flurazepam oder 20–30 mg Diazepam bzw. 12–18 mg Bromazepam zur Nacht einnehmen, nachdem tagsüber bereits 6–12 mg konsumiert worden sind.

Speziell von diesen Patienten stammen denn auch endlose Klagen bei der empfohlenen Verordnung kleiner Packungsgrößen. Hier anzusiedeln ist ferner der lebhafteste innerfamiliäre und sonstige Austausch von Benzodiazepinen als Schlafmittel, was dem Hausarzt auch noch als Akt sozialer Hilfestellung verkauft wird, um in den Genuß der nächsten Verordnung, aber bitteschön der größten Packung, zu gelangen.

Allgemeinärzte und Praktiker erleben täglich mehrfach, in welch nachgerade querulatorischer Kritikbesessenheit die Packungsbeilagen angeordneter Medikationen studiert werden mit der Konsequenz von Non-Compliance auf dem Boden gelesener und befürchteter, nicht jedoch erlebter unerwünschter Wirkungen.

Nicht so bei den Benzodiazepinen. Obwohl die überwiegende Mehrzahl dieser Fertigarzneimittel inzwischen die wahrlich apokalyptischen Warnhinweise der Sachverständigenkommission in ihre Packungsbeilagen übernommen hat, zeitigt dies nur eine geringe Wirkung. Entweder werden hier die Beipackzettel gar nicht erst angeschaut, oder ihr Inhalt wird verdrängt. Beide Möglichkeiten wären angesichts des sonst üblichen Patientenverhaltens, (sich nur zu ca. 45 % für den Nutzen eines Arzneimittels, aber zu 95 % für dessen theoretisch nachteilige Auswirkungen zu interessieren), ein wichtiges Indiz für die oft kritiklose Begehrlichkeit dieser Menschen nach ihrem nächtlichen Seelentröster als Ersatzkuschelobjekt in Gestalt von Tabletten, Dragees, Kapseln, Suppositorien etc. Dies sollte ein eklatanter Warnhinweis für das Mißbrauchpotential der Benzodiazepine sein.

Es sei daran erinnert, daß z. B. in New York Benzodiazepine inzwischen Verordnungsreglementierungen unterliegen, die unserem BTM-Gesetz vergleichbar sind. Aber hierzulande denkt man ausschließlich darüber nach, wie Benzodiazepine in zuzahlungsfreien Festbetragsgruppen unterzubringen sind. Widersprüchlicher kann es kaum zugehen.

Hinzukommt – als Folge der freien Arztwahl – daß GKV-Versicherte ihren individuellen Bedarf an Medikamenten mit Mißbruchspotential in Kassenarztpraxen fast sämtlicher Fachrichtungen unkontrolliert abdecken können.

Bezogen auf die alten Bundesländer kann also weder von einem rationalen noch von einem rationellen Einsatz der Benzodiazepine als Schlafmittel ausgegangen werden.

Gerade aus allgemeinärztlicher Sicht muß an dieser Stelle auch darauf verwiesen werden, daß die Entzugssymptomatik nach Benzodiazepinabusus ein außerordentlich schwieriges und langwieriges Problem ist, für dessen Lösung in vielen Fällen die Interventionsmöglichkeiten der hausärztlichen Praxis nicht ausreichen. Dies liegt teilweise an der Schwere der Entzugssymptomatik selbst, die sich mit massiven Beschwerden über Wochen hinziehen kann.

In diesem Zusammenhang ist anzumerken, daß die Kassenärzte in ihrem Bemühen um einen rationalen Umgang mit Benzodiazepinen kaum Unterstützung finden und daß es allerorten an Einrichtungen zur Langzeitentwöhnung mangelt.

Psychosoziale Ursachen von Schlafstörungen

Eine wichtige Rolle in der hausärztlichen Praxis spielen psychozoziale Faktoren des betroffenen Patienten selbst und/oder seines Umfeldes, die mit Schlafstörungen korrellieren und die Benzodiazepinabhängigkeit auslösen, unterhalten oder verschlimmern.

Die Bedeutung dieser psychoreaktiven Schlafstörungen ist daran abzulesen, daß bei mehr als einem Drittel aller Patienten einer Allgemeinpraxis psychische und psychosomatische Störungen von Krankheitswert vorliegen, die in weit mehr als der Hälfte der Fälle neurotischer Art sind [6].

Daraus können Einschlafstörungen resultieren, insbesondere dann, wenn es sich um bewußtseinsnahe Konflikte (unbewältigte Aktualkonflikte oder sog. Sandwich-Situationen mit dem Partner, mit der Familie oder am Arbeitsplatz) oder um Alltagssorgen, Überforderungen und Schicksalsschläge handelt.

Wiederholte, sich hinziehende Erfahrungen mit dem Unvermögen, einschlafen zu können, steigern sich bis zur Bettangst im Sinn anderer bekannter Versagensängste [3].

Die Therapie der Wahl ist hier das rechtzeitige Patient-Arzt-Gespräch, ggf. ergänzt durch das Einüben von Entspannungstechniken, und nicht die unreflektierte Schlafmittelverordnung. Die zukunftsweisende Gunst einer solch frühen hausärztlichen Interventionsstrategie sollte intensiv und systematisch genutzt werden.

Den Durchschlafstörungen liegen (sozusagen am Endpunkt einer neurotischen Entwicklung) meist bewußtseinsferne Konflikte zugrunde, die sich durch schlafbedingt realitätsbezogene Kontrollverluste bemerkbar machen. Betroffen sind insbesondere Patienten mit chronifizierten Konflikten. Dies trifft nach eigenen Untersuchungen für 55 % der neurotisch gestörten Patienten einer Allgemeinpraxis zu, die für eine Abhängigkeitsentwicklung in hohem Maß prädisponiert sind, und zwar hinsichtlich „Pille und Pulle“ sowie weiterer Fehlverhaltensweisen [6]. Ungeachtet der Schwere dieser Problematik sind auch hier qualifizierte allgemeinärztliche Interventionsstrategien erforderlich, um der sonst schicksalhaften Progredienz eines multifaktoriellen Mißbrauchs entgegenzuwirken.

Nur am Rande sei die auch heute noch vielfach unreflektierte Applikation von Benzodiazepinen als Schlafmittel unter stationären Bedingungen erwähnt, wodurch unter Ausblendung der realen Lebenssituation der Betroffenen manche einschlägige Patientenkarriere angestoßen wird.

Therapeutische Konsequenzen

Außer der gesprächsweisen Eruierung und Therapie psychoreaktiver Schlafstörungen zählt die anamnestische Fahndung nach exogenen Ursachen einer Schlafstörung zur Sorgfaltspflicht eines qualifizierten Allgemeinarztes. Dies setzt zweifellos den Mut zur Banalität voraus, denn im Prinzip geht es um nichts anderes als die Aufdeckung des Tagesablaufs und der häuslichen Umstände eines Patienten.

Beispiele:

1) Eine alleinstehende, ihrer früheren hausfraulichen Geschäftigkeit enthobene, sozial vereinsamte Patientin, verkriecht sich, des Fernsehens überdrüssig und frustriert von der Erfahrung, daß sich die Kinder ein weiteres Mal nicht gemeldet haben, gegen 21.00 Uhr ins Bett. Natürlich kann sie nicht einschlafen, denn sie ist ja gar nicht müde. Vom Schlaf schließlich eingeholt, schlummert sie bis in die späteren Vormittagsstunden. Dann wird das Nötigste erledigt. Mittags tritt das nächste Vakuum ein, das mit einem Mittagsschlaf überbrückt wird, bis z. B. die Geschäfte oder die Praxis wieder geöffnet sind. Die frühen Abendstunden werden mit gewisser Erwartungshaltung überbrückt. Damit landet man wieder bei 21.00 Uhr usw.

2) Die Arbeitsbedingungen eines Familienernährers , der im Laufe des späteren nachmittags heimkehrt, führt zur opulenten Aufnahme der Hauptmahlzeit in den frühen Abendstunden, begleitet vom TV, das rauchender-, trinkender- und naschenderweise verfolgt wird, bis die Uhr zum Schlafengehen mahnt. Der Mann kann nicht einschlafen, weil er einen vollen Magen und keinerlei körperliche Betätigung hat. Die Partnerin kann nicht einschlafen aus vergleichbaren Fehlverhaltensweisen und der Frustration, ihre spezifischen Alltagssorgen nicht verbalisiert zu haben.

3) Da sind überheizte, nicht durchlüftete, lärmdurchdrungene Schlafzimmer sowie Betten, die jeder Erkenntnis zeitgemäßer Schlafphysiologie widersprechen. Der Allgemeinarzt kann wie kein anderer ärztlicher Kollege aufgrund der Intensität seiner Hausbesuchstätigkeit solche Störfaktoren aufdecken und Anregungen zur Abhilfe geben.

Schließlich geht es – vor dem Griff zum Rezeptformular mit Verordnung – um den Ausschluß sekundärer bzw. organisch bedingter Schlafstörungen. Dies betrifft vorwiegend Patienten im Senium, die, wie geschildert, am großzügigsten mit diesen Substanzen versorgt werden [7].

Hierzu zählen u. a.:

- Schmerzzustände, v. a. auf dem Boden eines weichteilrheumatischen, eines degenerativen oder eines entzündlichen Rheumatismus oder einer Osteoporose;
- kardial oder pulmonal bedingte Dyspnoe;
- kardial bedingte Nykturie;
- Harn- und/oder Stuhlinkontinenz mit Angst vor nächtlichem Einnässen oder Einkoten;
- schmerzhafte Harnverhaltung, z. B. bei Prostataadenom;
- Hyperthyreose (mit steigendem Alter zunehmend oligosymptomatisch);
- nächtliche Hypoglykämie bei Diabetes mellitus;
- Herzrhythmusstörungen;
- Blutdruckschwankungen;
- Exsikkose;
- Pruritus;

- Hypoventilationssyndrome wie Schlafapnoe;
- Depression;
- beginnende Demenz bzw. Parasomnie.

Diese Auflistung zeigt, daß gerade der Allgemeinarzt eine Vielzahl von Schlafstörungen kausal behandeln und nicht – wie es mit dem unreflektierten Einsatz von Benzodiazepinen geschieht – symptomatisch kurieren sollte.

Mit zunehmendem Patientenalter müssen auch immer häufiger paradoxe Reaktionen der Benzodiazepine ins Kalkül gezogen werden, die von verstärktem Pruritus senilis über Unruhe- und Angstzustände bis hin zu halluzinatorischen und deliranten Zuständen führen können (oftmals von quälenden organischen Symptomen begleitet; [3]).

Die hier vorgestellten Daten und Praxisgegebenheiten mögen ausreichen, um den dringenden Handlungsbedarf für einen kritischen Einsatz von Benzodiazepinen zur Behandlung von Schlafstörungen zu veranschaulichen.

Literatur

1. Bundeverband der Pharmazeutischen Industrie e. V. (1991) Rote Liste 1991. Editio Cantor, Aulendorf/Württ.
2. Hamm H (1990, unveröffentlicht) Referat anläßlich des Deutschen Hausärztetages, Kiel, 22.09.1990
3. Luban-Plozza B, Pöldinger W, Kröger F (1989) Der psychosomatisch Kranke in der Praxis, 5. Aufl. Springer, Berlin Heidelberg New York Tokyo
4. Ray WA, Griffin MR, Downey W (1989) Benzodiazepines of long and short elimination half-line and the risk of hip-fracture. JAMA 262:3303–3307
5. Schwabe U, Paffrath D (eds) (1990) Arzneiverordnungsreport '90. Fischer, Stuttgart, New York
6. Sehrt U (1989) Psychosomatische Grundversorgung in der Allgemeinpraxis. In: Bergmann G (ed) Psychosomatische Grundversorgung. Springer, Berlin Heidelberg New York Tokyo
7. Sehrt U, Weber E (1986) Besonderheiten der Pharmakotherapie im Senium. Münch Med Wochenschr 35:595–598
8. Weber E (ed) (1988) Taschenbuch der unerwünschten Arzneiwirkungen, 2. Aufl Fischer, Stuttgart New York
9. Wissenschaftliches Institut der Ortskrankenkassen (WIdO) (ed) (1990) GKV-Arzneimittelindex: Arzneiverbrauch nach Altersgruppen

Muskel- und Gelenkbeschwerden in der Allgemeinpraxis: Therapiemöglichkeiten

Muscle Pain and Arthropathies in General Practice: Which Treatments are Possible?

Pharmakologische Gesichtspunkte

Gerhard Schmidt

Die Arzneitherapie von Muskel- und Gelenkbeschwerden ist vornehmlich eine symptomatische Therapie. Sowohl bei rheumatischen als auch bei degenerativen Erkrankungen ist kaum eine Möglichkeit gegeben, den Krankheitsverlauf an sich medikamtentös zu beeinflussen. Auch bei posttraumatischen Muskel- und Gelenkbeschwerden wird der Heilungsverlauf durch eine medikamentöse Therapie wenig verändert. Trotz dieses im wesentlichen rein symptomatischen Charakters der medikamentösen Therapie von Muskel- und Gelenkbeschwerden kommt ihr ein hoher Stellenwert zu, weil

- Schmerzen und die Bewegungseinschränkung erheblich vermindert werden können,
- bleibende Einschränkungen der Beweglichkeit von Gelenken als Folge längerbestehender Schonhaltung unterdrückt werden können,
- allgemeine gesundheitliche Nachteile als Folge verminderter Mobilität zurückgedrängt werden können.

Die in der Behandlung von Muskel- und Gelenkbeschwerden eingesetzte Arzneimittelgruppe der Analgetika/Antirheumatika nimmt in der Verordnungsstatistik der verschriebenen Arzneimittel seit vielen Jahren in der Bundesrepublik Deutschland die 1. Stelle ein. 1989 waren 11,7 % aller Arzneimittelverschreibungen aus diesem Sektor [13].

Therapieziel bei der medikamentösen Behandlung von Muskel- und Gelenkbeschwerden ist die Hemmung der entzündlichen Reaktion und ggf. auch eine über die Entzündungshemmung hinausgehende analgetische Wirkung. Für die *Entzündungshemmung* stehen prinzipiell zur Verfügung:

- nichtsteroidale Antiphlogistika (Übersicht bei [3]) und
- steroidale Antiphlogistika (Glukokortikoide) (Übersicht bei [6]).

Mit den Glukokortikoiden ist grundsätzlich eine stärkere Unterdrückung des Entzündungsprozesses erreichbar als mit den nichtsteroidalen Antiphlogistika; gleichzeitig wird aber – besonders bei längerdauernder Anwendung – auch ein größeres Risiko von schweren und schlecht reversiblen unerwünschten Wirkungen eingegangen. Aus diesem Grunde muß zunächst die entzündungshemmende Therapie auf die Stoffklasse der nichtsteroidalen Antiphlogistika beschränkt werden. Falls mit entzündungshemmenden Medikamenten keine ausreichende *Verminderung des Schmerzes* bei Muskel- und Gelenkbeschwerden erreicht werden kann, ist gelegentlich die zusätzliche Verwendung von Analgetika notwendig, entweder aus der Gruppe der

Rationale Pharmakotherapie in der Allgemeinpraxis
Rational Pharmacotherapy in General Practice
M. M. Kochen (Hrsg.)

- nichtopioiden Analgetika (Übersicht bei [5, 12]) oder der
- opioiden Analgetika (Übersicht bei [5]).

Auch hier gilt, daß die Substanzgruppe der Opioide zwar stärkere und zuverlässige analgetische Wirkungen ergibt als die nichtopioiden Analgetika, dieser Effekt aber wiederum mit einem sehr viel größeren Risiko unerwünschter Wirkungen erkauft wird.

Bei Gelenk- und Muskelbeschwerden werden häufig auch solche Medikamente eingesetzt, die durch eine spinale und supraspinale muskelrelaxierende Wirkung den Hartspann der Skelettmuskulatur vermindern [1]. Eine derartige Wirkung besitzen z.B. die Tranquilizer aus der Gruppe der Benzodiazepine. Die klinische Wirksamkeit bei Muskel- und Gelenkbeschwerden ist jedoch nicht zweifelsfrei gesichert.

Antiphlogistika

Nichtsteroidale Antiphlogistika

Hauptwirkungsmechanismus der nichtsteroidalen Antiphlogistika ist die Hemmung der Zyklooxygenase in der Arachidonsäurekaskade. Dadurch wird die Biosynthese der an der Entzüdungsgenese beteiligten Prostaglandine vermindert (Literaturübersicht bei [4]; Abb. 1).

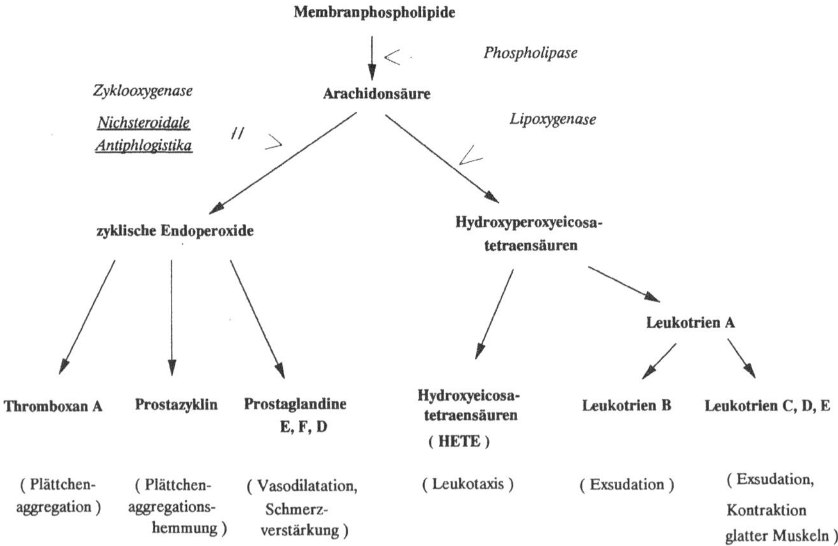

Abb. 1. Vereinfachtes Schema der Arachidonsäurekaskade mit dem Angriffspunkt der nichtsteroidalen Antiphlogistika

Durch die Einschränkung der Bildung von Prostaglandinen wird die durch sie vermittelte Empfindlichkeitssteigerung der Schmerzrezeption (= entzündliche Hyperalgesie) vermindert sowie die entzündliche Hyperämie und die z. T. dadurch vermittelte Ödementstehung eingeschränkt. Aus der Beeinflussung der Zyklooxygenaseaktivität durch die nichtsteroidalen Antiphlogistika ergibt sich aber auch ein umfängliches Wirkungsspektrum: So werden nicht nur die Prostaglandine in Anwesenheit von Zyklooxygenasehemmstoffen vermindert gebildet, es ergibt sich auch eine Abnahme der Biosynthese des thrombozytenaggregationfördernden Thromboxan A und des thrombozytenaggregationhemmenden Prostazyklins. Die Hemmung des Zyklooxygenaseweges durch nichtsteroidale Antiphlogistika fördert den Umsatz der Arachidonsäure im alternativen Lipoxygenaseweg. Dadurch können bei therapeutischer Anwendung nichtsteroidaler Antiphlogistika vermehrt Leukotriene gebildet werden.

Aufgrund dieses weitgehend identischen Wirkungsprinzips besitzen die verschiedenen nichtsteroidalen Antiphlogistika ein sehr ähnliches Wirkungsprofil. Es bestehen zwar innerhalb der nichtsteroidalen Antiphlogistika auch geringfügige Unterschiede in der Wirkungsqualität, die wesentlichen Differenzen betreffen aber die Pharmakokinetik.

Unterschiede in der Pharmakokinetik nichtsteroidaler Antiphlogistika

Während sich bezüglich der enteralen Bioverfügbarkeit und der Verteilung im Organismus nur geringe Unterschiede zwischen den einzelnen Substanzen ergeben, weisen die verschiedenen nichtsteroidalen Antiphlogistika außerordentliche

Tabelle 1. Halbwertzeiten ($t_{1/2}$) verschiedener nichtsteroidaler Antiphlogistika

Antiphlogistika	$t_{1/2}$ [h]
Kurz wirksame ($t_{1/2} < 4$ h):	
Acetylsalicylsäure (Aspirin, Generika)	0,25
daraus Salicylsäure	3–4 (in niedrigen Dosen)
Diclofenac (Voltaren, Generika)	1–2
Indometacin (Amuno, Generika)	2–3
Ibuprofen (Brufen, Generika)	2
Ketoprofen (Alrheumun, Orudis, Generika)	1,5–2,5
Mittellang wirksam ($t_{1/2}$ 6–15 h):	
Naproxen (Proxen)	14
Azapropazon (Prolixan, Tolyprin)	11
Lonazolac (Argun, Irritren)	6
Lang wirksame ($t_{1/2} > 48$ h):	
Piroxicam (Felden, Generika)	50
Tenoxicam (Tilcotil, Liman)	80
Phenylbutazon (Butazolidin)	70

und therapeutisch sehr wichtige Unterschiede in der Verweildauer und damit der Wirkungsdauer auf (vgl. Tabelle 1).

Da es sich bei den zu behandelnden Gelenk- und Muskelerkrankungen meist um längerdauernde Prozesse handelt, leuchtet ein, daß mit einem langwirkenden Arzneimittel ein gleichmäßigerer und auch zuverlässigerer therapeutischer Effekt erzielt werden kann als mit einer nur kurzwirkenden Verbindung. Es gibt allerdings 2 wichtige Argumente, die gegen die grundsätzliche Verwendung langwirkender Antiphlogistika sprehen:

1. Bei nicht ausreichender Berücksichtigung der langen Verweildauer reichern sich die Substanzen im Organismus an (Kumulation). Es muß bedacht werden, daß – bei regelmäßiger Zufuhr – erst nach 4 Halbwertszeiten ein Gleichgewicht erreicht wird. Es kommt hinzu, daß besonders bei älteren Patienten die Elimination erheblich verzögert sein kann.
2. Bei einer gleichmäßigen Hemmung der Zyklooxygenase über die Zeit ergeben sich besonders ausgeprägte Effekte, die auf einem Ausfall der physiologischen Funktion der Zyklooxygenaseprodukte aus der Arachidonsäurekaskade beruhen (z. B. Natrium- und Wasserretention in der Niere).

In der Therapie von Muskel- und Gelenkerkrankungen wird hierzulande z. Z. eindeutig Diclofenac präferiert; 1989 wurde in der Bundesrepublik Deutschland mehr Diclofenac verordnet als alle anderen nichtsteroidalen Antiphlogistika zusammen genommen. Durch eine Substanz mit einer Halbwertszeit von 1–2 h läßt sich die kurzzeitig wechselnde Entzündungssymptomatik auch besser steuern als mit einem langwirkenden Prinzip.

Die nichtsteroidalen Antiphlogistika sollten in der Regel über den Magen-Darm-Kanal zugeführt werden. Die parenterale Injektionsbehandlung vermindert zwar Unverträglichkeitsreaktionen am Gastrointestinaltrakt, dafür ergeben sich akute Gefahren durch anaphylaktoide Reaktionen und Schocksymptome.

Unerwünschte Wirkungen der nichtsteroidalen Antiphlogistika

Das gemeinsame Wirkungsprinzip der Zyklooxygenasehemmung ist auch die Ursache der meisten unerwünschten Wirkungen dieser Substanzklasse. Aus diesem Grunde sind die unerwünschten Wirkungen bei allen nichtsteroidalen Antiphlogistika ähnlich. Es gibt allerdings auch hier substanzspezifische Besonderheiten.

Gastrointestinaltrakt:
Die Störungen reichen von leichten Oberbauchbeschwerden bis hin zur Aktivierung peptischer Ulzera mit Blutungen. Ein wesentlicher Teil dieser Veränderungen geht auf die Hemmung der Zyklooxygenase in der Magenwand und den daraus resultierenden Wegfall der zytoprotektiven und säuresekretionshemmenden Wirkung von Prostaglandin E und Prostazyklin zurück. Aufgrund der hohen Konzentrationen und der guten Penetrationsfähgikeit im sauren Magen ist bei oraler Anwendung auch eine lokale Wirkung beteiligt, der Effekt tritt aber auch bei systemischer Wirkung auf. Man hat versucht, diese Lokalwirkung durch Verwendung solcher

Substanzen, die erst nach Resorption in der Leber in die aktive Form überführt werden („pro drug"), auszuschalten. Die Inzidenz von Magenläsionen ist jedoch bei allen Substanzen ähnlich und liegt bei längerdauernder Anwendung etwa bei 30% [14].

Niere:
Prostaglandine besitzen an der Niere eine schwache diuretische Wirkung und einen vasodilatatorischen Effekt in der renalen Strombahn. Der Ausfall dieser physiologischen Prostaglandinwirkung ist der Hauptgrund für die Natrium- und Wasserretention der nichtsteroidalen Antiphlogistika und damit der Ödementstehung. Ein besonderes Risiko besteht bei den längerwirksamen Substanzen, bei älteren Patienten, bei Herzinsiffizienz und bei bestehenden Nierenerkrankungen [9].

Bronchialsystem:
Nichtsteroidale Antiphlogistika können einen akuten Bronchospasmus und andere anaphylaktoide Reaktionen auslösen (Urtikaria, angioneurotische Ödeme). Es liegt keine immunologisch vermittelte Sensibilisierung, sondern eine Reaktion auf die ganze Stoffklasse der nichtsteroidalen Antiphlogistika vor. Bronchospastische Wirkungen treten besonders bei Patienten mit einer Asthmaanamnese und bei vasomotorischer Rhinitis und Nasenpolypen auf.

Uterus:
Nichtsteroidale Antiphlogistika hemmen durch Störung der Synthese wehenauslösender Prostaglandine den Geburtsverlauf. Die Prostaglandinsynthesehemmung beim ungeborenen Kind kann einen vorzeitigen Verschluß des Ductus arteriosus (Botalli) verursachen.

Blutungen:
Die Störung der Thromboxansynthese bewirkt eine Verlängerung der Blutungszeit durch verminderte Plättchenaggregation und lokale Vasokonstriktion. Acetylsalicylsäure ist ein besonders effektiver Hemmstoff der Zyklooxygenase in den Thrombozyten, weil die kernlosen Thrombozyten die Azetylierung der Zyklooxygenase nicht rückgängig machen können und die Wirkung schon in erheblichem Umfang präsystemisch, d. h. im Pfortaderblut vor Blutdurchfluß durch die Leber zustande kommt [7]. Die gesteigerte Blutungsneigung ist besonders bei posttraumatischen Gelenk- und Muskelaffektionen mit der Gefahr von Nachblutungen von Bedeutung.

Zentralnervensystem:
Höhere Dosen von nichtsteroidalen Antiphlogistika können unerwünschte Wirkungen im ZNS mit Kopfschmerzen, Hör- und Gleichgewichtsstörungen, Schlafstörungen, Konfusionen und psychotische Symptome besonders bei älteren Patienten auslösen (Indometacin!).

Lokale Verwendung nichtsteroidaler Antiphlogistika

Die Situation, daß zum einen eine Vielzahl unerwünschter Wirkungen die systemische Anwendbarkeit einschränkt und zum anderen die zu therapierenden Muskel- und Gelenkveränderungen meist peripher an den Extemitäten oder auch nahe unter der Haut lokalisiert sind, hat dazu geführt, diese Substanzen lokal an der Haut aufzutragen und eine perkutane Penetration durch die Haut auszunutzen. Ein grundsätzliches Problem ergibt sich dabei aus der Situation, daß Substanzen mit einer guten Penetrationsfähigkeit durch die Haut auch schnell resorbiert und mit dem kutanen und subkutanen Blutstrom abtransportiert werden. Unstrittig ist, daß nichtsteroidale Antiphlogistika die Haut durchdringen können. Die kutane Bioverfügbarkeit ist allerdings gering und liegt in Abhängigkeit vom Hautareal (besonders wegen der unterschiedlichen Dicke der Haut) und der Anwendungsart (Okklusivverbände ergeben höhere Resorptionsquoten) bei 10–20 %. Die gemessenen Plasmaspiegel betragen bei kutaner Anwendung nur wenige Prozent der bei enteraler Anwendung der gleichen Substanzmenge gefundenen Werte. Dies gilt sowohl für Diclofenac als auch für Ibuprofen, Indometacin, Tolmetin und Etofenamat (Literaturübersicht bei [10]). In neuerer Zeit ist die Gewebskonzentration von nichtsteroidalen Antiphlogistika im anwendungsnahen Gewebsbereich, z. B. Faszien, Gelenkkapseln und Muskulatur, gemessen worden. Dabei fanden sich in diesen Geweben z. T. höhere Gewebskonzentrationen, z. B. von Ibuprofen [8], als in der Subkutis. Bei der Interpretation dieser Befunde muß berücksichtigt werden, daß sich nichtsteroidale Antiphlogistika auch bei systemischer Anwendung im entzündlich veränderten Gewebe anreichern.

Die entscheidende Frage nach der klinischen Wirksamkeit der kutanen Anwendung nichtsteroidaler Antiphlogistika kann nur aufgrund kontrollierter klinischer Studien beantwortet werden. Einer großen Zahl von nichtkontrollierten Erfahrungsberichten stehen nur wenige Doppelblindstudien gegenüber. In einigen wurden statistisch gesicherte Effekte auf die Schmerzsymptomatik, Beweglichkeit und Gelenkschwellung berichtet. Der erreichbare Effekt steht hinter denen bei systemischer Anwendung zurück. Auch die kutane Anwendung der nichtsteroidalen Antiphlogistika ist nicht frei von unerwünschten Wirkungen, besonders an der lokalen Anwendungsstelle.

Die am häufigsten verordneten Externa in der Behandlung von Gelenk- und Muskelschmerzen waren in den letzten Jahren in der Bundesrepublik Deutschland Kombinationspräparate mit entzündungshemmenden und gefäßerweiternden Bestandteilen, bei denen die Zunahme der Hautdurchblutung mit einem Anstieg der Hauttemperatur ein wichtiger Vermittler der schmerzlindernden Wirkung zu sein scheint.

Steroidale Antiphlogistika (Glukokortikoide)

Eine systemische Verwendung von Glukokortikoiden kommt bei Gelenk- und Muskelbeschwerden nur in Ausnahmefällen in Betracht. Die vielfältigen und schwerwiegenden unerwünschten Wirkungen rechtfertigen trotz überzeugender Wirksamkeit ihren Einsatz meist nicht. Die früher oft verwendeten Kombinationspräparate aus Glukokortikoiden und nichtsteroidalen Antiphlogistika sind aus der Therapie praktisch verschwunden. Die Präparate sind nicht mehr im Handel.

Eine besondere Bedeutung besitzt die Möglichkeit, Glukokortikoide lokal in den entzündlich veränderten Bereich zu applizieren. Die Verwendung von Kristallsuspensionen erlaubt eine – bei den einzelnen Präparationen unterschiedlich lang anhaltende – Depotwirkung bei intraartikulärer oder infiltrativer Anwendung. Es muß jedoch berücksichtigt werden, daß die Glukokortikoide aus diesem lokalen Anwendungsbereich resorbiert werden und bei ausreichenden Gesamtdosen systemische Wirkungen auslösen können. Lokale Komplikationen ergeben sich aus der Infektionsgefahr, aus Knorpelschäden und katabolen Veränderungen im Sehnenbereich.

Analgetika

Die Anwendung nichtsteroidaler Antiphlogistika führt über eine Verminderung der entzündlichen – über Prostaglandine vermittelten – Hyperalgesie zu einer Reduktion von Muskel- und Gelenkschmerzen. Wenn durch diese Entzündungshemmung keine ausreichende Schmerzunterdrückung erreichbar ist, kann es erforderlich sein, zusätzlich analgetisch wirkende Medikamente einzusetzen.

Nichtopioide Analgetika

Während die Acetylsalicylsäure neben ihrer analgetischen Wirkung auch entzündungshemmend wirkt und beim entzündlich ausgelösten Schmerz besonders gut wirksam ist, hat Paracetamol in therapeutisch verwendbarer Dosierung keine antiphlogistischen Wirkungen. Die fehlende antiphlogistische Wirksamkeit von Paracetamol muß zunächst überraschen, weil auch Paracetamol ein Hemmstoff der Prostaglandinbiosynthese ist. Der Grund für die fehlende entzündungshemmende Wirkung ist einmal darin zu sehen, daß Paracetamol nicht wie die sauren, nichtsteroidalen Antiphlogistika im Entzündungsgewebe angereichert wird und daß es im Gegensatz zu diesen die Prostaglandinsynthese im ZNS stärker hemmt als im peripheren Gewebe [2]. Ein ähnliches Verhalten zeigen die Pyrazolanalgetika (z. B. Metamizol, Propyphenazon).

Opioide Analgetika

Muskel- und Gelenkbeschwerden sind keine Indikationen für die Verwendung opioider Analgetika. Gelegentlich kann es sinnvoll sein, für einen begrenzten Zeitraum eine nicht ausreichende Wirkung nichtopioder Analgetika durch das schwach wirksame Opioid Codein zu verstärken. Dieser in klinischen Versuchen nachgewiesene Effekt (Literaturübersicht bei [11]) hat sich in dem Stufenplan der allgemeinen analgetischen Therapie bewährt. Eine grundsätzliche Verwendung analgetischer Kombinationspräparate ist dagegen in der Therapie von Muskel- und Gelenkbeschwerden nicht vertretbar.

Spinal und supraspinal wirkende Muskelrelaxanzien

Bei Muskel- und Gelenkaffektionen treten häufig Muskelverspannungen auf, die den schmerzhaften Prozeß verstärken und die Bewegungseinschränkung weiter stabilisieren können. Durch eine spinale und supraspinale, im wesentlichen auf einer Verstärkung des inhibitorischen Überträgerstoffes γ-Aminobuttersäure (GABA) beruhenden zentralen muskelrelaxierenden Wirkung können diese Steigerungen des Muskeltonus beseitigt werden. Zu diesem Zweck werden Tranquilizer aus der Gruppe der Benzodiazepine [z. B. Diazepam, (Valium, Generika)], aber auch andere zentral muskelrelaxierende Substanzen wie Carisoprodol (Sanoma), Chlormezanon (Muskel-Trancopal) und das Anticholinergikum Orphenadrin (Norflex) verwendet. Der therapeutische Wert ist mangels ausreichender, kontrollierter Untersuchungen umstritten. Den Substanzen kommt eine ausgeprägte sedative Wirkung mit Einschränkung der Fahrtüchtigkeit und Verstärkung von Alkoholwirkungen zu. Für die Benzodiazepine besteht naturgemäß auch bei dieser Anwendung ein erhebliches Abhängigkeitsrisiko.

Aus dem Gesagten ergeben sich für die medikamentöse Therapie von Muskel- und Gelenkbeschwerden folgende Grundsätze:

- Die Standardtherapie mit nichtsteroidalen Antiphlogistika sollte in Form einer Monotherapie erfolgen. Man sollte sich auf die Verwendung weniger Verbindungen beschränken.
- Kürzer wirksame Substanzen sollte in der Regel der Vorzug vor länger wirksamen Antiphlogistika gegeben werden, weil sie der schwankenden Symptomatik besser adjustiert werden können und weniger Auswirkungen auf den Elektrolythaushalt besitzen.
- Es ist nicht sinnvoll, eine völlige Beschwerdefreiheit anzustreben, weil dann das Risiko unerwünschter Wirkungen stark zunimmt. Es geht darum, die Symptomatik auf ein erträgliches Maß zurückzudrängen.
- Wenn mit den nichtsteroidalen Antiphlogistika keine ausreichende Schmerzunterdrückung gelingt, kann es notwendig werden, zusätzlich Analgetika zu verwenden. Dies sollte immer gezielt und *nicht* durch Verwendung fixer Arzneimittelkombinationen erfolgen.

- Bei starken Muskelverspannungen kann der Einsatz von zentralen Muskelrelaxanzien sinnvoll sein. Auch hier gilt, daß eine solche Zusatztherapie individuell verwendet werden muß und nicht als Teil einer allgemeinen Kombiantionstherapie verstanden werden darf.

Literatur

1. Elenbaas JK (1980) Centrally acting oral skeletal muscle relaxants. Am J Hosp Pharm 37 : 1313–1323
2. Engelhardt G (1985) Zur Pharmakologie der schwachwirksamen Analgetika. Braun, Karlsruhe
3. Huskisson EC (1983) Anti-rheumatic drugs. Praeger, Eastburne
4. Insel PA (1990) Analgesic-antipyretics and antiinflammatory agents: Drugs employed in the treatment of rheumatoid arthritis and gout. In: Goodman Gilman A, Rall TW, Nies AS, Taylor P (eds) The pharmacological basis of therapeutics, 8th edn. Pergamon, Oxford, pp 638–681
5. Kahl GF, Schmidt G (1988) Schmerzbehandlung. In: König B (Hrsg) Allgemeinmedizin. Perimed, Erlangen, S 1697–1735
6. Kaiser H (1987) Cortisonderivate in Klinik und Praxis, 8. Aufl. Thieme, Stuttgart
7. Pedersen AK, Fitzgerald GA (1985) Dose-related kinetics of aspirin: presystemic acetylation of platelet cycloocygenase. N Engl J Med 312 : 1388–1389
8. Peters H, Chlud K, Berner G, Wagener HH, Staab R, Melchiar E, Zimmermann P (1987) Zur perkutanen Kinetik von Ibuprofen. Aktuel Rheumatol 12 : 208–211
9. Rieger J (1984) Nicht-steroidale Antiphlogistika und Niere. Arzneiverodnung in der Praxis 2
10. Sandholzer H, Kochen MM (1991) Perkutane Rheumatherapie. Pharmakritik 13 : 13–16
11. Schmidt G (1986) Arzneimittel für die Indikation Schmerzen. In: Dölle W, Müller-Oerlinghausen B, Schwabe U (Hrsg) Grundlagen der Arzneimitteltherapie. Wissenschaftsverlag, Mannheim, S 187–195
12. Schmidt G (1987) Pharmakologische Grundlagen der Therapie mit antiphlogistisch und antipyretisch wirkenden Analgetika. In: Friedberg KD, Rüfer R (Hrsg) Antiphlogistisch und antipyretisch wirkende Analgetika. Fischer, Stuttgart, S 1–10
13. Schmidt G (1990) Antirheumatika und Antiphlogistika. In: Schwabe U, Paffrath D (Hrsg) Arzneiverordnungsreport 90. Fischer, Stuttgart, S 97–113
14. Vrhovac B (1988) Antiinflammatory analgesics and drugs used in gout. In: Dukes MNG (ed) Meyler's side effects of drugs, 11th edn. Elsevier, Amsterdam, pp 151–182

Moderne Phytotherapie

Medicinal Plants

Möglichkeiten und Grenzen einer modernen Phytotherapie

Volker Fintelmann und Claus-Peter Siegers

Eine moderne Phytotherapie, die Behandlung mit Arzneimitteln aus Heilpflanzen, Teilen oder Zubereitungen derselben, muß Bestandteil einer modernen Medizin sein. Zwar wurde durch die Novellierung des Arzneimittelgesetzes (AMG) 1976 durch Festschreibung eines therapeutischen Pluralismus in der Medizin die Phytotherapie als besondere Therapierichtung benannt, doch darf sie, gerade in der Entwicklung des letzten Jahrzehnts, nicht als Alternative zu einer naturwissenschaftlich definierten Pharmakotherapie gesehen werden, sondern als deren *Ergänzung*.

Natürlich existiert die Schwierigkeit, daß die heutigen naturwissenschaftlich-pharmakologischen Methoden nicht ausreichen, um therapeutische Wirkungen und Wirksamkeiten von Phytopharmaka umfassend zu bewerten, da erstere mehr auf Einzelstoffuntersuchungen ausgerichtet sind, Phytopharmaka aber praktisch immer Vielstoffgemische darstellen. Der isolierte, aus einer Pflanze gewonnene Wirkstoff zählt definitionsgemäß nicht mehr zu den Phytopharmaka. Das in der skizzierten Frage auftretende wissenschaftliche Problem kann auch so charakterisiert werden:

Geht die analytisch-beweisende (naturwissenschaftliche) Methode immer auf das Verständins von Wirkungen der Einzelstoffe aus, muß zum richtigen Erfassen des „Vielstoffgemisches Heilpflanze“ eine mehr synthetisierend-beschreibende Methode entwickelt werden, die neben den einzelnen pharmakologisch erfaßbaren Wirkungen auch Wirksamkeit als Ganzheit erfaßt.

Dabei kann davon ausgegangen werden, daß die Wirksamkeit sich zunächst deutlicher in den Befindensänderungen zeigt, was auch zu der mißverständlichen Formulierung führte, Phytopharmaka wären vorzüglich für Befindlichkeitsstörungen geeignet.

Die Beobachtung zeigt, daß primär die Wirksamkeit Veränderungen der Befindlichkeit hervorruft, bei ausreichender Beobachtungsdauer aber auch die Befundebene im Sinne der objektiven Besserung erfaßt wird. Zielen moderne, chemisch definierte, synthetische Pharmaka möglichst exakt auf einen umschriebenen Wirkort (Rezeptor), erzielen damit definierte Wirkungen, sind Phytopharmaka offensichtlich mehr darauf gerichtet, körpereigene Steuerungs- und Regulationssysteme zu beeinflussen, sowohl zu stimulieren wie auch zu bremsen und somit als ihren Wirkort körpereigene Selbstheilungssysteme zu haben. Ärztliche Erfahrungen und auch zahlreiche experimentelle Daten lassen eine solche Arbeitshypothese aufstellen, wobei es zukünftiger intensivierter Forschung vorbehalten ist, die unwiderlegbare Bestätigung der Hypothese wissenschaftlich zu belegen.

Die *Möglichkeiten der Therapie* mit Phytopharmaka sind vielfältig, ihre Grenzen deutlich:

Rationale Pharmakotherapie in der Allgemeinpraxis
Rational Pharmacotherapy in General Practice
M. M. Kochen (Hrsg.)

Sie werden in der Akut- und Notfallmedizin, wo praktisch immer Soforteffekte erforderlich sind, keinen oder nur einen sehr geringen Stellenwert haben.

Ihre *Stärke* liegt in einer *Langzeitwirkung*, wobei Umstimmung oder Induktion körpereigener Systeme als eigentlicher Zielort bereits angesprochen wurden. Das schließt die Möglichkeit rascher Wirkungseintritte durch Phytopharmaka nicht aus, wofür als Beispiele die intravenöse Injektion von Crataegus-Präparaten vorzüglich bei rechtsführender Herzinsuffizienz oder auch die so einfache Einreibung der Bauchhaut mit Kümmelöl (Oleum carum carvi) bei quälendem Meteorismus dienen mögen.

Grenzen für Phytopharmaka:
Grenzen setzen auch solche Krankheitszustände, in denen bereits irreversible organische Schäden eingetreten sind, z. B. fortgeschrittene Stadien der Arteriosklerose und deren Folgekrankheiten.

Grenzen setzt schließlich bisher auch das Spezialgebiet der Onkologie, da spezifisch auf die Krebskrankheit einwirkende Phytopharmaka bisher nicht existieren, wobei die aus der anthroposophischen Medizin stammende Therapie der Krebskrankheit mit Mistelpräparaten in jüngster Zeit durch die Lektinforschung neues Interesse geweckt hat und hier mit großer Wahrscheinlichkeit auch standardisierte Phytopharmaka Anwendung finden werden.

**Diabetes mellitus:
Therapiestandard in der Allgemeinpraxis**

**Diabetes mellitus:
Treatment Standard in General Practice**

Die Versorgung von Typ-II-Diabetikern in Hausarztpraxen

Joachim A. Szecsenyi und Michael M. Kochen

Die Bedeutung des Diabetes mellitus in der hausärztlichen Praxis

Der Diabetes mellitus gehört mit einer geschätzten Prävalenz von 2–4 % zu den häufigsten Erkrankungen in den westlichen Industrienationen. Diese Häufigkeitsschätzungen gelten auch für die Bundesrepublik Deutschland, genaue Zahlenangaben sind jedoch erstaunlicherweise nicht verfügbar [17, 37]. Bei einer Untersuchung aus 14 Allgemeinpraxen in der ehemaligen DDR [21], die einen bevölkerungsbezogenen Rückschluß erlaubt, lag der Diabetes mellitus bei 14 841 Patienten, die ihren Hausarzt über den Zeitraum von einem Jahr aufsuchten, auf Rang 12 aller Diagnosen. Insgesamt waren 3,6 % der Bevölkerung Diabetiker. Bei über 65 Jahre alten Patienten hatten 13 % aller Frauen und 19 % aller Männer einen Diabetes mellitus.

Die Behandlung des nicht insulinabhängigen Diabetes mellitus ist nach wie vor eine Domäne des Hausarztes, der auch die Mehrheit der (insbesondere oralen) Antidiabetika verschreibt.

Betrachtet man die Zahl der kassenärztlichen Verordnungen von Antidiabetika, so fällt auf, daß im Jahre 1989 für ambulante in der gesetzlichen Krankenversicherung versicherte Patienten 158,1 Mio. definierte Tagesdosen (DDD) Insulinpräparate und 477,6 Mio. DDD orale Antidiabetika verschrieben wurden. Letztgenannte

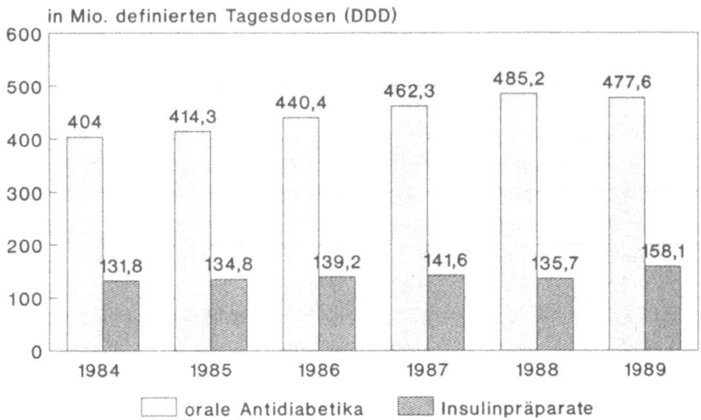

Abb. 1. Verordnungen von Antidiabetika 1984–1989 (nur ambulante Patienten der GKV; *DDD* definierte Tagesdosen). Zahlen für 1984 geschätzt, für 1985–1989 real. (Nach [18])

Rationale Pharmakotherapie in der Allgemeinpraxis
Rational Pharmacotherapy in General Practice
M. M. Kochen (Hrsg.)

Zahl würde ausreichen, um mehr als 1,3 Mio. Typ-II-Diabetiker mit diesen Medikamenten zu versorgen [18]. Dabei unterlagen die Verordnungen für orale Antidiabetika in den letzten 6 Jahren einer Steigerun um ca. 20% oder 72,4 Mio. DDD (Abb. 1). Selbst wenn Hintergrundeffekte, z. B. Veränderungen der Altersstruktur, die ein Ansteigen der Zahl der Diabetiker bedingen, berücksichtigt werden, muß man annehmen, daß ein erheblicher Anteil der Typ-II-Diabetiker mit hohen Dosen oraler Antidiabetika eingestellt ist. Nur im Jahre 1989 ließ sich ein leichtes Absinken dieser Verschreibungen verzeichnen.

Wie gut muß die Stoffwechselkontrolle beim Typ-II-Diabetes sein?

Die Lebensqualität und die Lebenserwartung des Diabetikers werden heute im wesentlichen durch Folgeerkrankungen wie Makroangiopathien, Mikroangiopathien (z. B. diabetische Retinopathie), Neuropathien sowie das Auftreten der seltenen diabetischen Katarakt bestimmt.

Bisher weiß man noch zu wenig darüber, ob selbst durch optimale Stoffwechseleinstellung das Auftreten dieser Komplikationen vollständig verhindert werden kann.

Die epidemiologische Forschung hat sich deshalb darauf konzentriert, die Güte der Blutzuckereinstellung als Prädiktor des Auftretens diabetischer Spätkomplikationen zu untersuchen. Leider gibt es auf diesem Gebiet nur wenige prospektive Kohortenstudien, in denen größere Gruppen von Diabetikern über einen längeren Zeitraum beobachtet wurden.

Pirart stellte in seiner 25 Jahre dauernden Kohortenstudie fest, daß eine über mehrere Jahre bestehende schlechte Stoffwechseleinstellung mit einer höheren Prävalenz und Inzidenz diabetischer Komplikationen (Neuropathie- und Mikroangiopathie, speziell schwere Retinopathie) gekoppelt ist. Die jährliche Inzidenz der diabetischen Neuro-, Retino- und Nephropathie korreliert nach dieser Studie auch eindeutig mit der Qualität der Einstellung im Jahr vor der jährlichen Untersuchung – unabhängig davon, wie gut oder schlecht der Patient in früherer Zeit eingestellt war [25].

Auch Alberti u. Home vertreten die Ansicht, daß eine gute Stoffwechseleinstellung Spätschäden verhindern bzw. hinauszögern kann [1].

Die kumulative Inzidenz eines schweren, dialysepflichtigen chronischen Nierenversagens beträgt beim Typ-II-Diabetes innerhalb von 25 Jahren 6,2% und beim Typ-I-Diabetes 8%. Typ-II-Diabetiker, die bei Diagnosestellung eine persitierende Proteinurie zeigen, haben ein 12fach höheres Risiko, ein chronisches Nierenversagen zu erleiden, als Patienten, bei denen dies nicht der Fall ist [12].

Im Bereich der ophthalmologischen Komplikationen zeigte sich bei einer Screeningstudie, daß unter 145 Patienten Typ-II-Diabetikern, die bisher nach eigenen Angaben nie augenärztlich untersucht wurden, 61% eine diabetische Retinopathie, ein Glaukom oder eine Katarakt hatten.

Dieser kurze Überblick kann nur andeuten, welche Bedeutung eine optimale Stoffwechselkontrolle für den Patienten mit Diabetes mellitus hat. Für den Typ-II-

Diabetes sind in den letzten Jahren auf nationaler [4] und internationaler [24] Ebene Empfehlungen zu Stoffwechselkontrolle, Selbstkontrolle, Schulung und Durchführung von klinischen Untersuchungen erarbeitet worden. Diese Empfehlungen sind als eine wichtige Grundlage für die Erarbeitung allgemeinmedizinischer Standards zur Versorgung von Diabetikern anzusehen.

Forschungsergebnisse über die Versorgung von Diabetikern in Hausarztpraxen

Die Forschung über die Qualität der Versorgung von Diabetikern in Hausarztpraxen hat besonders in Großbritannien und den Niederlanden Tradition.

Schon zu Beginn der 70er Jahre wurden sog. „diabetic-mini-clinics", spezielle Sprechstundenzeiten für Diabetiker, in englischen Allgemeinpraxen eingeführt. Zudem wurden spezielle Patientenkarten für Diabetiker geschaffen. Eine Untersuchung aus dem „Wolverhampton-Care-Scheme" zeigte schon 1973, daß durch diesen Ansatz ein mit Spezialambulanzen vergleichbarer Qualitätsstandard erreicht werden kann [38]. Dies konnte später auch durch eine kontrollierte Studie bestätigt werden [30].

Muir et al. wiesen nach, daß in Allgemeinpraxen mit Hilfe eines *strukturierten Behandlungs- und Kontrollschemas* eine *signifikante Verbesserung* verschiedener Stoffwechselparameter innerhalb eines Jahres möglich ist [19]. Ähnliche Erfolge wurden auch in anderen Untersuchungen erzielt [5,39].

Demgegenüber zeigte eine kontrollierte randomisierte Studie, daß die *routinemäßige Behandlung* von Typ-II-Diabetikern in Allgemeinpraxen in bezug auf die Blutzuckereinstellung und die regelmäßige Durchführung von Kontrolluntersuchungen der Behandlung in einer Spezialambulanz *unterlegen* waren [9].

Eine bevölkerungsbezogene Studie über die Versorgung eines ländlichen Bezirks in Wales ergab, daß Hausärzte gegenüber Gebietsärzten seltener Gewichts-, Blutglukose-, Blutdruck- und Augenhintergrundsuntersuchungen bei den von ihnen behandelten Diabetikern durchführen [6]. Vergleichbare Mängel wurden auch in anderen Untersuchungen nachgewiesen [2,4,14].

Studien im Rahmen von Qualitätssicherungsprogrammen in niederländischen Allgemeinpraxen kamen zu dem Ergebnis, daß die Dokumentation von klinischen Untersuchungsergebnissen und Laborwerten stark verbesserungswürdig war. Bei 27 % der Patienten wurde zu keinem Zeitpunkt das Körpergewicht registriert, und bei immerhin knapp 10der Patienten wurde kein einziger Blutzuckerwert dokumentiert [29]. Die Autoren kommen deshalb zu der Empfehlung, spezielle Dokumentationskarten für Diabetiker zu entwickeln und in den Praxen einzusetzen.

Trotz dieser Dokumentationsprobleme konnten einzelne Praxen, die einen systematischen Versorgungsansatz für Diabetiker wählten, gute Qualitätsstandards erreichen [27,28].

Aus der Bundesrepublik Deutschland gibt es bisher nur wenige Arbeiten zur Qualität der Versorgung von Diabetikern in Hausarztpraxen. In einer Querschnittstudie aus 25 Allgemeinpraxen [16] konnte gezeigt werden, daß dort in einem

Quartal 1304 Diabetiker (davon 10 % vom Typ I) versorgt wurden. Diese Studie hat jedoch ebenso wie die Studie von Karg [13] den Mangel, daß die jeweiligen Patientenpopulationen völlig unsystematisch und über kurze Zeiträume erfaßt wurden und Aussagen über die Frequenz der durchgeführten Kontrollen entweder aus den Angaben der Hausärzte abgeleitet oder gar nicht verfügbar waren.

Mehr Erfahrungen liegen hierzulande aus Projekten zur Evaluation von Gruppenschulungsprogrammen für Typ-II-Diabetiker vor. Diese Studien zielen jedoch vom Untersuchungsansatz her auf die Beobachtung von Subpopulationen von Typ-II-Diabetikern aus Hausarztpraxen [15, 34].

Zur Zeit wird in einem Düsseldorfer Modellprojekt die Effektivität einer von Hausärzten durchgeführten Einzelschulung für nichtinsulinspritzende Typ-II-Diabetiker erprobt [32]. Bisher liegen jedoch noch keine Untersuchungsergebnisse vor.

Eine kürzlich veröffentlichte Langzeitstudie [35, 36], in der alle 1272 Diabetiker (davon 8,6 % Typ-I-Diabetiker) aus 18 Hausarztpraxen über einen Zeitraum von 5 Quartalen beobachtet wurden, kam zusammenfassend zu folgendem *Ergebnissen für Typ-II-Diabetiker:*

- Das Durchschnittsalter der Typ-II-Diabetiker beträgt 69,5 Jahre (SD = 12 Jahre).
- 60 % sind Frauen; sie haben regelmäßiger Kontakt zur Praxis als Männer.
- Nur ca. die Hälfte der Diabetiker hat in jedem Quartal Kontakt zur Praxis.
- Gut eingestellte Patienten gehen regelmäßiger zum Hausarzt als schlecht eingestellte.
- Fast jede zweite Frau im Alter zwischen 50 und 70 Jahren ist übergewichtig, dies ist nur bei jedem vierten Mann der Fall.
- Etwa 44 % der Diabetiker sind mit einem oralen Antidiabetikum eingestellt, davon ist jede zweite Frau, unabhängig vom Alter, übergewichtig (bei Männern nur jeder vierte).
- Mit einem oralen Antidiabetikum eingestellte Patienten weisen signifikant häufiger schlechte Stoffwechselparameter auf als diätetisch eingestellte Diabetiker.

In unserem Gesundheitssystem hat der Hausarzt nur bedingt die Möglichkeit, Patienten regelmäßig zu Kontrolluntersuchungen einzubestellen. Nimmt der Patient einen vereinbarten Untersuchungstermin nicht wahr, hat der Hausarzt erst beim nächsten Praxiskontakt des Patienten, der u. U. ein anderes Gesundheitsproblem zum Anlaß hat, eine erneute Gelegenheit, eine Bertung bzw. Kontrolle durchzuführen. Es hängt dann sowohl von der Praxisorganisation (wird die Chance zur Stoffwechselkontrolle wahrgenommen, auch wenn der Patient erst nach Monaten erstmals wieder wegen eines Rezepts kommt?) als auch vom Willen des Patienten ab (wird vom Problem Diabetes abgelenkt und die Aufmerksamkeit des Hausarztes auf das aktuelle Gesundheitsproblem gerichtet?), ob gerade den schlechteingestellten Patienten auch eine verstärkte Aufmerksamkeit seitens der Praxis gewidmet wird.

Auffällig ist, daß mehr als 70 % aller im Längsschnitt gut eingestellten Patienten regelmäßig kontrolliert werden und daß dieser Prozentsatz bei den schlecht eingestellten Patienten nur unwesentlich höher ist (Tabelle 1). Dagegen gibt es bei den

Tabelle 1. Werden die „richtigen" Typ-II-Diabetiker kontrolliert? [36]

Kontakte zur Hausarztpraxis[a]	Qualität der Stoffwechseleinstellung im Längsschnitt über 5 Quartale			
	gut	[%]	schlecht	[%]
Selten Kontakt	34	6,0	14	3,9
Regelmäßiger Kontakt und regelmäßige Kontrollen	408	71,6	292	82,0
Regelmäßiger Kontakt und seltene Kontrollen	128	22,5	50[b]	14,0
Gesamt (n = 926)	570	100,0	356	38,4

[a] Nur Patienten mit einem Kontakt in mindestens 3 von 5 Quartalen.
[b] „Vergessene Diabetiker".

schlecht eingestellten Diabetikern eine Gruppe, die trotz bekannt schlechter Stoffwechsellage und trotz Kontakt zur Praxis (z. B. wegen eines anderen Gesundheitsproblems) kaum noch kontrolliert wird. Für diese Gruppe wurde die Hypothese des „vergessenen Diabetes" entwickelt [36]. Sie trifft jedoch nicht pauschal für alle Hausartzpraxen in gleicher Weise zu, sondern ist vermutlich Ausdruck eines multifaktoriellen Geschehens. Dabei könnten z. B. Interesse und Erfahrungshintergrund des Hausarztes, Organisationsgrad der Patientendokumentation und gemeinsame Behandlungserfahrung zwischen Arzt und Patient eine Rolle spielen. Das Thema Diabetes mellitus wird vermutlich in Form einer „stillschweigenden Einigung" aus der Beratung ausgeklammert.

Die oben aufgeführten Studien weisen auf strukturelle Mängel in der Betreuung von Diabetikern in Hausarztpraxen hin: Für eine große Zahl von Patienten, denen „nichts weh tut", von denen aber eine große Selbstdisziplin gefordert wird, ist ein Mindestmaß an Bewertung, Stoffwechselkontrolle und Zuwendung über einen jahrzehntelangen Zeitraum zu gewährleisten. Dabei ist es – wie es das Beispiel der vergessenen Diabetiker zeigt – von besonderer Wichtigkeit, daß der Hausarzt gerade die Patienten nicht aus dem Blickfeld verliert, denen Komplikationen drohen. Zur Durchsetzung dieses Ziels kann es schon hilfreich sein, ein einfaches Dokumentationsverfahren in der Praxis einzuführen und anhand der eigenen Praxisdaten zu überprüfen, ob bestimmte Mindestanforderungen hinsichtlich Stoffwechselkontrollen, körperlichen Untersuchungen und Schulungsmaßnahmen durchgeführt wurden.

Vor diesem Hintergrund wurden in einigen Ländern Standards für die Qualität der Versorgung von Diabetikern in Hausarztpraxen entwickelt, von denen hier beispielhaft der niederländische Entwurf vorgestellt wird.

Allgemeinmedizinische Standards: Das niederländische Modell

Ein Standard für den Typ-II-Diabetes wurde hier bereits im Jahre 1989 von der „Nederlands Huisartsen Genootschap" (NHG) eingeführt. Mittlerweile sind – basierend auf den Erfahrungen in „Qualitätszirkeln" niedergelassener Ärzte [8] und durch Arbeitsgruppen der NHG – Standards für 15 verschiedene Erkrankungen formuliert worden.

Sips [31] faßt die dabei gemachten Erfahrungen folgendermaßen zusammen:

a) Die wissenschaftliche Begründbarkeit eines Standards reicht nicht für seine Einführung aus, die formulierten Ziele müssen unter Praxisbedingungen auch erreichbar sein.
b) Standards sollten Teil einer nationalen Initiative sein.
c) Die Protokolle sollten durch ein unabhängiges wissenschaftliches Kommitee autorisiert werden.
d) Standards sollten durch Teilnahme möglichst vieler Hausärzte entstehen und nicht „von oben" verordnet werden.

Der NHG-Standard für den Typ-II-Diabetes zielt auf eine Stärkung der Eigeninitiative des Patienten, auf Schulung und Selbstkontrolle. Nur wenige Kontrol-

Tabelle 2. Diabetes mellitus Typ II – NHG[a]-Standard

a Diagnostik

	Glukose im Kapillarblut [mmol/l] nüchtern	2 h p.p.
Normal	$\leq 5,5$	$\leq 7,7$
Gestörte Glukosetoleranz	$< 6,7$	7,8–11
Diabetes mellitus[b]	$\geq 6,7$	$\geq 11,1$

[a] *NHG* Nederlands Huisartsen Genootschap, Utrecht.
[b] Diagnose Diabetes mellitus steht fest bei:
bestehender Symptomatik und einem abnormalen Glukosewert bzw.
fehlender Symptomatik und 2 pathologischen Glukosewerten.

b Behandlung

Ziele	Gut	Ausreichend	Schlecht
Gewichtsoptimierung (Quetelt-Index)[c]	< 25	25–27	> 27
Blutglukose			
nüchtern:	< 6,7	6,7–8	> 8
2 h p.p.	< 9	9–10	> 10

Schritte:
1. Gewicht[c] optimieren – Diätberatung, Schulung, Körperliche Bewegung[c]
   wenn *nach 6 Monaten* Glukosewerte schlecht bleiben:
2. Medikamentöse Therapie erwägen[c]

Tabelle 2 (Fortsetzung)

Ziele		Gut	Ausreichend	Schlecht
Medikamentöse Therapie:				
Beginn mit:	Tolbutamid	(z. B. Rastinon) Versuch mit 500 mg tgl. für 4 Wochen, maximal 2mal 1 g		
Wenn ohne Erfolg:	Glibenclamid	(z. B. Euglucon) Versuch mit 2,5 mg[d] tgl. für 4 Wochen, maximal 15 mg tgl.		
	oder Gliclazid	(Diamicron) Versuch mit 80 mg tgl. für 4 Wochen, maximal 3mal 80 mg		
	oder Glipizid	(Glibenese) Versuch mit 5 mg tgl. für 4 Wochen, maximal 20 mg tgl.		
Wenn ohne Erfolg:	Metformin	(z. B. Glucophage) Versuch mit 500 mg tgl. für 4 Wochen, maximal 3mal 850 mg		
Wenn ohne Erfolg:		Insulintherapie erwägen		

[c] Gewicht in kg/(Körperlänge in m^2).
[d] In der Bundesrepublik Deutschland in dieser Dosierung nicht im Handel.

c Kontrollen

Anamnese	Klinische Untersuchung/Labor
Vierteljährlich:	
Wohlbefinden	Gewicht
Beschwerden	Blutglukose (nüchtern)
Gewichtsentwicklung	
Diätprobleme	
Probleme mit Medikamenten	
Jährlich:	
Genitalpruritus	Gewicht
Parästhesien/-algien der Extremitäten	Fußkontrolle
Störungen des Sexuallebens	A. dorsalis predis
Sehstörungen	Blutdruck
pektanginöse Beschwerden	Augenärztliche Kontrolle alle 1–2 Jahre
Claudikatio	Blutglukose (nüchtern)
Gewicht, Diäte	Kreatinin
Körperliche Bewegung	(Cholesterin)
Nikotin	Eiweiß im Urin
Medikation	

len sollen durch die Praxis in vierteljährlichem Abstand durchgeführt werden. Die jährliche Untersuchung zielt besonders auf diabetische Komplikationen und Compliancefragen ab [20, 23]. In Tabelle 2 wird der NHG-Standard (geringfügig geändert) wiedergegeben [22].

Grol [7] führte 6 Wochen nach Einführung des NHG-Standards für den Typ-II-Diabetes eine Repräsentativbefragung niederländischer Hausärzte über den Einsatz des Standards in den Praxen durch. Zuvor waren die Grundlinien dieses Standards allerdings schon monatelang in der Fachpresse diskutiert worden:

Dabei stimmten die Hausärzte den Anforderungen des NHG-Standards zwar weitgehend zu. Hinsichtlich der Durchführung einzelner im Standard geforderter Untersuchungsmaßnahmen (z. B. jährliche Fußkontrolle und Einführung eines Dokumentationssystems) gab es jedoch erhebliche Abweichungen zwischen der Wirklichkeit in den Praxen und den Zielvorstellungen des Standards.

59 % der befragten Allgemeinmediziner sahen als Problem der Einführung von Standards die Gefahr, einzelnen Patienten nicht mehr gerecht werden zu können. Außerdem wurde es vielfach als schwierig angesehen, eine bestehende Praxisrou-

Tabelle 3. NHG-Standard für Typ-II-Diabetiker

a Ergebnisse einer Repräsentativbefragung unter 453 Allgemeinärzten zum NHG-Standard für Typ-II-Diabetiker. (Nach [8])

Anforderung	Einverstanden mit NHG Standard [%]	Durchführung in der eigenen Praxis [%]
Blutzuckerbestimmung alle 3 Monate	92	89
Definition:		
Blutzucker (nüchtern) $\geq 6,7$ mmol/l	82	62
Gewichtskontrolle alle 3 Monate	79	62
Fußinspektion einmal jährlich	84	44
Dokumenationssystem für Diabetiker	71	33

b Probleme der Durchsetzung des NHG-Standards für Typ-II-Diabetiker

Probleme	453 befragte Allgemeinärzte % der Antworten[a]
„Jeder Patient ist anders"	59
Kontrollen in der Regel durch Gebietsarzt	46
Praxisroutine läßt sich schwer ändern	44
Keine Belohnung für Änderung der Praxisroutine	38
Braucht mehr Zeit und Energie	33
Patienten wollen keine Änderung	25
Zweifel, ob für die Patienten dabei etwas Positives herauskommt	24
Fehlende Informationen und Fertigkeiten, um Standard umzusetzten	13

[a] Mehrfachantworten möglich.

tine zu ändern, zumal für den erwarteten Mehraufwand keine finanzielle Gratifikation zu erwarten war (Tabelle 3).

Ein Jahr nach Einführung des NHG-Standards erbracht eine Untersuchung in 11 computerisierten Praxen, daß noch mehr als ein Drittel aller Typ-II-Diabetiker nicht zufriedenstellend eingestellt war [11]. Nach einer anderen in 18 Praxen durchgeführten Studie waren 70% der Typ-II-Diabetiker schlechter eingestellt, als es der NHG-Standard vorschreibt [26]. Dies galt auch für die gleichzeitig von Internisten mitbetreuten Diabetiker. Diese Ergebnisse sind jedoch wegen der grundsätzlichen Unterschiede der Gesundheitssysteme nicht vorbehaltslos übertragbar: In den Niederlanden hat der Allgemeinarzt eine zentrale Verteilerfunktion im Gesundheitswesen. Es gibt in der Regel keinen freien Zugang zu gebietsärztlicher Versorgung. Außerdem sind die Hausarztpraxen meist als Gruppenpraxen ausgelegt, oft mit Anschluß an universitäre Abteilungen für Allgemeinmedizin.

Mittlerweile gibt es in den Niederlanden eine Diskussion, ob die im NHG-Standard aufgestellten Richtlinien hinsichtlich der Stoffwechselparameter nicht zu scharf sind oder sogar kontraproduktiv wirken [33]. Ziel der Entwicklung sollten ja verbindliche, wissenschaftlich fundierte und praktisch haltbare Richtlinien für Hausärzte sein. Wenn die in der Praxis mit vertretbarem Aufwand erreichbaren Werte erheblich von den Richtwerten abweichen, kann dies nach den niederländischen Erfahrungen zum verstärkten Einsatz von Medikamenten führen. Auch ethische und juristische Konsequenzen, z. B. die Einklagbarkeit einer guten Stoffwechseleinstellung durch den Patienten, sollten mit in die Entwicklung eines Standards einbezogen werden [7].

Trotzdem halten wir die Entwicklung eines allgemeinärtzlichen Standards für Versorgung von Typ-II-Diabetikern in der Bundesrepublik Deutschland für sinnvoll. Die Qualität der Versorgung von Diabetikern in Hausarztpraxen ist bei uns sicher nicht schlechter als in den gezeigten niederländischen und britischen Beispielen. Sie ist allerdings auch nicht so schlecht, wie dies häufig aus Sicht der Diabetologen im Vergleich zu deren Ambulanzen dargstellt wird, wenn man die grundsätzlichen Unterschiede der behandelten Populationen in Rechnung stellt. Hier gilt es, sinnvolle Kooperationsmodelle zu entwickeln. Für den Hausarzt kann ein Standard als Richtschnur dienen, an der er die Qualität der von ihm und seinem Praxisteam geleisteten Arbeit messen kann. Diese Arbeit könnte Grundlage für die Kooperation zwischen Hausärzten im Sinne eines Qualitätszirkels sein [10], in dem auf Praxisebene Lösungsansätze entwickelt werden.

Thesen für einen Therapiestandard zur Versorgung von Typ-II-Diabetikern in bundesdeutschen Hausarztpraxen

Bei der Entwicklung eines Standards sollten folgende Punkte beachtet werden:

- Der Standard muß unter maßgeblicher Beteiligung niedergelassener Ärzte entstehen.
- Der Standard sollte Handlungsleitlinie und nicht starres Kontrollinstrument sein. Der Gebrauch des Standards in der Praxis soll freiwillig erfolgen und darf

keinesfalls durch staatliche bzw. arztrechtliche Maßnahmen überwacht werden. Er muß deshalb für eine Mehrheit von Arztpraxen konsensfähig sein.

- Grundlage eines jeden Standards in unserem Gesundheitssystem sollte eine einfache, standardisierte Dokumentation sein. Die Dokumentation sollte so ausgerichtet sein, daß sie durchgeführte klinische Untersuchungen, Stoffwechselparameter und das Kontaktverhalten der Patienten zur Praxis miteinander in Beziehung setzten kann. Dadurch können „vergessene" Diabetiker und Inhomogenitäten in der Versorgung entdeckt werden.
- Ziel des Standards sollte die Stärkung der Eigenverantwortung des Patienten sein; allerdings sollte der Hausarzt eine gewisse Überwachungsfunktion behalten, um intervenieren zu können, wenn die Selbstkontrolle des Patienten nicht zustande kommt oder versagt.
- Nach der Entdeckung eines neuaufgetretenen Typ-II-Diabetes in der Praxis sollten – soweit vertretbar – mindestens 6 Monate vergehen, in denen der Hausarzt versucht, diätetische Maßnahmen, Gewichtsreduktion und geeignete Schulungsmaßnahmen einzuleiten, bevor er mit der medikamentösen Therapie beginnt.
- Besonderer Wert sollte auf die Durchführung von Untersuchungen zur Erfassung von Spätkomplikationen gelegt werden.
- Ergebnis der Behandlung muß die für den jeweiligen Patienten, in seiner jeweiligen körperlichen und psychosozialen Situation am besten erreichbare Stoffwechseleinstellung sein. Dabei sollte die unter der Therapie gegebene Lebensqualität jederzeit in Rechnung gestellt und gegen die rein medizinischen Zielvorstellungen abgewogen werden.

Literatur

1. Alberti KGMM, Home PD (1987) Diabetic complications: the importance of metaboliccontrol in man. Elsevier, Amsterdam, pp 8–15
2. Bury G, Duignan J, Finn A (1986) A survey of diabetic patients in general practice. Ir Med J 79:5–7
3. Deutsche Diabetes-Gesellschaft (1990) Grundlagen der Ernährung und Diätempfehlung für Diabetiker. Akt Endokr Stoffw 11:27–38
4. Dornan C, Fowler G, Mann JI, Markus A, Thorogood M (1983) A community study of diabets in Oxfordshire. J R Coll Gen Pract 33:151–155
5. Farmer A, Coulter A (1990) Organisation of care for diabetic patients in general practice: influence on hospital admissions. Br J Gen Pract 40:56–58
6. Gibbins RL, Saunders J (1989) Characteristics and pattern of care of a diabetic population in mid-Wales. J R Coll Gen Pact 39:206–208
7. Grol R (1990) National standard setting. Br J Gen Pract 40:361–364
8. Grol R, Mesker P, Schellevis F (1988) Peer review in general practice. Methods, standards, protocols. Dep of General Practice, Nijmegen
9. Hayes TM, Harris J (1984) Randomised controlled trial of routine hospital clinic care vs. routine general practice care for type II diabetes. Br Med J 289:728–730
10. Himmel W, Kochen MM (1991) Ärztliche Qualitätszirkel in der Allgemeinmedizin. MMW 133:200–204
11. Höppener P, Knotterus A, Grol R (1990) Praktijkautomatisiering en kwaliteitsbewaking. De bloedsuikerregulatie bij patienten met diabets emllitus type II onderzocht in het Registratienet Huisartspraktjken. Huisarts Wet 33:390–393

12. Humphrey LL, Ballard DJ, Frohnert PP, Chu C-P, O'Fallon WM, Palumbo PJ (1989) Chronic renal failure in non-insulin-dependent diabets mellitus. Ann Int Med 111:788–796
13. Karg T (1989) Qualität der Einstellung des Diabetes mellitus in der allgemeinärztlichen Praxis – Eine Bestandsaufnahme. (Vortrag 23. Jahrestagung der Deutschen Gesellschaft für Allgemeinmedizin, Göttingen)
14. Kratky AP (1977) An audit of the care of diabetes in one general practice. J R Coll Gen Pract 27:536–543
15. Kronsbein P, Jörgens V, Mühlhauser I, Scholz V, Venhaus A, Berger M (1988) Evaluation of a structured treatment and teaching programme on non-insulin-dependent diabets. Lancet II:1407–1410
16. Lamprecht K (19889 Einstellungsqualität, Therapie und epidemiologische Aspekte bei Diabetikern in Allgemeinpraxen. (Vortrag Int. SIMG Spring Congress 1988, Trondheim/Norway)
17. Mehnert H (1988) Der vernachlässigte Typ-II-Diabetes. MMW 130:59–60
18. Mengel K (1990) Antidiabetika. In: Schwabe U, Paffrath D (Hrsg) Arzneiverordnungs-Report '90. Fischer, Stuttgart New York, S 60–66
19. Muir A, Howe-Davies SA, Turner RC (1982) General practice care of non-insulin-dependent diabets with fasting blood glucose measurements. Am J Med 73:637–640
20. Mulder JD (1990) Dutch standard diabetes mellitus II. In: WONCA: Abstract I. WONCA European Conference on Family Medicine/General Practice, Barcelona, 10/14 December 1990. Pacifico S.A., Barcelona, p 106
21. Müller R (1989) Die Rostocker Studie. Universität Rostock
22. Nederlands Huisartsen Genootschap (ed) (1989) NHG Standaarden. Richtlinien voor het handelen en de praktijkvoering van de huisarts. NHG, Utrecht
23. Nederlands Huisartsen Genootschap (1989) Diabetes mellitus type II. Standard M01. Huisarts Wet 32:509–512
24. NIDDM Policy Group (1988) Häufige Kontrollen und Patientenschulung. MMW 130:22
25. Pirart J (1978) Diabetes mellitus and its degenerative complications: A prospective study of 4400 patients observed between 1947 und 1973, part 2. Diabetes Care 4:252–263
26. Reenders K, Rutten GEHM, Nobel E de, Hoogen HJM van den, Weel C van (1990) Meet de standaard als maatstaf. Diagnostiek en behandeling van diabetes mellitus in 19 huisartspraktijken. Huisarts Wet 33:379–383
27. Rutten GEHM, Eijk JThM van, Beek MML, Velden HGM van (1988) The type II diabetics: how are they doing? Huisarts Wet 31:124–129
28. Rutten GEHM, Cromme PVM, Zidweg J, Mulder JD (1989) Huisats en diabetes type II. Een verantwoording voor de NHG-standaard. Huisarts Wet 32:7–13
29. Rutten G, Eijk J van, Beek M, Velden H van der (1990) The quality of diabetes registration in eight general practice. Allgemeinmedizin 19:68–72
30. Singh BM, Holland MR, Thorn PA (1984) Metabolic control of diabets in general practice clinics: comparision with a hospital clinic. Br Med J 289:726–733
31. Sips AJBI (1990) Origin of Standards for GP's. In: WONCA: Abstract I. WONCA European Regional Conference on Family Medicine/General Practice. Barcelona, Pacifico S.A., p 105
32. Sohn W (1990) Typ II Diabetiker: wie betreuen? Ärztl Prax 42/22:5
33. Sprij B, Casparie AF, Grol R (1989) Interventemethoden om een verandering on de medische praktijkvoering te bewerkstelligen: wat is efectief? Ned Tijdschr Geneeskd 133:1115–1118
34. Standl R, Stiegler H, Rebell et al. (1990) Der Typ-II-Diabetes in der Praxis des niedergelassenen Arztes: – Konzept einer zentrumsunterstützten Betreuung und Ergebnisse einer Stichproben-Erhebung im Großraum München. Akt Endokr Stoffw 11:222–227

35. Szecsenyi J, in der Beek R (1990) Type-II-diabetics in general practice – how good are they treated? In: Zentralinstitut für die kassenärztliche Versorgung in der Bundesrepublik Deutschland (ed) Abstract Second European Conference on Health Services Research and Primary Health Care, Köln, December 14–15, p 85. Köln
36. Szecsenyi J, Köhle M, in der Beek R, Bormann M, Koc J (1990) Zur Qualität der allgemeinärztlichen Versorgung von Patienten mit Diabetes mellitus. Ein-Jahres-Ergebnisse aus 12 hausärztlichen Praxen. Allgemeinmedizin 19:99–108
37. Thefeld W, Hoffmeister H (1982) Sozialmedizinische Aspekte beim Diabetes Mellitus. Z Allg Med 58:1396–1403
38. Thorn A, Russel RG (1973) Diabetic clinics today and tomorrow: Mini-clinics in generals practice. Br Med J II:534–536
39. Williams DRR (1990) A three-year evaluation of the quality of diabetes care in the Norjwich community care scheme. Diabetes Care 7:74–79

Diabetes mellitus: Therapiestandards aus der Sicht eines Klinikers

Eberhard G. Siegel

Einleitung

In Ländern mit hohem Lebensstandard wie der Bundesrepublik Deutschland ist mit einer Diabeteshäufigkeit von ca. 4 % der Bevölkerung zu rechnen, d. h. rund 3 (+ DDR) Millionen Erkrankte. Hierbei ist zu berücksichtigen, daß die tatsächliche Zahl aufgrund einer gewissen Dunkelziffer sogar noch höher liegen dürfte. Die genannte Prozentzahl (4 %) hat sich gegenüber 1970 etwa verdoppelt, gegenüber 1960 verfünffacht [13] und ist sicher weiter im Ansteigen begriffen. Der Großteil der Diabetiker (ca. 75 %) ist über 60 Jahre alt und entspricht somit der Definition eines Altersdiabetes. Man schätzt, daß rund 20 % der über 60jährigen an einem Diabetes erkrankt sind. Die Betreuung gerade dieser Altersgruppe, aber auch der jüngeren Typ-II-Diabetiker, erfolgt sinnvollerweise vorwiegend in der Paxis des niedergelassenen Arztes, während Typ-I-Diabetiker häufig auch zusätzlich in Betreuung einer Spezialambulanz oder zunehmend auch einer diabetologisch orientierten, internistischen Praxis sind. Allgemein gültige Therapiestandards für die Behandlung des Diabetes können nur entworfen werden, wenn auch entspechende Therapieziele klar umrissen sind.

Therapieziele

Es gibt kaum eine andere internistische Erkrankung, bei der der Therapieerfolg so vom Patienten und seiner Mitarbeit abhängig ist wie beim Diabetes. Bei der Behandlung eines *jeden* Diabetikers ist es sinnvoll, ein individuell festzulegendes und möglichst mit dem Patienten abzusprechendes Therapieziel abzustecken. Hierbei sollte bewußt abgewogen werden zwischen dem, was wünschenswert ist, und dem, was realistischerweise erreicht werden kann. Die Bedeutung unterschiedlicher Therapieziele bei verschiedenen Gruppen von Diabetikern ist in Tabelle 1 wiedergegeben. Als weitere Therapieziele, die für alle Diabetiker gelten, sind zu nennen:

- Einsparung unnötiger Medikamente,
- Vermeidung von Krankenhausaufenthalten wegen diabetischer Komplikationen und Fußprobleme.

Ein individuelles Therapieziel sollte immer abgesteckt werden unter Einbeziehung des Alters, der sozialen Umgebung, der intellektuellen Fähigkeiten und insbesondere auch der beruflichen Möglichkeiten des Patienten. Ganz generell steht

Rationale Pharmakotherapie in der Allgemeinpraxis
Rational Pharmacotherapy in General Practice
M. M. Kochen (Hrsg.)

bei den über 70jährigen die Vermeidung von Akutkomplikationen, insbesondere auch Hypoglykämien, wesentlich stärker im Vordergrund als das Therapieziel der Normoglykämie zur Vermeidung von Spätkomplikationen. Dies darf jedoch nicht zu therapeutischer Nachlässigkeit verleiten, denn bei einer Diabetesmanifestation im Alter von 65–70 Jahren ist eine Lebenserwartung von 80 und darüber heutzutage durchaus realistisch. Somit besteht genügend Zeit zur Entwicklung von Sekundärkomplikationen. Zudem bestehen gerade bei Typ-II-Diabetikern nicht selten bereits bei Diabetesmanifestation Komplikationen im Sinne von Neuropathien und arteriellen Durchblutungsstörungen sowie häufig Pilzinfektionen und Dermatosen. Eine bessere Stoffwechseleinstellung bringt oft auch eine erstaunliche Besserung des Allgemeinbefindens mit sich.

Therapiestandards bei Typ-I-Diabetes

Auch wenn in den meisten Allgemeinpraxen die Typ-I-Diabetiker (in der BRD ca. 100 000–150 000) zahlenmäßig weniger als 10 % der Diabetiker ausmachen [18] seien doch einige wichtige Punkte kurz umrissen. Basis der Therapie des Typ-I-Diabetes sollte eine intensive Schulung des Patienten hinsichtlich seiner Krankheit sein [3]. Hierzu gehört, abgesehen von der intensiven diätetischen Anleitung, z. B. auch die Durchführung von Selbstkontrollen, Selbstanpassung der Insulindosen, das Verhalten in besonderen Situationen, das Wissen über Komplikationen. Da selbst eine relativ einfache Basisschulung sicher mehr als 20–40 h umfaßt, ist diese von einem Arzt in einer Allgemeinpraxis nur selten zu erbringen. Hier ist dann die Einweisung in ein entsprechendes Schulungszentrum zu befürworten; ideal wäre sicher, wenn ein solches in Wohnortnähe existiert, so daß dann eine weitere Zusammenarbeit zwischen Schulungszentrum und behandelndem Hausarzt möglich ist. Kann dies nicht realisiert werden, müßte auf ein wohnortfernes Schulungszentrum oder eine Diabetesklinik zurückgegriffen werden. Vorteile einer solchen, i. allg. als Gruppenschulung durchgeführten Unterweisung liegen auch darin, daß Diabetiker durch Austausch untereinander viele Dinge besser erlernen als allein durch die entsprechende Unterweisung. Zudem ist der Kontakt mit anderen Diabetikern hilfreich bei der Akzeptanz der eigenen einschneidenden Lebensveränderungen.

Wesentliches Therapieziel bei juvenilen Diabetikern, aber auch durchaus bei jüngeren Typ-II-Diabetikern, ist eine Blutzuckereinstellung, die möglichst im oder nahe dem normoglykämischen Bereich liegt [3, 14]. Es steht heutzutage außer Zweifel, daß mäßig oder schlecht eingestellte Diabetiker im Durchschnitt ihre Spätkomplikationen wesentlich früher entwickeln als gut eingestellte [12, 16]. Mit den neueren Entwicklungen der Diabetestherapie, insbesondere der intensivierten konventionellen Therapie und auch der Therapie mit extern getragenen Insulinpumpen, sind entscheidende Fortschritte im Sinne einer besseren Stoffwechselkontrolle erreicht worden. Erst mit den beiden letzteren Methoden, in Verbindung mit Selbstkontrolle und Selbstanpassung der Insulindosen, war es in den letzten Jahren möglich, auch größere Kollektive nahe dem normoglykämischen Niveau einzustellen. Dies gelingt in den meisten Fällen trotz der Möglichkeit eines we-

wesentlich freieren Tagesablaufs, was für viele, vorwiegend juvenile Diabetiker, ein wesentliches Therapieziel sein kann. Die durchschnittliche Verbesserung der Stoffwechsellage liegt im Bereich von 1–2 % HbA_1 (Hämoglobin A_1), d. h. rund 50–60 mg/dl Glukose [3, 14]. Aus diesen Gründen gilt die Empfehlung für eine Form der intensivierten Therapie beim jüngeren Typ-I-Diabetiker [3, 14].

Eine wesentliche Frage ist natürlich, was man als eine gute Einstellung bezeichnen kann. Richtet man sich nach den offiziellen Empfehlungen der Deutschen Diabetesgesellschaft [5], so beinhaltet dies normale Nüchternblutzuckerwerte, postprandiale Blutzuckerwerte bis 140 (ggf. 160–180 in Ausnahmefällen) sowie einen normalen HbA_1-Wert als Ausdruck der mittleren Blutglukosespiegel über 6 bis 8 Wochen vor dem Bestimmungszeitpunkt. Sieht man allerdings die Daten auch guter Diabeteszentren kritisch durch, sei es bezüglich nachverfolgter Patienten nach intensiver Schulung oder aber von Patienten, die in kontrollierte und randomisierte Studien aufgenommen wurden, so wird klar, daß dieses Therapieziel im Mittel vielleicht bei 20–30 % zu erreichen ist. Somit muß man auch unter den Bedingungen der intensivierten Therapie einen HbA_1-Spiegel, der 1–1,5 % über dem Normalwert Stoffwechselgesunder liegt, als zufriedenstellend ansehen [3, 14].

Hinsichtlich des wissenschaftlichen Standes weiterer therapeutischer Möglichkeiten zum Erreichen einer Normoglykämie (z. B. Pankreas- oder Inseltransplantation, künstliches Pankreas) sei auf andere Arbeiten verwiesen (z. B. [14, 15]).

Auch bei Typ-I-Diabetikern, bei denen die Krankheit noch nicht sehr lange besteht, sind regelmäßige Blutdruckkontrollen notwendig: Ein Hypertonus tritt bei 40–50 % der Typ-I-Diabetiker auf und begünstigt wesentlich Inzidenz wie Progression von Sekundärkomplikationen, (z. B. Retinopathie und Nephropathie) [8]. Typ-I-Diabetiker sollten regelmäßig (möglichst halbjährlich) augenärztlich untersucht werden. Zur Früherkennung einer beginnenden Nephropathie hat sich die Bestimmung der Mikroalbuminurie, die inzwischen auch über Urinstix (Micral) möglich ist, bewährt. Eine zumindest jährliche Kontrolle ist zu befürworten.

Therapiestandards bei Typ-II-Diabetes

Wie aus Tabelle 1 ersichtlich, sind die Therapieziele bei Typ-II-Diabetikern sehr unterschiedlich in Abhängigkeit vom Alter des Patienten. Abgesehen von der notwendigen Behandlung von Begleit- und Folgeerkrankungen, bestehen im wesentlichen folgende Behandlungsmöglichkeiten:

- Diät inklusive Schulung und ggf. Gewichtsreduktion,
- Diat und Sulfonylharnstoffe,
- Diät und Sulfonylharnstoffe und Biguanid (Metformin),
- Diät und Sulfonylharnstoffe und Insulin (Kombinationstherapie),
- Diät und Insulin,
- Diät und Hemmung der Glukosidase, ggf. mit Sulfonylharnstoffen oder Insulin.

Tabelle 1. Therapieziele bei Diabetikern

Therapieziel	Typ-I-Diabetes	Typ-II-Diabetes		Gravidität
		45–70 Jahre	über 70 Jahre	
Vermeidung von Akutkomplikationen	++	++	+++	+
Vermeidung von Hypoglykämien	+	++	++	+
Vermeidung von Spätkomplikationen (Normoglykämie)	+++	+	–	+++
Möglichst freier Tagesablauf	+(?)	+/–	+	+
Vermeidung von 1. oder 2. Injektion	–	–	++	–

Diät und Schulung

Ein großes Problem ist die adäquate Schulung des Typ-II-Diabetikers, insbesondere des Altersdiabetikers über 60 Jahre [10]. Die Gründe hierfür sind vielfach. Häufig sind die Patienten schwer zu motivieren; eine abrupte Änderung der Lebensgewohnheiten wird selten akzeptiert. Problematisch ist auch die Reaktion von Umwelt und Familie, die nicht bereit sind, die notwendige Änderung der Lebensgewohnheiten des Familienmitgliedes zu akzeptieren. Hinzu kommt nicht selten die mangelnde Motivation der behandelnden Ärzte: Diabetikerschulung ist aufwendig, die Abrechnungsmöglichkeiten nicht adäquat; oftmals sind die initialen Therapieziele zu hoch, was zu Mißerfolgen und damit mangelnder Compliance führt. Die Möglichkeit einer Initialschulung in einer spezialisierten Klinik ist zwar vielfach sinnvoll, oft allerdings trifft sie auf Ablehnung bei den vorwiegend älteren Patienten; ein anhaltender Effekt dieser Schulung ist längst nicht bei allen Patienten zu verzeichnen. In einer Zufallsstichprobe von 290 Typ-II-Diabetikern gaben nur 33 % an, eine Diät einzuhalten [17]; im Wissenstest bestanden besonders große Lücken im Bereich Diät und Fußpflege.

Obwohl Schulung als integraler Bestandteil der Diabetestherapie generell akzeptiert ist [10, 17], gibt es nur wenige strukturierte und angepaßte Schulungsprogramme für den Altersdiabetiker. Als beispielhaft für eine Gruppenschulung für Altersdiabetiker in der realen Situation der Praxis sei ein Programm vorgestellt, das von den Gruppen um Prof. Berger (Düsseldorf) und Prof. Standl (München) entwickelt wurde [10]. Es umfaßt die Unterweisung einer Arzthelferin sowie die Schulung der Patienten in der Arztpraxis durch die unterwiesene Arzthelferin in insgesamt 4mal 1,5–2 h, verteilt über 4 Wochen. Die Gruppengröße liegt bei 4–6 Patienten. Die erste Auswertung des Einsatzes wurde 1988 veröffentlicht [11]. Insgesamt waren 8 Praxen miteinbezogen, von denen 3 zustimmten, das Lernprogramm zunächst 1 Jahr zurückzustellen. Diese Patienten dienten als Kontrollgruppe. Die Schulung wird in der Arztpraxis selbst durchgeführt und umfaßt Diät, Selbstkontrolle, Bewegung, orale Antidiabetika und auch Spätschäden, insbesondere den diabetischen Fuß. Es werden keine unrealistischen Ziele wie Idealgewicht oder Normoglykämie gesetzt. Innerhalb eines Jahres wirkte sich bei dieser Auswertung das Lernprogramm hinsichtlich des Verbrauchs an Sulfonylharnstoffen und des Fortschreitens der Erkrankung im Sinne von Sekundärversagen (Insulinabhängigkeit) positiv aus. Zudem wurde eine Gewichtsabnahme erreicht. Bei den geschulten Patienten wurde innerhalb eines Jahres keiner insulinabhängig, in der Kontrollgruppe waren dies 10% [11]. Der HbA_1-Wert wurde bei diesen Diabetikern, deren HbA_1-Werte im Durchschnitt lediglich 1–2% über den Normalwert Gesunder lagen, nicht signifkant gesenkt.

Dieses Schulungsprogramm ist über den Deutschen Ärzteverlag erhältlich [4] und wurde bereits in über 2000 Arztpraxen eingeführt [10.]. Seit dem 1.7.1991 kann dieses Schulungsprogramm auch gegenüber den Kassen abgerechnet werden.

Diät und Sulfonylharnstoffe

Betrachtet man den Verbrauch an Sulfonylharnstoffen, so fällt auf, daß in der Bundesrepublik Deutschland der prozentuale Anteil von medikamentös behandelten Diabetikern an der Gesamtbevölkerung mit 2,4% wesentlich höher liegt als in anderen Ländern mit ähnlicher Prävalenz (USA 1%, Großbritannien 0,7%; [9]). In einer Zufallsstichprobe waren 2/3 der Diabetiker mit Medikamenten behandelt [8]. Diese Daten sprechen dafür, daß orale Antidiabetika häufig viel zu schnell verschrieben werden, ohne die Möglichkeiten der nicht medikamentösen Therapie (s. oben) voll auszuschöpfen. Erst wenn mit Diät, Schulung und ggf. Gewichtsreduktion keine ausreichende Einstellung erzielt werden kann, ist die Gabe eines oralen Antidiabetikums sinnvoll [7]. Hinsichtlich der Wirkweise der Sulfonylharnstoffe zeigen neuere Untersuchungen, daß die extrapankreatischen Effekte mit einer Verbesserung der Insulinempfindlichkeit eher sekundärer Natur sind, d.h. im wesentlichen durch die Änderung der Insulinsekretion und der Glukosespiegel bewirkt werden.

Aufgrund der Hypoglykämiegefahr, insbesondere bei Gabe der stärker wirkenden Sulfonylharnstoffe, sollte dem Patienten immer eine Diätvorschrift mitgegeben werden mit Verteilung der Kohlenhydrate über den Tag.

Therapie mit Biguaniden

Als einziges Biguanid ist in der Bundesrepublik Deutschland Metformin (Glucophage) als Zusatztherapie zur Medikation mit Sulfonylharnstoffen zugelassen. Dies steht im Gegensatz zur Praxis in Großbritannien und den USA, wo Biguanide auch als Monotherapie verwendet werden dürfen. Metformin ist besonders zur Therapie bei Übergewichtigen und sonst weitgehend Gesunden geeignet. Werden Kontraindikationen (wie Nephropathie, Herzinsuffizienz, respiratorische Insuffizienz, Krankheiten mit möglicher Gewebshypoxie, arterielle Verschlußkrankheit, Leberinsuffizienz, hoher Alkoholkonsum, konsumierende und schwere Erkrankungen, Reduktionskost sowie eine Zurückhaltung bei über 65jährigen) korrekt beachtet, kann die Therapie mit Metformin durchaus sinnvoll sein [7].

Diät, Sulfonylharnstoffe und Insulin

Hinsichtlich dieser als Kombinationstherapie bezeichneten Therapieform existiert eine große Anzahl an unkontrollierten Untersuchungen und Erfahrungsberichten, jedoch nur wenige gut kontrollierte Studien (insbesondere auch bezüglich der Nebenwirkungen). Ein Beispiel für die Probleme ist die deutsche Multicenter-Studie, die von der Rekrutierung von 500 Patienten ausging, von denen 256 über 6 Monate ausgewertet werden sollten. Dies gelang aber lediglich bei 68 [2]. Aufgrund der bisherigen Untersuchungen sollte man von folgenden Fakten ausgehen:

- Im Durchschnitt wird der Insulinbedarf um ca. 25 % gesenkt, d.h. 12–16 Einheiten pro Tag.
- Eine Verbesserung der Resistenz auf Insulin wird nicht erreicht, die Insulinspiegel scheinen nicht niedriger zu liegen.
- In den meisten Studien wird keine verbesserte Einstellung erreicht. Das Auftreten von Hypoglykämien scheint nicht wesentlich häufiger zu sein als bei der alleinigen Insulintherapie.

Hinsichtlich der Durchführung bestehen mehrere Möglichkeiten. Die Empfehlung der Deutschen Diabetesgesellschaft lautet folgendermaßen [1]:

1. Weiterhin maximale Dosierung von Glibenclamid (Euglucon, Generika);
2. vorsichtiger Beginn mit 4–8 Einheiten Intermediärinsulin morgens;
3. schrittweise und langsam erhöhen auf 20–24 Einheiten maximal;
4. Absetzen des Sulfonylharnstoffpräparates bei Überschreiten von maximal 24 Einheiten oder bei zusätzlicher Abendinsulingabe.

Andere Therapieformen sind durchaus möglich, z.B. die abendliche Gabe von Verzögerungsinsulin. Eine Alternative bei Leuten, die aus beruflichen Gründen nur 3 Mahlzeiten zu sich nehmen können, ist die Gabe von Altinsulin zu den Mahlzeiten [19]. Als Injektionshilfe haben sich für viele Patienten die Insulinpens bewährt, die seit dem letzten Jahr nicht nur für Altinsulin, sondern auch für Verzögerungs- und Mischinsuline angeboten werden. Sie sind allerdings lediglich als Injektionshilfe anzusehen; eine individuelle Zumischung ist mit keinem der Pens möglich.

Einstellung auf Insulin in der Praxis

Die Primäreinstellung von Typ-II-Diabetikern (reine Insulintherapie oder Kombinationstherapie) ist durchaus in der ambulanten Praxis möglich. Sie setzt allerdings voraus, daß der behandelnde Arzt und das Personal der Praxis ausreichend diabetologisch informiert und engagiert sind. Ähnlich wie bei den nicht insulinabhängigen Diabetikern existiert inzwischen ein strukturiertes Schulungsprogramm mit 5 Unterrichtseinheiten [10]. Auch hier ist die adäquate Schulung des Praxispersonals durch einen diabetologisch weitergebildeten Arzt Voraussetzung für die Anwendung.

Diät und Hemmung der Glukosidase

Ein gänzlich anderes Therapieprinzip eines oralen Antidiabetikums ist die Hemmung der Glukosidasen im Darm, das entsprechende Präparat ist seit Herbst 1990 auf dem Markt (Acarbose/Glucobay). Das Wirkprinzip der Acarbose, die nicht resorbiert wird, ist die Hemmung der α-Glukosidasen im Darm, was zu einer verzögerten Freisetzung von Glukose und damit verzögerter Resorption führt [19]. Die bisher vorliegenden Studien fanden, daß Acarbose die Blutglukose ähnlich oder stärker senkt als Biguanide bei Typ-II-Diabetikern, auch bei zusätzlicher Sulfonylharnstofftherapie [6]. Einige Untersuchungen zeigten, daß die blutzuckersenkende Wirkung sogar mit Glibenclamid vergleichbar ist. Zudem kann Acarbose auch bei Insulingabe eingesetzt werden. Wesentliche Nebenwirkungen, z. B. Hypoglykämien, sind in den zugelassenen Dosen nicht zu befürchten, jedoch sind aufgrund der Malabsorption insbesondere in den ersten Wochen der Therapie gastrointestinale Beschwerdesymptome wie Meteorismus, Flatulenz und Diarrhö häufig. Diese lassen zwar im Laufe von 4–6 Wochen deutlich nach, führen jedoch bei einem Teil der Diabetiker zum Absetzen der Medikation. Der endgültige Stellenwert dieses, im Vergleich zu den anderen oralen Antidiabetika wie Glibenclamid wesentlich teureren Präparats ist zum gegenwärtigen Zeitpunkt noch nicht definiert.

Einstellungskriterien bei Typ-II-Diabetes

Wie eingangs erwähnt, sind die Therapieziele individuell zu formulieren und sehen bei einem nichtschulbaren 85jährigen, bettlägerigen Patienten sicher anders aus als bei einem fast noch juvenilen Diabetiker von 40 Jahren. Als relativ gut formulierte Einstellungskriterien bei Typ-II-Diabetes können die der Amerikanischen und der Europäischen Diabetesgesellschaft gelten. Hierbei ist als einziger Unterschied zu vermerken, daß bei den Kriterien der Amerikanischen Diabetesgesellschaft auch eine „mäßig eingestellte" Kategorie mitgeführt wird [7]. Die entsprechenden Zahlen sind in Tabelle 2 angegeben.

Tabelle 2. Einstellungskriterien bei Typ-II-Diabetikern[a]

	Gut	Akzeptabel	Mäßig	Schlecht
Nü-Glukose [mg/dl]	80–120	−140	−180	> 180
pp Glukose [mg/dl]	80–140	−180	−235	> 235
HbA_1 [%]	< 7,2	7,2–9	9–10,8	> 10,8
Cholesterin	< 200	−220	−240	> 240
Triglyzeride	< 150	−200	−240	> 240
HDL-Cholesterin	> 40	35–40	30–35	< 30

[a] Die Einstellungskriterien entsprechen denen der Amerikanischen (mit „mäßig" eingestellter Kategorie) und Europäischen Diabetesgesellschaft (ohne „mäßig" eingestellte Subkategorie; [7]). Bei Verwendung von HbA_{1c} statt HbA_1 sind die Grenzwerte, je nach Methode, um 1–2,5 % niedriger anzusetzten.

Diabetes und Hypertonus

Als ein wesentlicher Punkt gerade für die Überwachung in der Arztpraxis ist die Therapie des Hypertonus zu erwähnen. Bei Typ-II-Diabetikern tritt auf lange Sicht in über 70 % ein Hypertonus auf [17], wobei dieser häufig schon bei Manifestation besteht. Da der Hypertonus entscheidend die Makroangiopathie, die bei über 50 % der Typ-II-Diabetiker besteht, verstärkt und der wichtigste Faktor für das Fortschreiten der Nephropathie ist, sollte eine antihypertensive Therapie frühzeitig begonnen werden [8]. Im Prinzip gelten auch bei Diabetikern die allgemeinen Richtlinien für die Hypertonustherapie. Wesentlich ist die nichtmedikamentöse Therapie durch Gewichtsreduktion, Kochsalzeinschränkung auf 5 g täglich, Einschränkung oder Einstellung des Alkohol- und Nikotinabusus und intensivere körperliche Bewegung [8]. Als empfohlene Antihypertensiva kommen, entsprechend den Empfehlungen der Deutschen Diabetesgesellschaft und der Deutschen Hochdruckliga [6] am ehesten in Frage: β-Blocker, Kalziumantagonisten, ACE-Hemmer und Diuretika.

Bei den *β-Blockern* sollten möglichst β_1-Blocker verwandt werden, z. B. Atenolol (Tenormin, Generika) und Metoprolol (Beloc, Generika). Im Gegensatz zu den nichtselektiven Subtanzen verschlechtern diese die Glukosetoleranz kaum, das Risiko der Verschleierung der Gegenregulation ist gering [8]. Der Einfluß auf die Lipide ist ebenfalls deutlich geringer; zudem besteht keine Beeinflussung der Perfusion. Bei Niereninsuffizienz ist Metoprolol besser steuerbar als das renal ausgeschiedene Atenolol.

Kalziumantagonisten werden bei zusätzlichen kardiovaskulären Erkrankungen als besonders günstig angesehen. Thiazide sollten wegen der Stoffwechselnebenwirkungen auf die Glukosetoleranz nur in niedriger Dosierung angewandt werden. Hinsichtlich der *ACE-Hemmer* scheinen einige Untersuchungen einen positiven Effekt auf das Fortschreiten der Nephropathie zu belegen [8].

Typ-II-Diabetes und Sekundärkomplikationen

Beim Typ-II-Diabetes tritt typischerweise eine Häufung von Risikofaktoren für Herz-Keislauf-Erkrankungen auf wie Hypertonie, Hyperinsulinämie, Erhöhung der VLDL-, Verminderung der HDL-Lipoproteine und Adipositas vom androiden Typ [8]. Da es sich meist um ältere Patienten handelt, bestehen in einem nennenswerten Prozentsatz bereits bei Diagnosestellung vaskuläre Schäden (z. B. bei 5 % eine Retinopathie). Dies trifft nicht nur auf die durch viele Faktoren beeinflußte Makroangiopathie (s. oben), sondern auch für die diabetesspezifische Mikroangiopathie zu.

Eine augenärztliche Untersuchung gehört somit unbedingt zum Therapiestandard. Diese sollte je nach Befund in 6- bis 12monatlichem Intervall wiederholt werden. Ebenso ist die halbjährliche bis jährliche Inspektion der Füße wesentlich, da diese häufig trophische Störungen, Interdigitalmykosen bzw. Fehlbelastungsstellen zeigen. Da die diabetische Gangrän mit ihren schlimmen Folgen ihren Ausgang oft von Bagatellverletzungen nimmt, muß Fußpflege und -inspektion ein wesentlicher Punkt der Behandlung und Schulung von Diabetikern sein.

Ebenso gehört hierzu die Untersuchung auf Nephropathie, als deren frühestes klinisches Symptom sich eine Mikroalbuminurie zeigt.

Wesentlich für die *Zukunft* ist sicher, daß gemeinsame Anstrengungen von niedergelassenen Ärzten, Diabeteszentren, Gesundheitsbehörden, Kostenträgern, wissenschaftlichen Gesellschaften und auch Laienorganistionen unternommen werden (wie in der 1989 abgefaßten St. Vincent-Deklaration), zur Verbesserung der Versorgung der Diabetiker, angepaßt an die individuellen Bedürfnisse.

Literatur

1. Bachmann W (1988) Kombinationstherapie mit Insulin und Sulfonylharnstoff. Dtsch Med Wochenschr 113 : 652–654
2. Bachmann W, Lotz N, Mehnert H, Rosak C, Schöffling K (1988) Wirksamkeit der Kombinationsbehandlung mit Glibenclymid und Insulin bei Sulfonylharnstoff-Sekundärversagen. Dtsch Med Wochenschr 113 : 631–636
3. Berger M (1989) Long-term efficacy and safety of intensified insulin treatment strategies. In: Creutzfeldt W, Lefèbre P (eds) Diabetes mellitus: Pathophysiology and treatment. Springer, Berlin Heidelberg New York Tokyo, pp 225–233
4. Berger M, Grüßer M, Jörgens V et al. (1987) Diabetesbehandlung in unserer Praxis – Schulungsprogramm für Diabetiker, die nicht Insulin spritzen. Deutscher Ärtzeverlag, Köln
5. Deutsche Diabetesgesellschaft (1985) Kriterien einer guten Einstellung. Dtsch Med Wochenschr 110 : 477–478
6. Deutsche Liga zur Bekämpfung des hohen Blutdrucks, in Zusammenarbeit mit der Deutschen Diabetesgesellschaft (1989) Empfehlungen für die Behandlung des Hochdrucks bei Diabets, 1. Aufl. (ggf. anzufordern Postfach 10 20 40, 6900 Heidelberg)
7. Gerich JE (1989) Oral hypoglycemic agents. N Engl J Med 321 : 1231–1245
8. Haslacher C, Ritz E (1990) Hypertonie und Diabetes mellitus. Internist 31 : 180–188
9. Haupt E, Landgraf R (1987) Verordnen wir zuviel Sulfonylharnstoffpräparate? Dtsch Med Wochenschr 112 : 1727–1729
10. Jörgens V, Berger M, Flatten G (1990) Diabetikerschulung in der Arztpraxis. Voraussetzung für eine effektive Behandlung. Dtsch Ärztebl 87 : 393–396
11. Kronsbein P, Jörgens V, Mühlhauser I, Scholz V, Venhaus A, Berger M (1988) Evaluation of a structured treatment and teaching programme on non-insulin-dependent diabetes. Lancet II : 1407–1411
12. Pirart J (1977) Diabéte et complications dégénertives. Presentation d'une étude prospectiveportant sur 4400 cas observés entre 1947 et 1973. Diabet Metab 3 : 97–107, 173–182, 245–256 (1978 in: Diabetes Care 1 : 168–188, 252–263)
13. Seige K (1987) Zur Epidemiologie des Diabetes mellitus. Internist 28 : 205–209
14. Siegel EG (1990) Normoglykämie als Therapieziel der Diabetesbehandlung – Konzept und Realisierung. Klin Wochenschr 68 : 306–312
15. Siegel EG, Creutzfeld W (1989) Pancreatic transplantation or intensive insulin therapy? Balliéres Clin Gastroenterol 3 : 877–886
16. Standl E (1987) Diabetische Mikroangiopathien. Internist 28 : 262–272
17. Standl R, Stiegler H, Rebell B et al. (1990) Der Typ II-Diabetes in der Praxis des niedergelassenen Arztes: Konzept einer zentrumsunterstützten Betreuung und Ergebnisse einer Stichproben-Erhebung im Großraum München. Akt Endokr Stoffw 11 : 222–227
18. Szecsenyi J, Köhle M, in der Beek R, Bormann M, Koc J (1990) Zur Qualität der allgemeinärztlichen Versorgung von Patienten mit Diabetes mellitus. Ein-Jahresergebnisse aus 12 hausärztlichen Praxen. Allgemeinmedizin 19 : 99–108
19. Willms B, Boustani A (1989) Insulin-Sulfonylharnstoff-Kombinationstherapie. Vergleich präprandialerAltinsulingabe mit spätabendlicher Gabe von Verzögerungsinsulin. MMW 131 : 67–71

Arzneimittelberatung durch Ärzte

Drug Counseling by Doctors

Peer Review Groups Concerned with the Quality Assessment of Pharmacotherapy in Primary Health Care: An Instrument for Educational Advancement and Quality Improvement*

Liselotte von Ferber, Luciano Alberti and Jutta Krappweis

Introduction

Drug therapy is the commonest and most important form of therapy. Annually, 20.6 billion German marks are spent on drugs used in ambulatory care in the Western part of Germany. This amount considerably exceeds the amount received by physicians who have their own private practice, for their diagnostic or therapeutic services (DM 16.9 billion [2]). Among the most frequently prescribed drugs, moreover, there are some whose mode of prescription does *not* accord with the recommendations of the experts, that is to say with rules of prescription as they have been formulated by pharmacologists or hospital physicians [7].

Our first thesis is the following: Physicians who have their own private practice know these basic principles of drug therapy. During everyday practice, however, this knowledge is frequently not applied. To show this discrepancy more clearly we should like to name some of the more prominent treatment problems in primary health care. Physicians know that:

- digitalis glycosides are only effective in cases of pronounced cardiac failure. Nevertheless a sizeable proportion of older patients in ambulatory care receive glycosides. Moreover, the doses are too small to achieve their (ostensible) purpose.
- Benzodiazepine compounds can be addictive. This fact notwithstanding, a considerable proportion of primary health care patients (25 %) receive these compounds.
- In most cases vasodilators are ineffective; in addition they carry the danger of a steal effect.
- The effectiveness of antivaricose drugs is open to doubt.

Despite all of this the prescription of these drugs forms a large part of prescription routine [7].

The question ist how the discrepancy between pharmacotherapeutic knowledge and actual pharmacotherapy, well known as the performance gap can be explained and diminished [4, 8, 9]?

* This investigation was supported by a grant from the ministry of research and technology under reference No 0706836A/5.

Rationale Pharmakotherapie in der Allgemeinpraxis
Rational Pharmacotherapy in General Practice
M. M. Kochen (Hrsg.)

Since Donabedian's fundamental work on medical evaluation, the scientific discussion of evaluation assumes a tripartite division of medical care into structure, process, and outcome. Drug therapy, with respect to evaluation and quality assurance, is divided up similarly, i.e. in the following manner:

1. Structure: The scientific principles of pharmacotherapy as well as the pharmacotherapeutic knowledge of such rules and principles in the minds of the physicians, attained through basic or advanced medical education, belong to the structure of pharmacotherapeutic care.
2. Process: Patient's therapy is an interactive process between physician and patient whose success is dependent upon both parties. Treatment (including drug therapy) by the physician and compliance on the part of the patient both belong to the process of therapy.
3. Outcome or result relates to the patient's state of health (according to the broad definition given by the WHO – the physical, psychic and social well-being of the patient) after treatment.

These three dimensions of medical care, especially as they apply to drug therapy, are comparatively independent of one another. This implies that a change in the structure of drug therapy, such as is constituted by improving knowledge on the part of the physicians, does not imply an equivalent change in another dimension, such as improved therapeutical behavior.

Our second thesis with respect to advanced education is therefore the following: only such a concept as will insure that newly acquired as well as dormant knowledge is actually applied in the treatment process stands a chance of improving treatment quality. Such an advanced medical education concept therefore must concentrate on the treatment process.

To diminish the performance gap and improve the treatment behavior our concept for advanced medical education is founded upon four basic principles derived from behavior-oriented adult education:

1. Observation of the physicians' treatment routines: creation of objective treatment data with the aid of prescriptions collected and supplied by the local statutory health insurance (Allgemeine Ortskrankenkasse, AOK). This implies observing
   - the individual physicians taking part in the advanced education group
   - the group as a whole
   - treatment data of other physicians' groups.
2. Recognition of quality problems through assessment of the practice routines of each individual member of the peer review group, critical observation and discussion of the treatment situation of primary care physicians in a climate of tolerance.
3. Joint search for solutions, i.e., for treatment concepts that take account of the needs of primary care patients, of the treatment situation of primary care physicians, and of the organization at framework of primary health care in the doctor's practice.

4. The evaluation of this form of continuing medical education takes account of its:
   - aceptability and
   - efficiency.

The "Concerted Action on Health Care"

The quality advancement program of the expert commission of the Federal Government's "Concerted Action on Health Care" divides the quality-securing process in the field of health care into five steps roughly equivalent to ours as listed above [6].

Observation of the Treatment Routine

To change routine behavior one has to be made aware of it. This can be done in Germany by collecting and processing the prescriptions stored in the archives of the statutory health insurance funds. The analysis of the prescription data of the individual physicians and the comparison between individual and group data makes prescription routines and the quality problems of drug therapy visible.

Example

Prescription of vasodilators in a peer review group composed of 13 primary care physicians. The physicians put in a request to the archives of their local statutory health insurance fund for copies of the prescriptions written by them during an annual quarter (II/1989), so as to have them collected, rendered anonymous, and analyzed by us in a patient-related fashion. The random sample for each physician was made up of 100 of his patients.

The analysis consisted of a descriptive statistical representation of the prescription frequency of specific drugs, the distribution of these drugs according to age, sex, and type of disease, as well as an investigation of the accompanying therapies. Analysis are undertaken for each physician individually and for the group as a whole.

Example

The prescribing of vasodilators. Vasodilators belong to the most frequently prescribed drugs. On average 15 % of the (1163) patients of the 13 physicians of the peer review group receive such drugs. Vasodilators are mostly prescribed in the geriatric field: whereas few people younger than 60 received them (7 %), the percentage of vasodilator recipients above 60 years of age was considerable (between 15 %, 60–65 years and 30 %, 75–80 years; Fig. 1).

To properly judge the quality of prescription behavior in the various practices it is necessary to take the prevalent age structure into account: the relative percentage

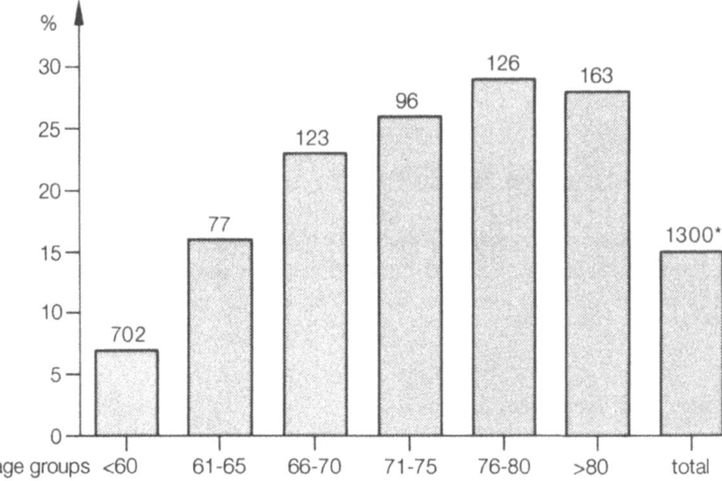

Fig. 1. Percentage of AOK-insured patients receiving prescriptions of antivaricose drugs (RL82) and/or vasodilators (RL36) according to age groups. *Numbers above bars*, indicate number of patients (13 patients without age data). Data from 13 physicians of the Peer Review Group Hessen, second quarter of 1989

of old patients in these practices ranged between 10% and 80% (Fig. 2). The proportion of vasodilator and antivaricose drug recipients among the patients of a physician rises with the average age of the physician's patients. Among the patients of only three physicians was there no such correlation (Fig. 2). These physicians with the largest shares of old patients treated the inhabitants of old people's homes.

Recognition of Quality Problems

Being confronted with descriptive statistical representations of one's drug prescription frequencies is a form of objectivized self-awareness for the individual physician. It is a way of being confronted with the objective data of one's actual everyday prescription behavior. This inevitably leads to the perception of a discrepancy between actual behavior and idealized ideas about behavior.

Example

Asked how many different vasodilating drugs they considered essential, the average answer of the physicians of the group was: 1 (min. 0, max. 4). In actual fact however, they prescribed an average of six different vasodilating drugs (min. 0, max. 9; Table 1).

The perception of this discrepancy, when linked to moral judgments, can lead to a loss of identity and a reduction in self-esteem. Therefore the discrepancy is frequently denied and the realization of it fended off.

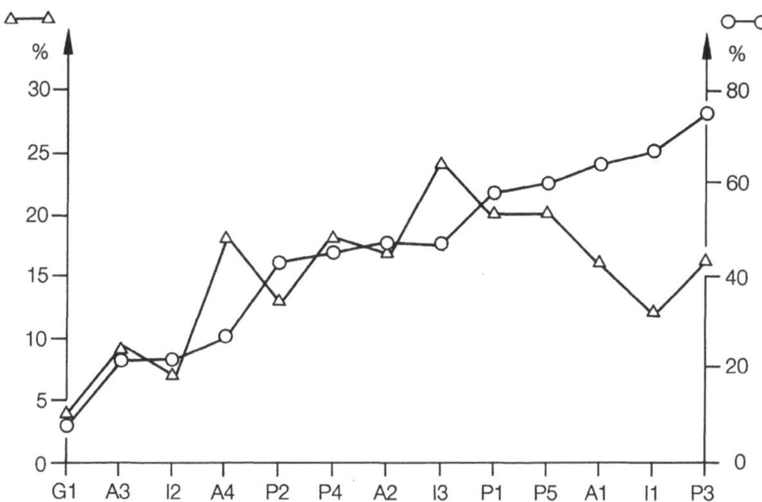

Fig. 2. Patients receiving vasodilators and/or antivaricose drugs (*triangels* and *left-side percentages*) and patients above 60 years of age (*circles* and *right-side percentages*) in 13 private practices in percent (%). 13 private practices of a Peer Review Group in Hessen arranged according to their percentage of patients above 60 years of age. *G*, gynecologist; *A, P*, general practitioner (*A*, Allgemeinarzt: *P*, praktischer Arzt); *I*, internist

Table 1. A comparison of pharmaceutical products prescribed with those considered indispensable by seven physicians

	Vasodilators (various products)		Antivaricose drugs (various products)			
Private practices	Objective number	Estimated indispensable number	Objective number[a]	Estimated indispensable number[b]		
				ext.	int.	total
A1	3	0	6	2	0	2
A3	0	0	5	0	0	0
P4	8	0	7	2	1	3
P5	7	1	10	0	2	2
I1	9	2	3	0	0	0
I2	3	0	3	0	0	0
I3	9	4	6	1/0	1/2	2
Total	39	7	40	5	4	9
Average number per physician	5.6	1.0	5.7	0.7	0.6	1.3

A, P general practitioner (A, Allgemeinarzt; P, Praktischer Arzt).

[a] Result of the analyses of the prescriptions of the second quarter 1989.

[b] Interview in November 1990.

Example

A physician is presenting his prescription frequencies of antivaricose drugs to the group. He had the group's highest incidence of prescription of these drugs. He says, whilst presenting his documentation: "I suppose these numbers are fairly low."

Peer Review Group QUADT*

Advanced medical education that works with objectivized self-awareness should take place in a peer review group setting so as a minimize the loss of professional identity among the participants. A peer review group in this sense is a group of equally affected physicians (a peer group) [4, 8]. The common realization of being equally affected is created and sustained by the objectivized self-awareness of the whole group. The routines of the individual participants are similar, and although the divergence between their behavior and the well-founded recommendations of pharmacologists or hospital physicians varies in degree and is frequently considerable, these routine are nevertheless comparable because similarly oriented.

The next step is to show that the phenomenon of disregard for clinical rules is widespread. The analysis of chronically ill patients registered with the AOK of Dortmund (period of observation, 4th quarter 1984–1st quarter 1986) shows that patients who receive dilators receive them from general practitioners and internists (Table 2).

Table 2. Which physicians prescribed vasodilators?

Patients receiving prescriptions from:	*n*	%	Type of doctor	%
One physician only	629	86	GP	54
			Internist	37
			Other specialist	9
Two physicians	93	13	GP and internist	39
			Internist and other specialist	34
			GP and other specialist	27
Three physicians	7	1	GP, internist and other specialist	

[a] Sample: chronically ill patients insured with the local statutory health insurance (AOK) in Dortmund, FRG. Period of observation: 4th quarter 1984–1st quarter 1986.
[b] Other specialists include: neurologists, dermatologists, ear-nose-throat specialists, orthopaedists, eye specialists, urologists, and surgeons.

The analysis of this sample enables one to discover the most important indication for prescribing vasodilating drugs the indication most frequently cited and the one whose frequency increases with the age of the patients is cerebrovascular disturbance (Table 3).

* Anality of outpatient drug treatment.

Table 3. Patients receiving prescriptions of vasodilators according to indication diagnoses[a]

Indication diagnoses	Age in years									
	20–50		51–60		61–70		>70		Totals	
	n	%	*n*	%	*n*	%	*n*	%	*n*	%
Cerebral circulat. disturbance	15	19	39	26	62	33	145	47	261	36
Cerebral and peripheral circulat. disturbance	1	1	15	10	16	9	22	7	54	7
Peripheral circulat. disturbance	8	10	15	10	15	8	13	4	51	7
General circulat. disturbance	9	11	23	15	42	22	71	23	145	20
Other indication diagnoses	27	34	28	19	18	10	23	7	96	13
No indication diagnoses	20	25	30	20	34	18	38	12	122	17
Totals	80	100	150	100	187	100	312	100	729	100

[a] Sample: Chronically ill patients insured with the local statutory health insurance (AOK) in Dortmund, FRG. Period of observation: fourth quarter 1984–first quarter 1986.
[b] Other indication diagnoses include: vertigo (disorder of balance), circulatory disturbance of the eye, circulatory disturbance of the ear, tinnitus, dementia, migraine, organic mental syndrome.

Working out Joint Suggestions for New Treatment Concepts that are Viable in Primary Health Care and Aim at Improving Prescription Behavior

Balint group-like rules of discussion ensure that openess and fairness prevail when individual behavior is jointly judged. These rules create a climate of tolerance in which the reasons for the divergence between ideal and actual behavior can be stated and suggestions for improved everyday prescription behavior can be made [1].

Balint group-like rules for team-work in a peer review group ensure that a climate:

- of tolerance: the opinions of each participant are important
- openness: opinions can be stated freely within the group because they remain confined to the group – they are treated as confidential
- and mutual understanding: the opinions voiced in the group are not judged as to their moral or political content

is created and maintained.

An important realisation that emerged from a discussion of primary care physicians in a peer review group was that pharmacotherapy cannot be based on a set of contex-free rules as formulated by clinical experts. Therapy and the disease to which it applies are part of the same psychosocial context.

Example

With regard to vasodilators the situation is as follows: Old people who tend to lose their sense of direction and feel that their short-term memory is playing tricks with them frequently live in dread of needing constant care and becoming dependent upon their caretakers. Consequently they frequently confront their physician with an outspoken desire to receive vasodilators. Their own subjective perceptions and those of the people taking care of them have raised expectations in them ... In a situations like this a physician must have a convincing alternative concept handy that does not dash the patient's hope. The following alternative responses with regard to such a request were suggested in the peer review group. To prevent a first prescription of vasodilators the doctor should to suggest (a) a memory jogging course, or (b) prescribe instead acetylsalicylic acid, which is cheap, in small doses therapeutically harmless, and has proved effective in recent American studies.

The Evaluation of this Form of Advanced Education

Two points must be checked in the assessment of this form of advanced education: the acceptability of its concept and its effectiveness with regard to the change and improvement of prescription behavior.

The *acceptability* of the continuing medical education concept: The group of twelve physicians habe by now been working together for about a year and have met seven times in the course of this period. The space between sessions has tended to diminish. The whole group considers its work to be meaningful and important. An expression of this attitude is a shared desire on the part of all the group members: each member intends to chair his or her own peer review group in the near future.

The evaluation of this form of continuing medical education with regard to *prescription behavior*: such advanced education must repeatedly allow for an objective insight into actual behavior (repeated documentation efforts) to be able to detect changes in prescription behavior. At the moment, after a year of peer review group work, we are now in the process of collecting and analyzing prescriptions of group members. After rendering them anonymous and analyse them we will proceed to compare this later batch with our first collection effort. Although no data are available so far the participants are convinced that they have changed their prescription behavior for the better.

Summary

Teaching which aims at changing levels of consciousness and modifying behavior to a considerable extent cannot take the form of a one-time passing on of information. Such advanced education must be "continuing medical education" [5]. The improvement of prescription behavior is the result of a learning process that needs to be reinforced continually. Such advanced education cannot be reduced to a transmission of knowledge from experts to docile pupils. It has to take place in a peer review group, in which equally affected physicians (peers) can discuss openly and with an appropriate measure of understanding the difficulties attending everyday prescription behavior. Such an atmosphere is guaranteed by Balint group-like rules of discussion.

References

1. Alberti L, v Ferber L, Krappweis H (1988) Qualitätsbewußte Arzneitherapie niedergelassener Ärzte. Rhein Ärztebl 42 : 1023–1026
2. Daten des Gesundheitswesens 1985 (1985) Schriftenreihe des Bundesministers für Jugend, Familie und Gesundheit, Stuttgart
3. Grol K, Schellevis F (1988) Qualitätskontrolle in der Allgemeinmedizin: Interkollegiale Überprüfung für Hausärzte. Allgemeinmedizin 17 : 1–7
4. Hulka BS, Romm FJ Pakerson GR, Russell IT, Clapp NE, Johnson FS (1979) Peer review in ambulatory care: use of explicit criteria and implicit judgments. Med Care 17 Suppl : 1–73
5. Manning P, Petit D (1987) The past, present, and future of continuing medical education. JAMA 258 : 3542–3546
6. Sachverständigenrat für die Konzertierte Aktion im Gesundheitswesen (1989) Qualität, Wirtschaftlichkeit und Persepktiven der Gesundheitsversorgung, Jahresgutachten, Bonn
7. Schwabe U, Paffrath D (eds) (1989) Arzneiverordnungsreport. Fischer, Stuttgart
8. Scharzt R, Soumerai St, Avron J (1989) Physician motivations for nonscientific drug prescribing. Soc Sci Med 28 : 577–582
9. Williamson J, Alexander M (1967) Continuing education and patient care research. JAMA 201 : 118–122

Factors Influencing GP Prescribing Habits

Henk G.A. Mokkink, Jan de Maeseneer, and Richard Grol

Introduction

In the past decade prescribing by general practitioners (GPs) has increasingly become an issue of interest for researchers. In this paper we will discuss the nature of GPs' prescribing habits and the factors influencing these habits. We will mainly make use of our own research findings from the Netherlands and from Belgium.

Aspects of GPs' Prescribing Habits

Prescribing by GPs has many aspects. In most research the quantity of overall prescriptions or of some group of medication (e.g., antibiotics) has been studied. A major methodological problem refers to the denominator: is the quantity of medication to be related to the number of consultations or to the number of patients (the doctor's personal list size)? Other reseachers are not only interested in quantity but also in quality: the rationality of prescribing. Maybe some GPs do better than others. Which criteria are available to measure the quality of prescribing? Another aspect is the cost of prescriptions. Are GPs conscious of the price of the medications they prescribe or not; does this influence their decisions? Next, "over the counter prescribing" is of interest: what is the percentage of prescriptions without direct doctor-patient contact?

Factors Influencing GPs' Prescribing Habits

In the literature three major categories of influencing factors are distinguished:

- Patient factors: one of the major reasons for prescribing is the health status of the patients. This is obvious. There must be a diagnosis leading to the prescription. Many factors are related to morbidity and therefore (indirectly) to prescribing: age, sex, education, occupation, social status, etc. Moreover the attitude of the patient towards medication and his/her style of coping with illnesses are factors of interest. A certain attitude and a certain coping behavior can induce demands for medication. Nevertheless within a certain diagnosis (e. g. cough) there are enormous differences between GPs in prescribing behavior. So a second group of factors can be discerned.

Rationale Pharmakotherapie in der Allgemeinpraxis
Rational Pharmacotherapy in General Practice
M. M. Kochen (Hrsg.)

- GP factors: The GP's attitude and performance probably influence his/her prescribing behavior. Several factors may correlate with attitude and practice style such as age and sex of the GP, education, and information from the pharmaceutical industry.
- Last but not least, factors related to the work setting: the social environment, the cultural health beliefs and customs of the region or the country that both doctor and patient are living in. It is known that there are typical national routines in medical practice, in which countries can differ very much (e.g., hysterectomy). Figure 1 shows the differences in the cost of drugs in several Western countries (excluding drug use in hospitals) in 1988. In France and in West Germany more than twice as much money was spent on drugs as in the UK or the Netherlands.

Making use of study data from Ghent and Nijmegen, we will deal with the following questions:

1. Which dimensions can be distinguished in the presribing habits of GPs?
2. What is the relationship between prescribing habits of GPs and patient and GP factors?

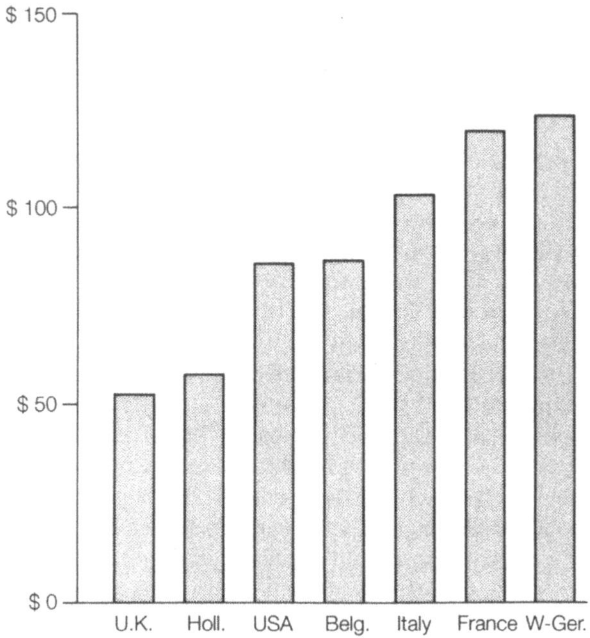

Fig. 1. Cost of drugs ($) per capita in some Western countries. (From [1])

Methods

In the Ghent study [2, 3] 5609 doctor-patient contacts of 94 GPs in Flanders were observed by trainees (during their vocational training in general practice) from October 1984 until September 1986. Information was collected on the reason for encounter, the diagnosis (ICPC codes) and prescriptions (ATC codes).

In Nijmegen two studies were done. In the first study (1980–1985) 57 GPs in Nijmegen and the surrounding area were observed. Medical and non-medical aspects of GPs' consultation behavior were measured. Moreover, health insurance data on prescriptions and referrals of the observed GPs were available and some relevant attitudes were measured by means of a questionnaire [4, 5]. In the second study (1986–1990) 75 GPs in Arnhem and the surrounding area were observed. The same method of observation and the same health-fund data were used. In addition a random sample of 20 female patients from each practice (age range 50–64 years) was investigated. Both studies took place in the east of the Netherlands [6]. (We thank BAZ Nijmegen and RZR Arnhem for placing their health fund data at our disposal).

Results

Dimensions in Prescription

Large prescribing differences between GPs were found. In the Ghent study one third of the GPs prescribed one drug per contact or less; 20 % prescribed more than 1.5 drugs per contact. In the Nijmegen study the annual number of prescriptions per patient was calculated. The 25 % of the GPs with the highest prescription rate prescribed about twice as many drugs as the 25 % of the GPs with the lowest prescription rate. The same variance was found in all the yearly figures from 1976 to 1986 and in the data from two different health funds in two different areas.

The next question is whether the prescribing behavior of GPs is one-dimensional. In other words, if a GP prescribes a lot, does he prescribe an array of different drugs or not? Factor analysis on the yearly prescription rates (15 categories of drugs) showed two independent dimensions in the prescribing behavior of GPs (Table 1). The first dimension consists of the prescription rates of analgesics, antibiotics, antihistamines, antirheumatics, corticosteroids, antitussives, tranquilizers, and sedatives. The second dimension consist of hypoglycemics, diuretics, antihypertensives, coronary drugs, and cardiac drugs. Looking at the first factor it was concluded that these drugs:

- Cover a wide range of indications
- Are mostly used in cases of minor ailments
- Are often precribed in cases of vague and uncertain diagnoses
- In general are not indispensable for the patient
- Are often prescribed as a symptomatic approach in cases of psychosocial problems (especially tranquilizers and sedatives).

Table 1. Mean factor loadings of the yearly prescription rates on 15 categories of drugs of 80 GPs (Nijmegen, BAZ) and of 150 GPs (Arnhem, RZR) on two orthogonal factors, varimax rotated

	BAZ 1976–1981	RZR 1982–1986
Factor I: nonspecific prescription		
Analgesics	.54	.69
Antibiotics	.58	.62
Antihistamines	.56	.59
Antirheumatics	.53	.63
Corticosteroids	.45	.60
Antitussives	.61	.59
Tranquillisers	.73	.67
Sedatives	.53	.61
Factor II: specific prescription		
Hypoglycemics	.74	.69
Diuretics	.89	.78
Antihypertensives	.41	.61
Coronary drugs	.83	.77
Cardiac drugs	.53	.83

For this reason, this dimension was interpreted as related to nonspecific prescription habits. Note that this denomination aims to characterize not the drugs but the prescription habits of GPs. Prescribing an antibiotic drug or a corticosteroid for example is not non-specific in all cases; however a very high level of prescription of these drugs might indicate a nonspecific prescribing habit.

Looking at the second factor the common features of the drugs in this cluster are that they:

- are used for clearly defined diagnoses
- indicate an active screening (of hypertension, diabetes)
- are prescribed with the intention to cure and prevent serious organic illness
- are generally prescribed to elderly people

This dimension was interpreted as the specific prescribing habit. High correlations were found between the yearly scores on both dimension ($r > .80$). This indicates that the prescription rates of individual GPs are quite similar year after year.

Patient Factors

One of the major reasons for prescribing medication is the health state of the patients. The Ghent study gives detailed information about which drugs are most prescribed per diagnosis. For example, Table 2 shows that antibiotics, benzodiazepines, and vitamins were prescribed in almost all chapters of ICPC codes.

Table 2. Prescription of antibiotics (n = 662 RFEs), benzodiazepines (n = 504 RFEs), and vitamins (n = 263 RFEs) per diagnosis (percentages)

General and unspecific	.8	10.1	11.9
Blood, blood-forming organs, lymphatics	.5	0.2	2.0
Digestive	4.2	5.0	5.7
Eye	.1		2.3
Ear	5.1	0.2	.4
Circulatory	.4	10.1	3.1
Musculoskeletal	1.1	4.6	27.0
Neurological		5.6	10.2
Psychological		43.2	9.8
Respiratory	73.6	1.4	8.0
Skin	10.1	.4	7.5
Endocrine, metabolic, nutritional	1.5	1.4	6.4
Urological		.2	1.2
Pregnancy, child-bearing, family planning			2.7
Female genital	1.2	.2	.4
Male genital	1.1		.1
Social		7.5	1.1

Morbidity is strongly correlated with age: there is more (serious) morbidity in older people [7]. Thus, more drug prescribing may be expected in the older population. This was found both in the Ghent and the Nijmegen studies. In the Ghent study the relation had the shape of a U curve: youngsters and to a greater extent older people received more drugs per contact than people 16–44 years of age. In the Nijmegen study a relationship was found between the yearly prescription rates (all drugs) and the percentage of aged people in the practice (r = .30). The older the population, the more drugs the GP prescribes. This correlation however was completely due to the specific prescription habit (r = .55 and r = .77, respectively), while the nonspecific prescription habit did not correlate with the percentage of elderly people. This was found in both Nijmegen studies (Table 3). Analysis of the observational data confirmed this finding. Nonspecific prescribing was not correlated with the age of the 1049 patients who visited their doctor during the observations; in all age categories about half of the patients received a drug related to the nonspecific prescription habit. In specific prescribing, however, there is a clear relationship with the age of the patients: the older the patient, the more drugs are related to specific prescribing habits.

Table 3. Pearson correlation between (non-)specific prescription and percentage of aged people in practice (NUHI, Nijmegen)

Non specific prescription	.08	−.02
Specific prescription	.55**	.77*

*p < .01, **p < .001.

The sex of the patient showed a less clear correlation with drug prescription. In the Ghent study women were prescribed a few more than men. In the Nijmegen study a slight difference was found the other way around; female patients received slightly fewer drugs (related to nonspecific as well as specific prescribing habits).

In some cases the patient visits the GP with the special aim of getting a prescription. In the studies in both countries a relationship was found. In the Ghent study in 78 % of the contacts the GP had the feeling that the patient expected a drug. In the Nijmegen study the patients were asked retrospectively whether the wish to get a prescription was a reason to visit the doctor or not. This turned out to have a strong correlation with nonspecific prescription, but not with specific prescription.

In the second Nijmegen study a random sample of patients (females, age 50–64) of the 75 observed GPs was asked which drugs, pescribed by their GPs, they used. Twenty percent of them used sedatives. In women with negative subjective feelings about their own health and with low notions about self-care for minor ailments the use of sedatives was significantly higher. More women with a low socioeconomic status and women without a paid job used sedatives.

Table 4. Pearson correlations between nonspecific prescription habit and patients characteristics (n = 75)

Feeling healthy	–.32**
Self-care for minor ailments	–.29*
Expectations in GP's care	.31**
Number of visits to GP	.28*

*p < .0.5, **p < .01.

GP Factors

The Ghent study showd that GPs with a defensive attitude and GPs who were receptive to commercial source of information prescribed significantly more antibiotics in respiratory infections, especially infections in the upper-respiratory system, and also more benzodiazepines when psychosocial problems are presented by the patients.

In the Nijmegen study the relationship between prescribing habits and other aspects of performance during consultation was studied. GPs who gave less information to the patients, who were less open to the patients' views, and GPs with poor diagnostic medical performance, scored higher on non-specific prescription habits (and/or on referral). A typology of four practice styles was constructed based on these findings. These practice styles correlated significantly with GPs' attitudes: GPs with a so-called integrated practice style (good doctor-patient relationship, adequate diagnostic medical performance, and low scores on referral and nonspecific prescribing habits) were more open to external control (e.g. by peer review), were more in favor of an egalitarian doctor-patient relationship, and were less inclined to always "stay on the safe side" in medical decisions.

Of the 57 Nijmegen GPs 43 participated in an extended program of peer review. One year after the program a significant increase in nonspecific prescription was found compared with the year before the program. The specific prescription behavior remained stable [8].

In the second Nijmegen study significant correlations were found between nonspecific prescribing habits and patients characteristics: in practices of GPs with a high score on nonspecific prescribing habits the average patient felt significantly less healthy, was less in favor of self-care, had high expectations of the GP with respect to minor ailments, and visited the doctor more often.

Differences between Belgium and the Netherlands

In the Belgian study a prescription was written in 77 % of the contacts (1.41 prescriptions per contact); 84 % were drugs related to nonspecific prescribing habits. In the Dutch study a prescription was written in 63 % of the consultations (.95 prescription per contact); 60 % were drugs related to nonspecific prescribing habits.

Discussion

In this short paper two studies on prescribing habits of GPs are presented. In the Ghent study GPs' prescriptions were investigated on the contact level, with detailed medical information on reasons for encounter (REFs), diagnoses and prescriptions. The Nijmegen study primarily focused on questions such as: how do GPs perform in general, what pescribing habits and practice styles are to be discerned, how does the doctor as a person with given attitudes and psychological background influence his/her medical performance, what is the correlation between GPs' practice styles and patients' health and illness behavior.

First we can conclude that drug prescribing is determined by habits: once a GP has developed specific habits, they will be preserved for years. Secondly, GPs differ widely in their prescribing habits. This was found in both the Belgium and the Dutch studies. On the one hand these habits are linked to the amount of morbidity in the population. The Ghent study gives detailed insight on this point. However, the notable differences between prescription rates of individual GPs and between countries indicate that the influence of other factors should not be underestimated. Prescribing habits are not isolated aspects of medical performance. They are part of the overall practice style of the general practitioner. They have their roots in the diagnostic routines of the GPs and their ways of relating to patients [9]. Drug prescribing by GPs is not only determined by their medical background and knowledge, but also by their attitudes and behavioral habits.

Finally, much drug research focuses on the effectiveness of particular drugs. Knowledge about the affectiveness or the lack of effectiveness is of course important. However, we think that the use and benefits of drugs not only depend on this knowledge but also on the prescribing habits, the practice styles, and the attitudes of the pescribers on the one hand and on the illness behavior, the (overly high) expectations of the users of drugs about the effectiveness of medication, the notions about self-care and those about the resources of patients to cope with problems themselves, on the other hand. The correlation between the nonspecific prescription habits of GPs and the attitudes of patients indicates that both patients and doctors influence each other in one way or another. Knowledge about these processes may help us to determine the rationality of different prescribing habits.

References

1. Anonymous (1988) Nederlande Associatie van de Farmaceutische Industrie. Nefarma Jaarverslag, Utrecht
2. De Maeseneer J (1989) Huisartsgeneeskunde: een verkenning. Een explorerend onderzoek bij huisarts-stagebegeleiders aan de R.U. Gent. Dissertation Ghent
3. De Maeseneer J (1990) Wat zit in de -50? Het voorschrijven van geneesmiddelen geanalyseerd met IC-Process-PC. Huisarts en Wet 33 : 300–307
4. Mokkink HGA (1986) Ziekenfondscijfers als parameter voor het handelen van huisartsen. Dissertation, Nijmegen
5. Mokkink HGA, Tielens VCL, Smits AJA, Grol RPTM (1986) Werkstijlen van huisartsen. Een explorerend onderzoek naar verschillende tijlen van huisartsgeneeskundig handelen. Huisarts en Wet 29 : 72–76
6. Smits AJA, Mokkink HGA, Meyboom WA, Van Son J, Van Eijk JThM (1990) Eindrapport Ophar-Outcome. NUHI, Nijmegen
7. Anonymous (1984) Morbidity figures in four general practices. NUHI, Nijmegen
8. Grol RPTM (1987) Kwaliteitsbewaking in de huisartsgeneeskunde. Effecten van onderlinge toetsing. Dissertation, Nijmegen
9. Grol RPTM (1985) Die Prävention somatischer Fixierung. Springer, Berlin Heidelberg New York Tokyo

Sachverzeichnis / Subject Index

Acarbose 297
ACE inhibitors 236
ACE-Hemmer 40, 298
Acetylsalicylic acid 13, 310
Acetylsalicylsäure 32, 42, 120, 132, 158, 244, 269
Acupuncture 227
Ademetionin 34
Adverse effects of drugs 5
Advertising, pharmaceutical 4
Aescin 146, 154
Akupunktur 113
Aldosteronantagonisten 53
Alpha-blockers 14
Alpha-Liponsäure 152
Alzheimer Erkrankung 156, 157, 244
Ambroxol 35
American Heart Association 84
Aminobuttersäure 270
Aminoglycoside 9
Aminopenicilline 59
Amiodarone 9
Amitriptylin 42, 214
Amlodipine 14
Amoxicillin 59, 132
Amphetamine 9
Ampicillin 59
Amytriptylinoxid 214
Anafranil 214
Analgesics 314
Analgetika 131, 209, 265, 269
  koffeinhaltige 47
  nichtopioide 264, 269
  opioide 270
Anexate 33
Angina pectoris 182
Angiotensin converting enzyme (ACE) inhibitors 14
Angstneurose 215
Aniflazym 34
Antazida 225
Antiarrhythmika 53
Antiasthmatics 7, 8
Antiasthmatika 52, 209
Antibiotics 9, 198, 230, 312, 314, 315
Antibiotika 52, 155, 209
Antidepressiva 211, 212, 214, 215, 217–219
Antidiabetika, orale 279, 280, 282, 294, 295
Antifibrillantien 42
Antihistamines 314
Antihistaminika 131
Antihypertensiva 32, 52
Antihypertensives 314
Antihypotonika 209
Antipyretika 131, 132
Antirheumatics 314
Antirheumatika 52, 61, 209, 265
Antitussiva 52, 131, 225
Antitussives 314
Antra 34
Anxiolytika 225
Aponal 214
Apothekenumsatz 44
Aromatherapy 227
Arthropathies 261
Arzneimittelgesetz 32, 202, 275
Arzneimittelkommission der Deutschen Ärzteschaft 5
Arzneimittelmarkt 31, 35, 36
Arzneimittelpreise 48
Arzneimittelsicherheit 42
Arzneimittelverbrauch 45
Arzneimittelverbrauchsanalyse 49, 209
Arzt-Patienten-Beziehung 225
Ärztebesucher 223
Asparaginsäure 152
Aspirin 235
Asthma 134, 136, 138, 182
Atenolol 298
Atosil 214
Atropine 181, 182
Audit, medical 167, 169, 174–177
Auranofin 9

Barbiturate 33, 181
Belgien 44, 45, 48
Belgium 163
Beloc 298
Bemetizid 147
Benzaron 153, 154
Benzodiazepinabhängigkeit 258
Benzodiazepine 42, 198, 212, 213, 215, 217, 219, 251, 253, 254–257, 260, 264, 270, 315
  low-dose-dependence 256, 257
Benzodiazepines 230
  addiction 249
Benzyclan 158
Berlocombin 58
Beta-Acetyldigoxin 42
Beta-blockers 12, 236
Betäubungsmittel (BTM) 117
Betäubungsmittelgesetz (BtMG) 117, 257
Betäubungsmittelrezept 119
Bifiteral 145, 152
Biguanid 293
Bilobalid 245
Bioäquivalenz 35
Bioavailability 9
Bioverfügbarkeit 35, 201
Bismutsubcitrat 33
Black-triangle drug 5
Brallobarbital 33
British National Formulary 41
Bromazepam 213, 254, 257
Bronchitis, chronische 134, 136, 138
Bronchodilatantien 134
Broncholytika 209
Brotizolam 254
Bucetin 42
Bufedil 158
Buflomedil 158
Bulgarien 41
Bundesgesundheitsamt (BGA) 35, 154, 157, 201
Bundesopiumstelle 118
Bundesrepublik Deutschland 44, 47
Buprenorphin 119
Butyrophenone 214

Caffeine 181
Calcium channel blockers 14
Calciumdobesilat 154
Captopril 10
Cardiac drugs 198, 314
Carisoprodol 270
Ceftriaxone 182
Cetal 158
Chemotherapeutika 52, 209
Chinidin 32, 42
Chinin 42
Chlordiazepoxid 42
Chlormezanon 270
Cholesterinbestimmung 70
Cholesterinscreening 67, 95, 101
Cholestyramine 13
Cholin 42
Chondroprotektiva 39
Chordotomie 113
Cicletanin 33
Cimetidine 14
Cinnarizin 42
Clarvisor 34
Clobazam 33
Clofezon 42
Clofibrat 74, 75
Clomipramin 214
Closing strategy 227, 229
Codein 132, 270
Codeine 20
Codeine-paracetamol combinations 10
Co-dergocrin 158
Coffein 131
Colestipol 13
Colestyramin 72, 79
Combination products 8
Committee on Safety of Medicines 5
Complamin 158
Compliance 172, 176, 204, 294
Contraceptives, oral 198
Contraception 182
Cordichin 42
Coronary drugs 314
Corticobiss 33
Corticoliberin 33
Corticosteroids 314
Co-trimoxazole 172
Crataegus 276
Cronassial 34
Crotamiton 42
Cyanacobalamin 230

Dalmadorm 253
Dantron 42
DDR 49, 51, 54
Dehydro sanol tri 147
Dermatika 209
Dexium 154
Dextropropoxyphene 9, 13
Diabetes mellitus 279
Diättherapie 84
Diazepam 35, 213, 254, 257, 270

Diclofenac 35, 57, 266, 268
Digitalisglykoside 40, 42, 52
Digitoxin 53,
Digoxin 53
Dihydroergotamin (DHE) 153, 154
Diltiazem 14
Diosmin 153, 154
Dipiperon 148, 214
Dipyridamol 42, 181
Disoprivan 33
Diterpenoide 245
Diuretics 314
Diuretika 52, 147, 153–155, 225, 298
Doppelblindstudie 30, 268
Double-blind randomised trial 228
Doxepin 214
Doxyzyklin 59, 132
Drug counseling 301
Drug expenditure 236
Drug Licensing Authorities 7, 8
Drug safety 3
Drugs for varicose veins 143
Dura Silimarin 145
Durchblutungsfördernde Mittel 156, 157, 209, 243, 244, 247
Dusodril 40, 158, 243

EEC 239
Enalapril 10
Encephabol 157
Equilibrin 214
Ergotamine tartrate 181
Ergotismus 154
Erypo 33
Erythromycin 59, 132
Erythropoietin 33
Essentiale forte 152
Ethikkommission 206
Etodroxinin 33
Etofenamat 268
Eukalisan 152
Eunerpan 148, 214
Europäische Gemeinschaft (EG) 44
European Formulary 239
European Formulary Group (EFG) 183–185
Expektoranzien 132

Famotidine 14
Feedback 186, 193
Felodipine 14
Fenfluramine 10
Fettleber 150–152
Fibrate 75, 77

Fiebersenkung 130, 131
Flavonoide 153, 154, 245
Fludilat 158
Flumazenil 33
Flunitrazepam 253, 254, 257
Fluspirilen 214
Folsäure 152
Food and Drug Administration (FDA) 205
Formulary 4, 21, 169, 170–172, 181–185, 198, 238, 239
Fragivix 154
Frankreich 31, 44, 45, 47, 48
Furosemid 53, 155

Gadopentetsäure 33
Ganglion-coeliacum-Blockade, perkutane 113
Ganglioside 34
Gemfibrozil 72, 79
Generic drugs 187, 188
Generika 35, 214, 224, 225, 245, 253, 254, 270, 298
  Markengenerika 224
  Wirkstoffgenerika 224
Geriatrika 155, 159
Germany 181
Ghent 163, 164
Gichtmittel 209
Gingko-biloba 158
Ginkolide 245
Ginseng 155
GKV-Arzneimittelindex 210, 251, 254
Glibenclamid 297
Glucobay 297
Glukosidase 293, 297
Glyceryl trinatrate 181, 182
Glyvenol 154
Griechenland 44, 45
GRIPS-Studie 87–89, 95, 99, 103
Großbritannien 31, 39, 41, 44, 45, 47, 48, 134, 159
Guide to Good Prescribing 21
Gumbaral 34

H_2-blockers 9, 236
Halcion 253
Haldol 214
Haloperidol 14, 214
HbA_1 293, 295
Helfergin 157
Helsinki Heart Study 72
Hepagrisevit Forte 152
Hepa Merz 152
Heparin 146, 155

Heparinoide 155
Hepatofalk 152
Herzglykoside, s. Digitalisglykoside
Hesperidinkomplex 147
Homoeopathy 227
Homöopathika 155
Hydergin 158
Hydrochlorothiazid-Kombination 53
Hypercholesterinämie 71, 72, 74, 77, 78, 82, 84, 87
Hypercholesterinämiebehandlung 67
Hypnotika 210, 211, 213, 218, 251, 253–255
Hypoglycaemics, oral 198
Hypoglycemics 314

Ibuprofen 35, 57, 268
Imap 214
Indometacin 57, 62, 267, 268
Infarktgefährdung 71
Infarktmortalität 75, 77, 79
Infarktrisiko 69
Insidon 214
Insulin 230, 279, 293, 296
Interferon 33
Interkantonale Kontrollstelle für Heilmittel (IKS) 222, 224
Ionenaustauschharze 75
Ipratropiumbromid 134, 138
Irland 31, 44, 45
Isotretinoin 10
Italien 44, 45, 47, 48
Italy 182, 239

Johanniskraut 155
Jugoslawien 41
Justar 33

Kalziumantagonisten 40, 55, 56, 62, 298
Kardiaka 37, 52
Kebuzon 57
Ketoconazole 9
Kielholz-Schema 214
Klinische Prüfung 201, 202, 204–206
Knoblauch 155
Koanalgetika 116, 117
Kombinationspräparate 32, 37, 131, 270
Kontrazeptiva, orale 32
Kortikosteroide 136, 140, 151, 155, 269
Krankenkassen 223, 224
Kümmelöl 276

Lactulose 145, 146, 152
Lactulose Neda 145, 152
Laevilac 152
Lanitop 40
Lasix 155
Lebensalter 209
Lebensqualität 205
Lebermittel 145, 150, 151, 152, 159
Leberschutztherapeutikum 145
Legalon 145, 152
Legitimation of 'Sick Role' 227, 229
Lendormin 254
Leukocianidol 154
Leukotriene 265
Levodopa 9
Levomethadon 119
Limbatril 42
Lipid Research Clinic 72
Lipidsenker 77, 79
Lipidtheorie 67, 70, 77
Lisinopril 10
Lithiumcitrat 32
Liver Disease 143
Lorazepam 254
Lormetazepam 253
Lovastatin 9, 13, 33
LRC-Studie 87

Magnevist 33
Marketing 31
Marketingstrategie 223
Meclofenoxat 157
Medical representatives 4
Medicinal plants 273
Melleretten 214
Melleril 214
Melperon 214
Meprobamate 181
Metamizol 269
Metformin 293, 295
Methadone 9
Methylfenidate 9
Metoprolol 298
Me-too-Präparate 35
Mevinacor 34
Migränemittel 210
Mistelkraut 155
Mogadan 253
Morphin 116, 119, 120
Morphine 9
MST 117
Mucolytics 182
Mukolytika 132
Multiinfarktdemenz 156
Multimorbidität 216

Muskel-Transcopal 270
Musterpräparate 223
Mykoplasma pneumoniae 130
Myocardon 181

Nachahmerpräparate, s. Generika
Naftidrofuril 158
National Cholesterol Program 84, 96
Nationale Cholesterin-Initiative 96, 99
Negativliste 41–43
Nervenblockade 113
Neuroleptika 211, 212, 214, 217–219
Neurolytika 113
NHG-Standard 286, 287
Nichtsteroidale Antiphlogistika 56, 155, 265, 267–270
Niederlande 31, 44, 45, 48, 134
Nifedipin 35, 56
Nifedipine 14
Nimodipine 14
Nitrazepam 253, 254, 257
Nitro-Novodigal 42
Noctamid 253
Nomifensin 33
Non-Compliance 29, 30, 257
Non-diseases 230
Nonsteroidal antiinflammatory agents 198, 228
Nootrop 157
Nootropika 145, 148, 149, 156, 157, 243, 244, 247
Nordic Drug Index 49
Northern Ireland 186
Norway 7, 181
Norwegen 41
Noscapine 20
Novodigal 41

Ödemprotektiva 153, 155
Oleum carum carvi 276
Omeprazol 9, 14, 34
Opiate 182
Opiates 228
Opioide 115–117, 264
Opipramol 214
Oralpenicilline 58
Orotsäure 152
Organextrakte 155
Ornithinaspartat 146, 152
Österreich 45
OTC (over the counter medication) 59, 131
Oxazepam 42, 181, 219, 254, 257

PACT (Prescribing Analysis and Cost) 175, 176
Papaverine 181, 182
Paracetamol 132, 169
Paralgin forte 8
Peer review 174, 302
Penicillamine 9
Penicillin 235
Penicillinallergie 132
Pentoxifyllin 158
Perkutane Penetration 268
Perphenazine 14
Persumbran 42, 181
Pervincamin 158
Pharmaceutical industry 235, 312
Pharmaindustrie 222–224
Pharmakokinetik 201
Phase-I-Studien 201
Phase-III-Studien 201, 202
Phenobarbitone 181
Phenothiazine 214
Phospholipide 151
Phytopharmaka 275, 276
Phytotherapie 275
Pipamperon 214
Piperacillin 182
Piracetam 148, 157
Pirenoxin 34
Piroxicam 57
Placebos 29, 30, 39, 227, 228, 244, 247
  Pseudoplacebos 29, 245
Planum 254
Polyferon 33
Polymedikation 29
Portugal 44, 45, 48
Positivliste 41, 43
Pößneck 49
Postgraduate Training 16
PRIND 156
Practolol 13
Prescribing
  analysis 186
  analysis visit 187, 198, 200
  feedback 187, 190
  habits 312
  specific 17–19, 191, 192
  symptomatic 191, 193
  tradition 235
Pro Dorm 254
Procain 155
Promethazin 214
Promethazine 20
Propofol 33
Propranolol 35

Propyrhenazon 269
Prostaglandine 264–267, 269
Prostazyklin 265, 266
Prüfplan 202, 205
Psychopharmaka 148, 157, 209–212, 215, 217, 254
  Geschlecht 209
Psyton 33
Pyrazolanalgetika 269
Pyritinol 157

Qualitätszirkel 284

Randomisierung 202, 203
Rantitidine 14
Reduktasehemmer 75, 79
Registration 8
Remestan 254
Repeat prescriptions 172, 229
Retinoid 10
β-Rezeptorenblocker 40, 53–56, 62, 298
Rhinitis medicamentosa 132
Rhizotomie, perkutane 113
Risikofaktoren 71, 74, 83, 87–89, 92, 95, 97
Risikofaktoren, kardiovaskuläre 82
Rohypnol 253
Rökan 158
Roßkastanienextrakt 147, 153, 154
Rote Liste 209
Royal College of General Practitioners 169
Rudolstadt 49
Rutin 146, 154
Rutoside 147, 154

Salbutamol 134, 138
Sanoma 270
Saponine 154
Saroten 214
Schlafmittel 225, 254, 256, 257
Schlafstörungen 256, 258–260
  Durchschlafstörungen 258
  Einschlafstörungen 258
Schmerzkontrolle 114
Schmerztherapie 109
Schweden 41
Schweiz 222
Screening 67, 77, 78
Secobarbital 33
Sedativa 210, 211, 213, 218, 251, 253–255
Sedatives 314
Sekretolytika 52
Selbstmedikation 131
Serrapeptase 34
Sexualhormone 155
Sibelium 243
Silibene 152
Silibinin 145, 152
Silymarin 152
Skandinavische Länder 159
Skorbut 74
Spalt N 46
Spanien 44, 45, 47, 48
Spasmolytika 225
Standards 176
Statens legemiddelkontroll (SLK) 8
Students 18, 19, 21
Sulfonamid-Trimethoprim-Kombination 58
Sulfonylharnstoffe 293, 295, 296
Surfactant 33
Survanta 33
Sympathikomimetika 132
β-Sympatomimetika 134
Symptom Relief 227

Talinolol 53
Taurolidin 33
Taurolin 33
Tavor 254
Teaching 18
Tebonin 40, 158, 243–247
Telen 33
Temazepam 253
Tenormin 298
Terminal care, analgesia in 106
Tetrazyklin 59, 132
Theophylline 181
  slow-release 198
Therapeutic habits 236
Therapeutics of doubtful efficacy 143
Therapiefreiheit 221
Therapiestandard 291, 293
Thiamin 147
Thiazide 53, 235, 298
Thioridazin 214
Thomapyrin 46
Throat infection 182
Thromboxan A 265
Thromboxansynthese 267
Thrombozytenaggregationshemmung 158
Thyroxine 230
TIA (transitorische ischämische Attacke) 156
Togal 32, 42

Tolmetin 268
Tranquilizer 264, 314
Tranquillanzien 211, 212, 219, 254, 255
Transkutane elektrische Nervenstimulation (TENS) 113
Trental 158, 243
Triampur 53
Triamteren 53, 147
Triazolam 253
Tribenosid 154
Tricyclics 230
Tuberkulostatika 151
Tumorschmerztherapie 107, 117
psychosoziale Probleme 122

Undergraduate medical training 163
Upper respiratory infection 127
Urinary tract infections 182
Urologika 209
USA 39, 48, 159
Utilization Research Group (DURG) 49

Valium 270
Vasodilatanzien 52, 158
Vasodilator 305, 310
Venalot 147
Venenmittel 145, 147, 150, 153, 159, 210 225
Venentonisierende Substanzen 154
Venoruton 147, 154
Venostasin 147, 154
Verapamil 14, 35, 42, 56
Vesparax mite 33
Vincamin 158
Virusinfekt 129, 130
Vitamine 146, 165, 315
B-Vitamine 152
Vitamin B^{12} defiency 230
Vitamin C 74, 131
Vitamin E 35, 152
Vocational Training 165
Voltaren Emugel 41
Vorhersagewert
negativer 70, 100
positiver 69, 100, 102
Weißdorn 155
Weizenkeimöl 155
WHO 18, 21, 40, 95, 184, 238
WHO-Stufenplan 14, 109, 110, 114, 116
Wirksamkeit, umstrittene 38, 159
Wirksamkeitsnachweis 201
WIdO (Wissenschaftliches Institut der Ortskrankenkassen 251, 254

Xantinolnicotinat 158
Xylometazolin 132

Zerebrales Jogging 243
Zuclopentixol 14
Zulassungsprüfung 34
Zyklooxygenase 266, 267